T0195197

Prostate Cancer Genetics: Changing the Paradigm of Care

Editors

LEONARD G. GOMELLA

VEDA N. GIRI

UROLOGIC CLINICS
OF NORTH AMERICA

www.urologic.theclinics.com

EDITOR-IN-CHIEF
KEVIN R. LOUGHLIN

August 2021 • Volume 48 • Number 3

ELSEVIER

1600 John F. Kennedy Boulevard • Suite 1800 • Philadelphia, Pennsylvania, 19103-2899

http://www.theclinics.com

UROLOGIC CLINICS OF NORTH AMERICA Volume 48, Number 3
August 2021 ISSN 0094-0143, ISBN-13: 978-0-323-79167-0

Editor: Kerry Holland
Developmental Editor: Diana Ang

Urologic Clinics of North America (ISSN 0094-0143) is published quarterly by Elsevier Inc., 360 Park Avenue South, New York, NY 10010-1710. Months of issue are February, May, August, and November. Business and Editorial Offices: 1600 John F. Kennedy Blvd., Suite 1800, Philadelphia, PA 19103-2899. Periodicals postage paid at New York, NY and additional mailing offices. Subscription prices are $395.00 per year (US individuals), $1033.00 per year (US institutions), $100.00 per year (US students and residents), $450.00 per year (Canadian individuals), $1059.00 per year (Canadian institutions), $100.00 per year (Canadian students/residents), $520.00 per year (foreign individuals), $1059.00 per year (foreign institutions), and $240.00 per year (foreign students/residents). Foreign air speed delivery is included in all *Clinics* subscription prices. All prices are subject to change without notice. **POSTMASTER:** Send address changes to *Urologic Clinics of North America*, Elsevier Health Sciences Division, Subscription Customer Service, 3251 Riverport Lane, Maryland Heights, MO 63043. **Customer Service: 1-800-654-2452 (US). From outside the United States, call 1-314-447-8871. Fax: 1-314-447-8029. E-mail: JournalsCustomerServiceusa@elsevier.com (for print support)** and **JournalsOnlineSupport-usa@elsevier.com (for online support).**

Reprints. For copies of 100 or more, of articles in this publication, please contact the Commercial Reprints Department, Elsevier Inc., 360 Park Avenue South, New York, New York 10010-1710. Tel.: 212-633-3874; Fax: 212-633-3820; E-mail: reprints@elsevier.com.

Urologic Clinics of North America is covered in MEDLINE/PubMed (*Index Medicus*), *Excerpta Medica, Current Contents/Clinical Medicine, Science Citation Index,* and *ISI/BIOMED.*

Printed in the United States of America.

Contributors

CONSULTING EDITOR

KEVIN R. LOUGHLIN, MD, MBA
Emeritus Professor of Surgery (Urology),
Harvard Medical School, Visiting Scientist,
Vascular Biology Research Program at Boston
Children's Hospital, Boston, Massachusetts

EDITORS

LEONARD G. GOMELLA, MD, FACS
The Bernard W. Godwin Professor of Prostate
Cancer, Chairman, Department of Urology,
Senior Director Clinical Affairs, Sidney Kimmel
Cancer Center, Thomas Jefferson University/
Thomas Jefferson University Hospital,
Philadelphia, Pennsylvania

VEDA N. GIRI, MD
Professor, Medical Oncology, Cancer Biology,
and Urology, Director, Cancer Risk
Assessment and Clinical Cancer Genetics,
Sidney Kimmel Cancer Center, Thomas
Jefferson University, Philadelphia,
Pennsylvania

AUTHORS

SAUD H. ALDUBAYAN, MD
Division of Genetics, Brigham and Women's
Hospital, Department of Medical Oncology,
Dana-Farber Cancer Institute, Harvard Medical
School, Boston, Massachusetts

ROHITH ARCOT, MD
Division of Urology, Duke University Durham,
North Carolina

ELIZABETH BARRETT, MS
Division of Genetics, Brigham and Women's
Hospital, Department of Medical Oncology,
Dana-Farber Cancer Institute, Harvard Medical
School, Boston, Massachusetts

TALA BERRO, MS, CGC
Division of Genetics, Brigham and Women's
Hospital, Harvard Medical School, Boston,
Massachusetts

YASIN BHANJI, MD
Department of Urology, The James Buchanan
Brady Urological Institute, Johns Hopkins
School of Medicine, Baltimore, Maryland

KELLY K. BREE, MD
The University of Texas MD Anderson Cancer
Center, Department of Urology, Houston,
Texas

LINDSEY BYRNE, MS
Clinical Assistant Professor, Department of
Internal Medicine, Division of Human Genetics,
The Ohio State University Comprehensive
Cancer Center, The Ohio State University
Wexner Medical Center, Columbus, Ohio

THENAPPAN CHANDRASEKAR, MD
Assistant Professor, Director of Abington-
Jefferson Urology, Department of Urology,
Sidney Kimmel Cancer Center, Thomas
Jefferson University, Philadelphia,
Pennsylvania

HEATHER H. CHENG, MD, PhD
Department of Medicine (Division of Oncology),
University of Washington, Clinical Research
Division, Fred Hutchinson Cancer Research
Center, Seattle, Washington

KATHLEEN A. COONEY, MD
Department of Medicine, Duke University School of Medicine and the Duke Cancer Institute, Durham, North Carolina

VEDA N. GIRI, MD
Professor, Medical Oncology, Cancer Biology, and Urology, Director, Cancer Risk Assessment and Clinical Cancer Genetics, Sidney Kimmel Cancer Center, Thomas Jefferson University, Philadelphia, Pennsylvania

LEONARD G. GOMELLA, MD, FACS
The Bernard W. Godwin Professor of Prostate Cancer, Chairman, Department of Urology, Senior Director Clinical Affairs, Sidney Kimmel Cancer Center, Thomas Jefferson University/ Thomas Jefferson University Hospital, Philadelphia, Pennsylvania

BRIAN T. HELFAND, MD, PhD
Program for Personalized Cancer Care, Division of Urology, NorthShore University HealthSystem, Evanston, Illinois

PATRICK J. HENLEY, MD
The University of Texas MD Anderson Cancer Center, Department of Urology, Houston, Texas

COLETTE HYATT, MS, CGC
The University of Vermont Medical Center, Familial Cancer Program, Burlington, Vermont

WILLIAM B. ISAACS, PhD
Department of Urology, The James Buchanan Brady Urological Institute, Johns Hopkins School of Medicine, Baltimore, Maryland

WILLIAM K. KELLY, DO
Professor, Medical Oncology and Urology, Director, Division of Solid Tumor Oncology, Department of Medical Oncology, Associate Director of Clinical Research, Sidney Kimmel Medical College, Thomas Jefferson University, Sidney Kimmel Cancer Center, Philadelphia, Pennsylvania

KAREN E. KNUDSEN, MBA, PhD
Executive Vice President of Oncology Services, Jefferson Health and Enterprise, Director of the Sidney Kimmel Cancer Center at Jefferson, Departments of Cancer Biology, Urology, Medical Oncology, and Radiation

Oncology, Thomas Jefferson University, Philadelphia, Pennsylvania

JAMES RYAN MARK, MD
Department of Urology, Thomas Jefferson University, Philadelphia, Pennsylvania

CAREY MCDOUGALL, MS, LCGC
Cancer Risk Assessment and Clinical Cancer Genetics, Departments of Medical Oncology and Cancer Biology, Sidney Kimmel Cancer Center, Thomas Jefferson University, Philadelphia, Pennsylvania

SUSAN MILLER-SAMUEL, MSN, RN, AGN-BC
Sidney Kimmel Cancer Center, Clinical Cancer Genetics, Philadelphia, Pennsylvania

TODD M. MORGAN, MD
Department of Urology, University of Michigan, Ann Arbor, Michigan

ALICIA K. MORGANS, MD, MPH
Division of Hematology/Oncology, Department of Medicine, Feinberg School of Medicine at Northwestern University, Chicago, Illinois

YAZAN NUMAN, MD
Division of Hematology/Oncology, Department of Medicine, Feinberg School of Medicine at Northwestern University, Chicago, Illinois

ELIAS I. OBEID, MD, MPH
Fox Chase Cancer Center, Philadelphia, Pennsylvania

CURTIS A. PETTAWAY, MD
The University of Texas MD Anderson Cancer Center, Department of Urology, Houston, Texas

THOMAS J. POLASCIK, MD, FACS
Division of Urology, Duke University Durham, North Carolina

JESSICA RUSSO, MS, LCGC
Sidney Kimmel Cancer Center, Clinical Cancer Genetics, Philadelphia, Pennsylvania

MATTHEW J. SCHIEWER, PhD
Assistant Professor, Departments of Urology and Cancer Biology, Director, Urology Research Laboratory, Thomas Jefferson University, Sidney Kimmel Cancer Center, Philadelphia, Pennsylvania

AISHA L. SIEBERT, MD, PhD, MPH
Department of Urology, Feinberg School of Medicine at Northwestern University, Chicago, Illinois

ALEXANDRA O. SOKOLOVA, MD
Department of Medicine (Division of Oncology), University of Washington, Clinical Research Division, Fred Hutchinson Cancer Research Center, VA Puget Sound Health Care System, Seattle, Washington

BRITTANY M. SZYMANIAK, PhD, CGC
Department of Urology, Feinberg School of Medicine at Northwestern University, Chicago, Illinois

AMANDA EWART TOLAND, PhD
Professor and Vice Chair, Department of Cancer Biology and Genetics, Division of Human Genetics, Department of Cancer Biology and Genetics, Comprehensive Cancer Center, The Ohio State University, Columbus, Ohio

JIANFENG XU, MD, DrPH
Program for Personalized Cancer Care, Division of Urology, NorthShore University HealthSystem, Evanston, Illinois

Contents

to controversy due to concerns of overdiagnosis and overtreatment. Advancements in molecular oncology have provided evidence for the inherited predisposition to prostate cancer, which could improve individualized, risk-adapted approaches to screening and mitigate the harms of routine screening. This review presents the current evidence for the genetic basis of prostate cancer and novel genetically informed, risk-adapted screening strategies for prostate cancer.

UROLOGIC CLINICS OF NORTH AMERICA

SERIES OF RELATED INTEREST
Surgical Clinics of North America
https://www.surgical.theclinics.com/

Foreword

Prostate Cancer Genetics: The Urologic Research Promissory Note Is Being Cashed

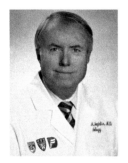

Kevin R. Loughlin, MD, MBA
Consulting Editor

In 2017, the Sidney Kimmel Cancer Center of Thomas Jefferson University held the First International Consensus Conference on The Role of Genetic Testing for Inherited Prostate Cancer Risk, which was organized by Leonard G. Gomella, Karen E. Knudsen, and Veda N. Giri.[1] This was followed by the 2019 Philadelphia Prostate Cancer Consensus Program: Implementation of Genetic Testing for Prostate Cancer by the same group.[2] These conferences, which were multidisciplinary and attended by national and international experts, were hugely successful. Future biennial meetings are being planned, and as many other successful endeavors, it is now referred to in its shortened form by prostate experts simply as the "Philadelphia Conference."

The Philadelphia Conference has achieved, in a meaningful way, the harvest of many years of prostate cancer genetics research. This issue of *Urologic Clinics*, "Prostate Cancer Genetics: Changing the Paradigm of Care," represents the practical, clinical applications of genetics research. Too many clinicians view medical research as a remote, abstract entity that has little relevance to their practice or patients. This issue reviews the direct clinical applications and benefits of prostate cancer genetic testing.

Personalized medicine, also referred to as precision medicine, has received increasing attention in both the medical and the lay press.[3,4] It is clear that the incorporation of personalized medicine into clinical practice will continue to accelerate. It is increasingly apparent that our genetic fingerprint not only influences our susceptibility to certain diseases but also modulates the natural history of those diseases as well. This issue, produced through the efforts of Drs Gomella and Giri, represents, in a tangible way, the cashing of the promissory note of years of basic science research. The reader should consider it a down payment of the future currency of "bench to bedside."

The reader will find, herein, articles that review a wide range of the applications of prostate cancer genetics in clinical practice. Prostate cancer genetics now plays a role in prostate cancer screening, intensity of follow-up, selection of patients suitable for active surveillance, genetic counseling for other family members, selection of treatment, and the management of some patients with metastatic disease.

A decade ago, prostate cancer genetics remained within the domain of academics; today it is emerging as a cutting-edge clinical tool. It will soon be the standard of care in prostate cancer management.

Kevin R. Loughlin, MD, MBA
Vascular Biology Research Program at
Boston Children's Hospital
300 Longwood Avenue
Boston, MA 02115, USA

E-mail address:
kloughlin@partners.org

Urol Clin N Am 48 (2021) xi–xii
https://doi.org/10.1016/j.ucl.2021.06.002
0094-0143/21/© 2021 Published by Elsevier Inc.

urologic.theclinics.com

REFERENCES

1. Giri VN, Knudsen KE, Kelly WK, et al. Role of genetic testing for inherited prostate cancer risk: Philadelphia Prostate Cancer Conference 2017. J Clin Oncol 2018; 36(4):414–24.
2. Giri VN, Knudsen KE, Kelly WK, et al. Implementation of germline testing for prostate cancer: Philadelphia Prostate Cancer Consensus Conference 2019. J Clin Oncol 2020;38(24):2798–811.
3. Jameson JL, Longo DL. Precision medicine-personalized, problematic and promising. N Engl J Med 2015;372:2229–34.
4. Kolata G. A path for precision medicine. New York Times 2015.

Preface

Prostate Cancer Genetics: Changing the Paradigm of Care

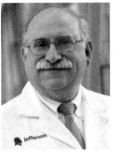
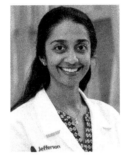

Leonard G. Gomella, MD, FACS   Veda N. Giri, MD
Editors

Our understanding the genomic landscape of prostate cancer has greatly expanded over the last few years. The Human Genome Project initiated by the NIH in 1990 and completed in 2003 accelerated the application of genetic testing in daily patient care for many diseases, including prostate cancer. We are increasingly learning how these genetic studies may inform all aspects of prostate cancer care from screening and diagnosis, through the treatment of early-stage disease, to life-threatening metastatic castration-resistant disease.

To fully understand how rapidly the field of prostate cancer genetics is evolving, the National Comprehensive Cancer Network (NCCN) guidelines provide some context. Before 2016, prostate cancer genetic testing and genes such as *BRCA 1/2* were only discussed in Genetic/Familial High-Risk Assessment: Breast and Ovarian Cancer NCCN Guidelines. For many years, these guidelines instructed women with hereditary breast and ovarian cancer to inform their close male relatives about the potential for an increased risk of prostate cancer, male breast cancer, and other linked malignancies. In 2016, the NCCN Prostate Cancer Early Detection Guidelines made the first mention of prostate cancer genetics, stating that a family history of mutations in *BRCA1/2* should be considered in prostate cancer screening decisions. In 2017, the NCCN Prostate Cancer Guideline, focused primarily on the treatment of prostate cancer, made mention of the importance of knowledge of germline mutations in family members. In 2018, these NCCN Prostate Cancer Guidelines noted that germline testing be "considered" based on risk assessment. With rapidly evolving supportive data, these germline testing "considerations" had become firmly established as "recommendations" just 2 years later in the 2020 updated NCCN guidelines.

In order to bring some clarity to this rapidly evolving area of prostate cancer genetic testing, we convened the first Philadelphia Prostate Cancer Consensus meeting in 2017. This meeting was hosted by the Sidney Kimmel Cancer Center and the Department of Urology at Thomas Jefferson University and brought together a diverse multidisciplinary group to address a genetic evaluation framework for inherited prostate cancer in the multigene testing era. A second consensus meeting took place in Philadelphia in 2019 that focused on implementation of germline testing for prostate cancer across practice settings, addressing topics such as the incorporation of genetic testing and genetic counseling in prostate cancer risk and management, delivery of genetic counseling, alternate genetic evaluation models, and provider education.

In 2020, FDA approvals of the poly(ADP-ribose) polymerase inhibitors olaparib and rucaparib for metastatic castrate-resistant prostate cancer in patients with identified alterations in DNA repair genes firmly established the need for genetic testing in treatment decision making for men with

Urol Clin N Am 48 (2021) xiii–xiv
https://doi.org/10.1016/j.ucl.2021.06.001
0094-0143/21/© 2021 Published by Elsevier Inc.

urologic.theclinics.com

advanced disease. Thus, the field has entered a new phase of genetic testing in prostate cancer for precision medicine necessitating broad-scale understanding of genetic testing and genetic counseling for men with prostate cancer.

This issue of *Urologic Clinics of North America,* entitled "Prostate Cancer Genetics: Changing the Paradigm of Care" has been designed to provide the reader with a comprehensive overview of the current state-of-the-art in prostate cancer genetic testing. The spectrum of topics presented includes basic principles and how genetic alterations contribute to prostate cancer development, the approaches and tools available for genetic testing at various stages of the disease, and how genetic testing informs treatment or management across the stage and risk spectrum. We are most appreciative that many of the researchers and clinicians that have made significant contributions to our understanding of the genetics of prostate cancer have contributed to this issue of the *Urologic Clinics of North America*. Our thanks to Editor-in-Chief, Dr Kevin Loughlin, for this opportunity gather these outstanding contributors for this issue.

Leonard G. Gomella, MD, FACS
Department of Urology
Thomas Jefferson University and Hospital
Sidney Kimmel Cancer Center
Thomas Jefferson University
1025 Walnut Street, Suite 1100
Philadelphia, PA 19107, USA

Veda N. Giri, MD
Medical Oncology, Cancer Biology, Urology
Cancer Risk Assessment and Clinical Cancer
Genetics
1025 Walnut Street, Suite 1015
Philadelphia, PA 19107, USA

E-mail addresses:
leonard.gomella@jefferson.edu (L.G. Gomella)
veda.giri@jefferson.edu (V.N. Giri)

Overview of Prostate Cancer Genetic Testing

Thenappan Chandrasekar, MD[a],*, William K. Kelly, DO[b], Leonard G. Gomella, MD, FACS[c]

KEYWORDS

- Prostate cancer • Germline • Genetic testing • BRCA2 • HOXB13 • Lynch syndrome

KEY POINTS

- The understanding of prostate cancer (PCa) inherited risk has drastically improved over the past decade.
- Established hereditary cancer syndromes associated with PCa include hereditary PCa, familial PCa, hereditary breast and ovarian cancer, and Lynch syndrome.
- Current National Comprehensive Cancer Network guidelines recommend germline testing for men with high-risk or very high-risk localized PCa, metastatic PCa, or intraductal carcinoma on histology, as well as men with Ashkenazi Jewish ancestry, family history of high-risk germline mutations and known germline variants, or a positive strong history of PCa.
- Panels for PCa germline testing are offered in multiple different formats, ranging from focused guidelines-based panels to PCa-specific panels to comprehensive cancer panels.
- The increasing gap between the number of men with PCa being referred for germline genetic testing and the availability and access to genetic counselors represents a critical gap in health care delivery; novel delivery models are required to help bridge that gap.

Prostate cancer (PCa) remains the most common solid malignancy in men in the United States. Contributing to 33,330 deaths in 2020 in the United States, it is second to only lung cancer as a cause of cancer death in men in 2020.[1,2]

Established risk factors for PCa have included family history of PCa, African ancestry, and increasing age. Knowledge of family cancer history and risk for PCa has expanded to include cancers linked with hereditary cancer syndromes in which PCa is associated, such as breast cancer, ovarian cancer, pancreatic cancer, colorectal cancer, uterine cancer, along with other potential cancers.

Prior epidemiologic studies have consistently demonstrated the impact of a family history of first-degree relatives with PCa on an individual's PCa risk. Men with a first-degree relative of PCa have 2- to 4-fold increased risk of developing PCa, and the risk increases with the number of affected individuals.[3,4] Importantly, there also appears to be a genetic predisposition to lethal PCa: men with first-degree relatives who died of PCa have a 2- to 3-fold increased risk of death

Funding Source: None.

Conflicts of interest: All authors report no conflict of interest.

[a] Department of Urology, Sidney Kimmel Cancer Center, Thomas Jefferson University, 1025 Walnut Street, Suite 1100, Philadelphia, PA 19107, USA; [b] Medical Oncology and Urology, Division of Solid Tumor Oncology, Department of Medical Oncology, Sidney Kimmel Medical College, Thomas Jefferson University, Sidney Kimmel Cancer Center, 1025 Walnut Street, Suite 700, Philadelphia, PA 19107, USA; [c] Department of Urology, Thomas Jefferson University and Hospital, Sidney Kimmel Cancer Center, Thomas Jefferson University, 1025 Walnut Street, Suite 1100, Philadelphia, PA 19107, USA

* Corresponding author.

E-mail address: thenappan.chandrasekar@gmail.com

Twitter: @tchandra_uromd; @JEFFUrology (T.C.); @LeonardGomella; @JEFFUrology (L.G.G.)

from PCa themselves.[5] Based on the above family history associations, hereditary prostate cancer (HPC) and familial prostate cancer (FPC) were defined.[3,6,7]

Initial genome-wide association studies through 2010 identified more than 100 potential loci, which in aggregate, are thought to account for ∼33% of FPC risk.[8–11] Nevertheless, many of these variants, although highly prevalent in the population, had low penetrance and therefore were not clinically useful in risk stratifying aggressive and indolent PCa.[11] This area is an area of active investigation with polygenic risk scores emerging for testing.

Over the past decade, we have begun to understand the impact of high- and moderate-penetrance germline mutations on PCa risk and treatment. One of the most significant contributions was the identification of the germline variant *HOXB13 G84E*, which normally interacts with the androgen receptor (AR) and modulates PCa development. This variant was strongly associated with families with multiple cases of PCa.[12–14] Men with PCa were 20-fold more likely to harbor this variant than the general population (1.4% vs 0.1%), and it was especially predominant in men with a family history of PCa (3.1%).[12] Subsequent analyses, including a 2013 meta-analysis, have established that being a *HOXB13 G84E* carrier is associated with a 4- to 4.5-fold risk of developing PCa, especially early-onset PCa.[14,15] HOXB13 has therefore emerged as an HPC gene with significant clinical impact.

The role of pathogenic variants (mutations) in DNA repair genes has been an exciting story in PCa risk and precision therapy. Robinson and colleagues,[16] as part of the Stand Up To Cancer–Prostate Cancer Foundation Dream Team, clinically sequenced (whole-exome and transcriptome sequencing) bone or soft tissue tumor biopsies from 150 men with advanced metastatic castration-resistance PCa (mCRPC). Importantly, they found that 29 men (19.3%) had an alteration in BRCA1, BRCA2, or ATM, and 12 men (8%) had pathogenic germline mutations, which is significantly higher than in localized disease. Pritchard and colleagues[17] specifically isolated germline DNA and assessed mutations in 20 DNA-repair genes, all of which were associated with autosomal dominant cancer-predisposition syndromes. Of the 692 men with documented metastatic PCa, 11.8% had germline DNA-repair gene mutations, primarily in BRCA2 (5.3%), ATM (1.6%), CHEK2 (1.9%), BRCA1 (0.9%), RAD51D (0.4%), and PALB2 (0.4%). Of note, even in 499 men with localized PCa, the prevalence (4.6%) was higher than previously reported.

These seminal papers led to an improved understanding of the role of high-penetrance germline mutations on PCa risk and, more importantly, treatment. Specifically, in the setting of advanced PCa, men with germline mutations in DNA damage repair genes, such as BRCA2, BRCA1, ATM, appear to be sensitive to poly-ADP ribose polymerase (PARP) inhibitors.[7,18,19] This sensitivity has led to important phase 2 and 3 clinical trials establishing the efficacy of PARP inhibitors in late-stage advanced PCa, ultimately resulting in the approval of olaparib and rucaparib, and incorporation into the 2020 American Urological Association/American Society for Radiation Oncology/Society of Urologic Oncology 2020 guidelines.[18–20] The National Comprehensive Cancer Network (NCCN) guidelines now recommend that clinicians offer a PARP inhibitor to patients with deleterious or suspected deleterious germline or somatic homologous recombination repair gene-mutated mCRPC following prior treatment with enzalutamide or abiraterone acetate and/or a taxane-based chemotherapy.[21]

A recent international consensus conference published by Giri and colleagues[22] streamlined recommendations for genetic testing and management. Current NCCN guidelines[21] recommend germline testing for an increasing number of men with PCa, including men with high-risk or very high-risk localized PCa, men with metastatic PCa, men with intraductal or cribriform histology, men with Ashkenazi Jewish ancestry, men with family history of high-risk germline mutations and known germline variants (BRCA1/2, Lynch syndrome, ATM, PALB2, CHEK2), or men with a positive strong history of PCa (first-degree relative with PCa death or diagnosed < age 60) and cancers associated with hereditary breast and ovarian cancer or Lynch syndrome.[21] Based on reported data on candidate genes, the NCCN guidelines recommend testing specifically for homologous recombination genes (BRCA1/2, ATM, PALB2, CHEK2) and Lynch syndrome–associated genes (MLH1, MSH2, MSH6, and PMS2).

The challenge in practice is implementing NCCN guidelines, incorporating multiple testing capabilities appropriately, and collaborating with genetic counseling. Multiple genetic testing panel options are available; it is important to understand the benefits and limitations of various panel testing options when considering germline testing of men with PCa and at risk for PCa. The expanding role of germline testing in precision medicine, PCa screening, and potentially active surveillance now impacts urology and oncology practice. As such, current NCCN guidelines highlight the importance of both pretest and posttest genetic counseling with a trained genetic counselor (GC),[21] and practices must consider how best to implement pretest and posttest counseling and delivery approaches. Guidance has been provided by professional efforts.[22] Numerous studies emphasize the importance of counseling regarding test results before testing and after testing to help address delivery of comprehensive genetically based and family history–based recommendations and the uncertainty surrounding some test results.[22–29]

In addition, as germline genetic testing for all malignancies continues to rapidly increase, the traditional model of genetic counseling care delivery needs to be adapted.[30–32] The current care model depends on referral from a nongenetics provider (clinician), who identifies an at-risk individual, to an in-person GC for pretest counseling, genetic testing, and posttest counseling.[30] With only a limited number of GC at any given institution, the current cohort of GC will not be able to meet the demands of projected genetic testing. The increasing gap between the number of men with PCa being referred for germline genetic testing and the availability and access to GC represents a critical gap in health care delivery.[30,33] Novel delivery models are required to help bridge that gap.[33–36]

Given the increasing role of germline testing in PCa care, the accompanying review articles in this special issue delve into the nuances of genetic predisposition for PCa, current guidelines and considerations regarding PCa germline testing, precision therapy and genetically based PCa screening, and the practical aspects of PCa genetic counseling and testing. Specific articles address disparities in PCa germline knowledge, biologic understanding of PCa aggressiveness, and how providers can obtain greater working knowledge of germline testing for PCa in this rapidly growing field.

DISCLOSURE

L.G. Gomella is a consultant for Ambry and Strand.

REFERENCES

1. Siegel RL, Miller KD, Jemal A. Cancer statistics, 2020. CA Cancer J Clin 2020;70(1):7–30.
2. Taitt HE. Global trends and prostate cancer: a review of incidence, detection, and mortality as influenced by race, ethnicity, and geographic location. Am J Mens Health 2018;12(6):1807–23.
3. Carter BS, Bova GS, Beaty TH, et al. Hereditary prostate cancer: epidemiologic and clinical features. J Urol 1993;150(3):797–802.
4. Kicinski M, Vangronsveld J, Nawrot TS. An epidemiological reappraisal of the familial aggregation of prostate cancer: a meta-analysis. PLoS One 2011; 6(10):e27130.
5. Brandt A, Sundquist J, Hemminki K. Risk for incident and fatal prostate cancer in men with a family history of any incident and fatal cancer. Ann Oncol 2012; 23(1):251–6.
6. Stanford JL, Ostrander EA. Familial prostate cancer. Epidemiol Rev 2001;23(1):19–23.
7. Brandão A, Paulo P, Teixeira MR. Hereditary predisposition to prostate cancer: from genetics to clinical implications. Int J Mol Sci 2020;21(14):5036.
8. Eeles RA, Olama AA, Benlloch S, et al. Identification of 23 new prostate cancer susceptibility loci using the iCOGS custom genotyping array. Nat Genet 2013;45(4):385–91.
9. Gudmundsson J, Sulem P, Gudbjartsson DF, et al. A study based on whole-genome sequencing yields a rare variant at 8q24 associated with prostate cancer. Nat Genet 2012;44(12):1326–9.
10. Amin Al Olama A, Kote-Jarai Z, Schumacher FR, et al. A meta-analysis of genome-wide association studies to identify prostate cancer susceptibility loci associated with aggressive and non-aggressive disease. Hum Mol Genet 2013;22(2):408–15.
11. Goh CL, Schumacher FR, Easton D, et al. Genetic variants associated with predisposition to prostate cancer and potential clinical implications. J Intern Med 2012;271(4):353–65.
12. Ewing CM, Ray AM, Lange EM, et al. Germline mutations in HOXB13 and prostate-cancer risk. N Engl J Med 2012;366(2):141–9.
13. Norris JD, Chang CY, Wittmann BM, et al. The homeodomain protein HOXB13 regulates the cellular response to androgens. Mol Cell 2009;36(3): 405–16.
14. Xu J, Lange EM, Lu L, et al. HOXB13 is a susceptibility gene for prostate cancer: results from the International Consortium for Prostate Cancer Genetics (ICPCG). Hum Genet 2013;132(1):5–14.
15. Shang Z, Zhu S, Zhang H, et al. Germline homeobox B13 (HOXB13) G84E mutation and prostate cancer risk in European descendants: a meta-analysis of 24,213 cases and 73,631 controls. Eur Urol 2013; 64(1):173–6.
16. Robinson D, Van Allen EM, Wu YM, et al. Integrative clinical genomics of advanced prostate cancer. Cell 2015;161(5):1215–28.
17. Pritchard CC, Mateo J, Walsh MF, et al. Inherited DNA-repair gene mutations in men with metastatic prostate cancer. N Engl J Med 2016;375(5):443–53.
18. de Bono J, Mateo J, Fizazi K, et al. Olaparib for metastatic castration-resistant prostate cancer. N Engl J Med 2020;382(22):2091–102.
19. Abida W, Patnaik A, Campbell D, et al. Rucaparib in men with metastatic castration-resistant prostate

cancer harboring a BRCA1 or BRCA2 gene alteration. J Clin Oncol 2020;38(32):3763–72.

20. Lowrance W, Breau R, Chou R, et al. Advanced prostate cancer: AUA/ASTRO/SUO guideline 2020. 2020. Available at: https://www.auanet.org/guidelines/advanced-prostate-cancer. Accessed October 23, 2020.

21. NCCN clinical practice guidelines in oncology (NCCN guidelines®): prostate (version 2.2020). 2020. Available at: https://www.nccn.org/professionals/physician_gls/pdf/prostate.pdf. Accessed October 23, 2020.

22. Giri VN, Knudsen KE, Kelly WK, et al. Implementation of germline testing for prostate cancer: Philadelphia prostate cancer consensus conference 2019. J Clin Oncol 2020;38(24):2798–811.

23. Park J, Zayhowski K, Newson AJ, et al. Genetic counselors' perceptions of uncertainty in pretest counseling for genomic sequencing: a qualitative study. J Genet Couns 2019;28(2):292–303.

24. Biesecker BB, Woolford SW, Klein WMP, et al. PUGS: a novel scale to assess perceptions of uncertainties in genome sequencing. Clin Genet 2017;92(2):172–9.

25. Newson AJ, Leonard SJ, Hall A, et al. Known unknowns: building an ethics of uncertainty into genomic medicine. BMC Med Genomics 2016;9(1):57.

26. Doyle DL, Awwad RI, Austin JC, et al. 2013 review and update of the genetic counseling practice based competencies by a task force of the Accreditation Council for Genetic Counseling. J Genet Couns 2016;25(5):868–79.

27. Gray SW, Martins Y, Feuerman LZ, et al. Social and behavioral research in genomic sequencing: approaches from the clinical sequencing exploratory research consortium outcomes and measures working group. Genet Med 2014;16(10):727–35.

28. ACMG Board of Directors. Points to consider in the clinical application of genomic sequencing. Genet Med 2012;14(8):759–61.

29. Giri VN, Hegarty SE, Hyatt C, et al. Germline genetic testing for inherited prostate cancer in practice: implications for genetic testing, precision therapy, and cascade testing. Prostate 2019;79(4):333–9.

30. Szymaniak BM, Facchini LA, Giri VN, et al. Practical considerations and challenges for germline genetic testing in patients with prostate cancer: recommendations from the Germline Genetics Working Group of the PCCTC. JCO Oncol Pract 2020;16(12):811–9.

31. Maiese DR, Keehn A, Lyon M, et al, Working Groups of the National Coordinating Center for Seven Regional Genetics Service Collaboratives. Current conditions in medical genetics practice. Genet Med 2019;21(8):1874–7.

32. Hoskovec JM, Bennett RL, Carey ME, et al. Projecting the supply and demand for certified genetic counselors: a workforce study. J Genet Couns 2018;27(1):16–20.

33. Boothe E, Greenberg S, Delaney CL, et al. Genetic counseling service delivery models: a study of genetic counselors' interests, needs, and barriers to implementation. J Genet Couns 2020;30(1):283–92.

34. Greenberg SE, Boothe E, Delaney CL, et al. Genetic counseling service delivery models in the United States: assessment of changes in use from 2010 to 2017. J Genet Couns 2020;29(6):1126–41.

35. Stoll K, Kubendran S, Cohen SA. The past, present and future of service delivery in genetic counseling: keeping up in the era of precision medicine. Am J Med Genet C Semin Med Genet 2018;178(1):24–37.

36. Kubendran S, Sivamurthy S, Schaefer GB. A novel approach in pediatric telegenetic services: geneticist, pediatrician and genetic counselor team. Genet Med 2017;19(11):1260–7.

Prostate Cancer Predisposition

Yasin Bhanji, MD[a], William B. Isaacs, PhD[b],*, Jianfeng Xu, MD, DrPH[c], Kathleen A. Cooney, MD[d]

KEYWORDS

- Prostate cancer • Hereditary cancer syndrome • Cancer susceptibility gene • Polygenic risk score

KEY POINTS

- Three risk factors for prostate cancer (PCa), namely family history, increasing age, and African ancestry, have been consistently recognized.
- Recently, rare pathogenic variants/mutations (RPMs) in several genes with moderate to high penetrance, such as *BRCA2*, *ATM*, *PALB2*, *CHEK2*, and *HOXB13*, and more than 160 common single nucleotide polymorphisms (SNPs), have been associated with PCa risk.
- The 3 inherited risk factors (family history, RPMs, and polygenic risk score) each affect the risk for PCa and may act independently. For example, most men carrying RPMs and high polygenic risk score in the general population do not have positive family history. Although family history and RPMs can identify 11% of men at higher PCa risk in the general population, adding polygenic risk score can identify an additional 22% of men at increased PCa risk.
- Although pathogenic mutations in *BRCA2*, *ATM*, and *PALB2* are associated with more aggressive PCa, the roles of mutations in other candidate PCa genes and SNP-based polygenic risk scores in PCa aggressiveness and progression is unclear.
- Pathogenic mutations in genes responsible for several hereditary cancer syndromes are likely relevant for PCa.
- For largely unexplained reasons, men of African ancestry are affected disproportionately by PCa; mutations in rare cancer susceptibility genes may contribute but cannot account for this disparity. Ancestry-specific risk SNPs may be more important.
- Two clinical strategies for germline testing in the setting of PCa are supported by available evidence: (1) testing RPMs in several genes (eg, *BRCA2*, *ATM*, *PALB2*, *CHEK2*, and *HOXB13*) and race-specific polygenic risk score among unaffected men to identify men at increased risk for early PCa development; and (2) testing RPMs in a subset of genes (eg, *BRCA2*, *ATM*, and *PALB2*) at time of diagnosis of high-grade and/or metastatic PCa for developing personalized treatment approaches.

INTRODUCTION

The 3 most important recognized risks for prostate cancer (PCa) are increasing age, ancestry, and family history of the disease. The clustering of PCa within families can be attributed to genetic factors, environmental factors, and/or random chance. Multiple lines of evidence support the hypothesis that genetic factors underlie much of the inherited predisposition to PCa. In a recent report

[a] Department of Urology, The James Buchanan Brady Urological Institute, Johns Hopkins University School of Medicine, Marburg 134, 600 North Wolfe Street, Baltimore, MD 21287, USA; [b] Department of Urology, The James Buchanan Brady Urological Institute, Johns Hopkins University School of Medicine, Marburg 115, 600 North Wolfe Street, Baltimore, MD 21287, USA; [c] Program for Personalized Cancer Care, NorthShore University HealthSystem, 1001 University Place, Evanston, IL 60201, USA; [d] Department of Medicine, Duke University School of Medicine and the Duke Cancer Institute, 2301 Erwin Road, DUH 1102, Durham, NC 27710-3703, USA
* Corresponding author.
E-mail address: wisaacs1@jh.edu

Urol Clin N Am 48 (2021) 283–296
https://doi.org/10.1016/j.ucl.2021.03.001

urologic.theclinics.com

from the Nordic Twin Study of Cancer (NorTwin-Can) comparing cancer risks between monozygotic and dizygotic twins, PCa showed one of the highest estimates of heritability and no measurable contribution of environmental factors.[1] Over the last 30 years, significant progress has been made in defining the genetic factors that contribute to PCa risk and aggressiveness. This article focuses on describing the impact of family history, rare pathogenic mutations (RPMs), and single nucleotide polymorphisms (SNPs) on the understanding of inherited forms of PCa.

EPIDEMIOLOGY OF PROSTATE CANCER RISK

PCa is the most common noncutaneous malignancy in the United States among men, and an estimated 13% of all men alive now can expect to be diagnosed with the disease, with approximately 2.5% expected to die of the disease. The incidence of PCa varies by ancestry and ethnicity, with African Americans experiencing a 73% higher incidence than European Americans. According to the American Cancer Society, for 2020, an estimated 191,930 new cases of PCa will be diagnosed in the United States, and the age-adjusted incidence rate is 104.2 per 100,000 men per year. The average age at diagnosis is 66 years, with 55% of all deaths occurring after the age of 65 years.[2,3] A detailed review of the incidence and mortality patterns, lifestyle, and dietary factors for PCa has been recently presented by Pernar and colleagues.[4]

The observation that the number of men dying of PCa is less than one-fifth the number of diagnosed cases emphasizes the low malignant potential of most PCa cancers. This situation creates significant challenges for optimal patient management. This problem is compounded by the observations made at autopsy that between 30% and 70% of men more than 70 years of age have lesions that, if detected by biopsy, result in a cancer diagnosis.[5] Most of these lesions, often termed latent cancers, are small-volume, low-grade tumors that do not become clinically manifest. Knowing which men are more likely to develop a high-risk, potentially lethal PCa that requires early detection and aggressive treatment versus more ubiquitous latent cancers, which can be safely monitored by active surveillance, is a critical goal that can be reached through better identification and understanding of molecular risk factors associated with tumor progression to lethal disease.

IMPLICATION OF GENETIC RISK FACTORS

Increasing age, family history, and ancestry/ethnicity are 3 of the most important factors associated with risk of PCa. Increasing age, although associated with risk of virtually all common human cancers, is perhaps the strongest risk factor for PCa, because the exponential rate at which both diagnosis and mortality increase for PCa far exceeds that of virtually all other cancers.[6] Although several hypotheses have been put forth, including prostate-specific deficiencies in DNA damage response, the underlying mechanistic basis for the age-related basis for PCa is unknown.[7]

Several different epidemiologic approaches have been used to detect and understand the genetic contribution to PCa risk. Investigations of family history and twin studies have been particularly informative in providing data consistent with a genetic cause for PCa. Twin studies of cancer in a population can provide valuable inferences regarding the variable contributions of inherited factors to a particular disease cause by taking advantage of the increased genetic likeness of monozygotic versus dizygotic pairs of twins. In NorTwinCan, time-to-event analyses were used to estimate familial risk of cancer given a twin's development of cancer as well as heritability or the proportion of variance in cancer risk caused by interindividual genetic differences.[1] A total of 27,156 cancers were diagnosed in 23,980 individuals who were included in the study, of which PCa had the highest estimated cumulative incidence (10.5%) with a heritability estimate of nearly 57%. This percentage was substantially higher than the corresponding estimates for other common cancers, including those of the breast, colon, and kidney, 3 types of cancers with multiple, known, well-established genetic risk factors.

Relatedly, family history was one of the first risk factors identified for PCa, and remains a consistent and robust marker of increased risk.[8] In general, the relative risk of developing PCa increases as (1) the number of affected family members increases, (2) the closer in relatedness the affected relatives are, and (3) the age of diagnosis of the affected decreases.[9] The recognition of the importance of these 3 characteristics led to the first operational definition of hereditary PCa (HPC), which was defined as a family with (1) 3 generations affected with PCa, and/or (2) 3 first-degree relatives affected, and/or (3) 2 relatives affected before age 55 years.[10]

Although all professional screening guidelines, including the National Comprehensive Cancer Network (NCCN), recommend an assessment of family history, family history used by itself has important limitations for assessing PCa risk.[11] Family history is based on the current disease status of related family members and not on the individual's genetic makeup. Furthermore, it is limited by recall and screening bias.[12] Although having an affected first-degree relative is consistently associated with increased risk for PCa, the magnitude of this increase varies substantially, ranging from less than 1.5 to more than 2, depending largely on the intensity of disease screening in the population studied, and the extent to which a positive family history increases this screening.[10] Differential screening intensity for PCa in different settings and populations likely plays an important role in shaping many of the demographic characteristics of PCa. Although the operational definition of HPC has been useful for framing gene mapping studies and other investigations of familial clustering, the lack of inclusion of any clinical variable to assess tumor aggressiveness has diluted its translational utility. As an example of this, a comparison of 324 patients with PCa with HPC, who fit the operational definition of HPC listed earlier, with 1664 patients with sporadic PCa (ie, with no family history) was performed using the Netherlands Cancer Registry. Patients with HPC were on average 3 years younger at diagnosis, had lower prostate-specific antigen (PSA) values, lower Gleason scores, and more often had locally confined disease, with 35% having high-risk disease compared with 51% of patients with sporadic PCa. Despite the favorable clinical phenotype in patients with HPC, they were less likely to receive active surveillance, and instead were more likely to receive radical treatment.[13]

Familial Prostate Cancer versus Hereditary Prostate Cancer

Familial PCa (FPC) and HPC both imply a heightened risk for development of the disease, but these two terms carry very different implications. FPC refers to a constellation of disease within families, whereas HPC implies a familial inheritance pattern consistent with the passage of a major susceptibility gene in a mendelian fashion. An early segregation analysis of patterns of familial clustering of PCa provided evidence in support of the existence of 1 or more rare (mutation allele frequency of 0.30%), high-penetrance mutations in genes inherited in an autosomal dominant, mendelian fashion.[14] These alleles were proposed to account for only 9% of PCa overall but had penetrance of 88% by age 85 years. Presciently, these numbers are strikingly similar to the characteristics of HOXB13, ATM, and BRCA2 described later.

Regarding epidemiologic studies of risk for more aggressive disease, there are data to suggest that patients with PCa are more likely to die of the disease if their fathers died of PCa.[15] Using a population-based database that includes approximately 3 million families to analyze the relationship of survival between sons and their fathers, Lindström and colleagues[16] found the hazard ratio (HR) for PCa death in an affected son was 2.1 (95% confidence interval [CI], 1.1–3.8) if there was poor survival in the father. In addition, when a father's survival was categorized as good, intermediate, or poor, a significant trend of increasing HR estimates for death of affected sons with a worsening survival outcome in fathers was observed. Furthermore, Albright and colleagues[17] provided population-based estimates of lethal PCa risk based on lethal PCa family history. Many family history constellations associated with 2 to greater than 5 times increased risk for lethal PCa were identified. These results support a genetic susceptibility to lethal PCa.

Although many genetic factors, including the large number of common SNPs discussed later, contribute to familial clustering, in PCa, like other cancers, mutations in a very small number of major genes have been identified that have the degree of penetrance required to generate strict mendelian inheritance patterns in PCa families. This feature is compounded by the high prevalence (and thus high phenocopy rate) of PCa, particularly low-grade disease, and the heterogeneous genetic influences that contribute to this common disease. As the genetics underlying familial clustering and inheritance of PCa in general become more well elucidated, the further refinement of the terms sporadic, familial, and hereditary with respect to PCa, and their relevance in terms of clinical application and utility, might be expected. Furthermore, by having a better genetics-based definition of HPC that incorporates a clinicopathologic component to address disease aggressiveness, it may be possible to reduce the overdiagnosis and overtreatment among men with a family history of the disease.

LINKAGE ANALYSIS, HOXB13

Providing evidence through segregation analysis for the possible existence of a large-effect PCa susceptibility allele set the stage for PCa family collection and linkage-based gene mapping efforts. The International Consortium for Prostate Cancer Genetics (ICPCG) was formed in 1996 to address this question. This group performed a genome-wide linkage scan of 1233 families that fit HPC criteria.[18] Although suggestive, 5 moderate linkage signals were observed, including 1 at 17q21. Sequencing candidate genes under this linkage peak led to the identification of a recurrent but rare missense change, G84E, in HOXB13, a gene highly expressed and intimately involved in prostate biology. In an analysis of germline DNA from more than 5000 patients with PCa and controls, our group reported that the frequency of the G84E allele was significantly higher in patients with PCa (1.4%) than controls (0.1%–0.4%).[19] An enrichment of G84E was found in patients with PCa who were diagnosed at early age (eg, <55 years) and with a positive family history of PCa. These finding have been consistently confirmed by many laboratories around the world, with odds ratios for PCa varying from 2-fold to 15-fold. Through combined analyses of international study populations by the ICPCG, the most common mutation in HOXB13 in US men, G84E, had the highest frequency in individuals of Nordic descent.[20] As many as 8% to 10% of Swedish and Finnish men with family history positive for PCa diagnosed at an early age carry a G84E HOXB13 mutation, compared with ~1% or less in unaffected men.[21,22] A critical additional finding was that nearly all G84E mutation carriers shared a common haplotype, meaning they are all descended from a common founder, presumably of Nordic ancestry.[20] Potential founder mutations in HOXB13 have subsequently been found to be associated with PCa risk in other distinct populations, including the G132E mutation in Japanese, and the G135E mutation in Chinese.[23,24] Along with G84E, these 3 changes, substituting a glutamic acid for glycine at amino acid positions 84, 132, and 135, respectively, lie in 1 of 2 highly conserved domains in the HOXB13 protein that are responsible for binding to the homeobox cofactor, MEIS, suggesting an alteration of this binding as a mechanistic feature of the cancer-promoting action of these variants.[25,26] More recently, a rare (minor allele frequency 0.2%) but recurrent stop loss mutation in HOXB13 (Ter285-Lys, c.853delT) has been found in a collection of PCa cases of African ancestry in Martinique.[27] In ClinVar, this change is listed as a variant of unknown significance.[28]

HOXB13 is a prostate-specific homeobox transcription factor that plays a crucial role in the normal embryonic development of the prostate through its modulation of the prostate transcriptome via interaction with other key prostate transcription factors, including the androgen receptor (AR), FOXA1, and NKX3.1.[29–31] HOXB13 expression is maintained through adulthood and is generally maintained throughout initiation and progression of PCa. As indicated earlier, 3 critical factors affect the frequency, and thus importance, of G84E as a susceptibility gene: (1) early age of PCa diagnosis, with men diagnosed before age 55 years having the highest frequency of G84E;

(2) family history, with the frequency of G84E increased in men with first-degree relatives affected with PCa; and (3) ancestry, with individuals of Nordic ancestry having the highest population frequencies of G84E (as mentioned earlier). In men of African and eastern European descent, G84E is extremely rare. Although not uniform, most studies do not find any differences in PCa clinicopathologic variables between carriers and noncarriers of G84E. The association of G84E and PCa seems to be equally strong in men with high-risk and low-risk PCa (ie, carriers of G84E are at increased risk of the full spectrum of PCa, including high-risk, lethal disease). The G84E mutation can be highly penetrant and the penetrance seems to vary with ancestry, age at diagnosis, family history, and year of birth.[32] Penetrance estimates range from 40% to 60% by age 80 years, and almost complete penetrance in men who have a strong family history of early-onset PCa.[21,32] Penetrance of G84E may also be modified by genetic risk score (GRS) derived from multiple PCa risk-associated SNPs. In a large Swedish population-based study, the cumulative PCa risk by age 80 years was 33% for G84E carriers. This risk increased to 48% if carriers also had higher polygenic risk score (top quartile).[21,33] In addition, recent analyses of other cancers have implicated G84E as a risk factor for both rectosigmoid cancer (odds ratio [OR] = 2.25 [1.05–4.15]; P = .05) and nonmelanoma skin cancer (OR = 1.40 [1.12–1.74]; P = .01). Curiously, these findings were only observed in men.[34]

INHERITED DNA-REPAIR GENE MUTATIONS IN MEN WITH AGGRESSIVE PROSTATE CANCER

It has been widely established that germline mutations in DNA-repair genes (DRGs) are major contributors to the inherited risk for multiple common human cancers, including those of the breast and colon. However, until approximately 5 years ago, the frequencies of pathogenic DRG mutations in PCa were uncertain or reported to be low, leading to a poor appreciation of the potential importance of this class of genes to PCa genetic risk. The understanding of the contribution of DRGs in PCa susceptibility changed dramatically when next-generation sequencing studies began to focus on men with metastatic disease with the goal of identifying therapeutic targets. In 2015, Robinson and colleagues[35] analyzed 150 patients with metastatic, castration resistant PCa by whole-exome sequencing. Eight percent of these patients were found to have rare pathogenic germline mutations in DRGs such as BRCA2, a frequency 4 to 5 times higher than observed in previous studies of patients with PCa. These findings were expanded on in another critical article, by Pritchard and colleagues,[36] who showed that the incidence of germline mutations in genes mediating DNA-repair processes in men with metastatic PCa was 11.8%, much higher than the incidence among men with localized disease. Mutations were identified in 16 different genes, with the most frequent in *BRCA2* (44% of total mutations), *ATM* (13%), and *CHEK2* (12%). **Table 1** shows the relative risk for metastatic PCa in 8 DRGs by comparing the mutation frequency in the Pritchard report with control data from the Exome Aggregation Consortium. Interestingly, the frequency of germline mutations in DRGs in men with metastatic PCa did not vary significantly when stratified by age at diagnosis or based on a positive family history of the disease.

To directly compare the ability of mutations in *BRCA* genes and *ATM* to distinguish risk for lethal disease, Na and colleagues[37] sequenced *BRCA1*, *BRCA2*, and *ATM* in a set of men who died of PCa and a set of men who had radical prostatectomy and had Gleason grade group (GG) 1, pathologically localized, low-risk disease. The rate of pathogenic mutations in these 3 genes was found to be 4-fold higher in men who had died of PCa. In addition, mutations in these genes, in particular *BRCA2*, were associated with decreased age at death, and decreased time to death from the time of diagnosis. Carter and colleagues[38] further showed the association of mutations in these 3 genes with more aggressive disease in an analysis of more than 1200 men undergoing active surveillance for PCa. Although the frequency was low, men who carried mutations in these genes were significantly more likely to undergo grade reclassification, with the OR for grade reclassification from GG1 to GG3 being more than 4.

CHEK2 is among the DRGs that are most commonly found to harbor germline loss-of-function mutations in PCa, although the association of these mutations with increased risk of high-risk disease is less consistent.[39] Likewise, *NBN*, along with *BRCA2* and *ATM*, was reported to be associated with high-risk disease in a recent study of Polish men, although this result is also less consistent in other populations.[40]

Because not all DRGs are associated with aggressive PCa risk, when interpreting panel testing in the PCa realm, it is important to understand which genes harbor mutations that are associated with tumor aggressiveness and which do not. Results from a study of 1694 radical prostatectomy patients with pathologically verified tumor grade indicate the strong association of mutations in 3 genes, *ATM*, *BRCA2*, and *MSH2*, and high risk as assessed by tumor grade.[41]

For example, men carrying a loss-of-function *BRCA2* or *ATM* mutation were more than 5 times more likely to have GG4 or GG5 tumors than GG1. *MSH2* showed a significant association as well. Although multiple other genes showed higher mutation rates in GG5 versus GG1 disease, including *BRCA1*, *CHEK2*, *MSH6*, *NBN*, *PALB2*, and *TP53*, none of the other genes tested showed a significant association with tumor grade. These results must be tempered by the rarity of mutations and thus power to detect association. Although none of the non-*ATM/BRCA2/MSH2* genes showed significant evidence of association with high tumor grade, it should be pointed out

Table 1
Genes associated with metastatic prostate cancer

Gene	Metastatic Prostate Cancer(N = 692)		Exome Aggregation Consortium (N=53,105)		Relative Risk	95% CI	P Value
	Carriers (N)	%	Carriers (N)	%			
ATM	11	1.59	133	0.25	6.3	3.2–11.3	<.001
BRCA1	6	0.87	104	0.22	3.9	1.4–8.5	.005
BRCA2	37	5.35	153	0.29	18.6	13.2–25.3	<.001
CHEK2	10	1.87	314	0.61	3.1	1.5–5.6	.002
MSH2	1	0.14	23	0.04	3.3	0.1–18.5	.26
MSH6	1	0.14	41	0.08	1.9	0.05–10.4	.41
NBN	2	0.29	61	0.11	2.5	0.3–9.1	.19
PALB2	3	0.43	65	0.12	2.7	0.3–6.6	.17

Data from Pritchard CC, Mateo J, Walsh MF, et al. Inherited DNA-repair gene mutations in men with metastatic prostate cancer. *N Engl J Med.* 2016;375(5):443-453. https://doi.org/10.1056/NEJMoa1603144.

that, in a combined analysis with all genes other than these 3, a significant association was still observed. This signal suggests that other genes in this panel may associate with tumor grade, but larger studies are needed to detect this effect. **Table 2** presents a summary of estimates of the importance of various DRGs as risk-affecting genes for both PCa diagnosis and advanced cancer development.

To further understand and explain the hereditary risk of PCa, the identification of additional genetic variants associated with PCa risk could be very helpful in the identification of at-risk individuals and provide more insight into the mechanisms of aggressive disease and potentially, novel targeted therapies. In a unique, 2-stage study of affected men who had a strong family history of disease or more aggressive disease, Schaid and colleagues[42] identified genes in stage 1 and screened them in stage 2 using a custom-capture design among 2917 cases and 1899 controls. In addition to HOXB13 and several other previously identified genes including BRCA2 and ATM, 10 novel genes, including MYCBP2 and RNASEH2B, were implicated as prostate cancer associated genes in this study.[42] Confirmatory studies are needed to address the significance of these novel candidates.[42]

Germline testing is recommended by the NCCN for the subset of patients with PCa with high-risk, very-high-risk, regional, or metastatic disease, or with a family history of hereditary breast and ovarian cancer and Lynch syndrome (discussed later). Beyond the substantial screening value that the identification of specific germline variants

has on identifying disease early and predicting its course, this type of knowledge also has profound therapeutic implications. For example, treatment with olaparib, a poly-(ADP-ribose) polymerase (PARP) inhibitor, in patients who had highly pre-treated PCa and who had defects in DRGs had high response rates to therapy. Mateo and colleagues[43] performed next-generation sequencing in a cohort of these patients and 33% had mutations in BRCA1/2, ATM, or CHEK2 and, of these, 88% had a response to olaparib, including 100% of patients with BRCA2 loss, and 4 of 5 with ATM mutations.

Most cancer susceptibility genes function as tumor suppressors and are active as such as long as at least 1 of the 2 inherited copies of the gene are intact and expressed. Referring to the 2-hit hypothesis, inheriting 1 copy of a mutated ATM, for example, does not elicit a phenotype unless the remaining copy becomes inactive through deletion, mutation, or gene expression silencing. Correspondingly, this second hit, which can be difficult to discern in some clinical settings, can determine whether or not a mutation in a gene such as ATM, BRCA2, and most other genes that act in a tumor-suppressing manner contribute causally to tumor formation or, in the case of PARP inhibitor treatment, to treatment response.[44]

AFRICAN AMERICAN GERMLINE PREDISPOSITION TO PROSTATE CANCER

As described earlier, there is substantial evidence regarding the role of high-penetrance genes and

Table 2
Estimates of DNA-repair gene importance in susceptibility for all prostate cancer and for more aggressive disease

Gene	PCa Susceptibility	Risk for Aggressive/ Metastatic/Lethal Disease
ATM	++	++++
BRCA1	+	+
BRCA2	+++	++++
HOXB13	++++	+/−
CHEK2	+	+/−
MSH2	+	+++
MSH6	+	++
NBN	+	+/−
PALB2	+	++
RAD51C-DI	+/−	+/−
BRIPl other Fanconi Anemia genes	—	—

Increasing numbers of plus signs indicates increasingly strong evidence as a risk factor; +/− indicates no significance evidence to support a role as a risk factor.

their significance in the increased risk of disease and as drivers of lethality. However, most of the studies documenting these findings have largely focused on men of European ancestry. This point is against the backdrop that African American men have the highest incidence and mortality from PCa in the world. Although several factors are likely contributing to the excess PCa mortality in African American men, some studies show that the difference in clinical outcomes continues to persist for African American men even after controlling for socioeconomic differences, suggesting the presence of biological factors driving this disparity.[45]

In a large recent study of African American and Ugandan PCa patients and controls, pathogenic variants of DRGs were found in 3.6% of patients compared with 2.1% in controls, and the highest risk of aggressive disease was seen in men with variants in *ATM*, *BRCA2*, *PALB2*, and *NBN* genes.[46] For single genes, significant results were seen for *BRCA2* and *ATM* mutation frequencies in patients versus controls, with ORs of 3.92 and 3.83, respectively, for the combined group of Ugandan and African American patients. The combined frequencies of pathogenic mutations in *BRCA2* and *ATM* in metastatic disease were 1.4% and 4.8% for African American and Ugandan patients, respectively. These results indicate that *BRCA2* and *ATM* mutations are significant risk factors for high-risk disease in men of African descent, although the frequencies of mutation in both genes are lower than has been observed in European Americans with high-risk disease. This finding suggests that, as in men of European ancestry, the prevalence of DNA-repair mutations remains low. An increased frequency of these potent, high-risk-inducing genes in African American men does not seem to explain the increased mortalities observed in men of African descent.

PROSTATE CANCER AS PART OF KNOWN CANCER SYNDROMES

PCa risk can be increased in men who carry a mutation in genes related to several known cancer syndromes. This finding is expected because cancer gene mutations typically increase the risk of more than 1 type of cancer in a family.

Hereditary breast and ovarian cancer

Several studies of families with hereditary breast and ovarian cancer (HBOC) conducted in the 1990s revealed that this syndrome can be attributed in some families to deleterious mutations in one of the 2 genes, namely *BRCA1* on chromosome 17 and *BRCA2* on chromosome 13.[47,48] Studies of HBOC families segregating *BRCA1* or *BRCA2* mutations confirm that there is an increased risk of male *BRCA1* and *BRCA2* mutation carriers compared with non–mutation carriers within HBOC families and compared with the general population (data from the Breast Cancer Linkage Consortium).[49,50] In these studies, the overall relative risk (RR) of PCa in men with *BRCA1* mutations was 1.07 (95% CI, 0.75–1.54) and the RR of PCa in men with *BRCA1* mutations younger than 65 years was 1.82 (95% CI, 1.01–3.29). In comparison, men with *BRCA2* mutations had a higher RR of PCa (4.65; 95% CI, 3.48–6.22) as well as a higher RR of PCa for male mutations carriers younger than 65 years (7.33; 95% CI, 4.66–11.52). Note that these risk estimates may be inflated because they are based on information from highly selected HBOC families and may not apply to the general population. Furthermore, studies of PC-only families have not found a significant number of *BRCA1/2* pathogenic mutations, indicating that these mutations likely contribute to a small portion of hereditary PC defined as families with multiple cases of PCa.[51,52]

Studies of the Icelandic founder *BRCA2* mutation, which is a 5-bp deletion beginning at nucleotide 999 (999del5), provided the initial insights into the relationship between mutations in genes associated with HBOC and aggressive and/or lethal PC.[53] Sigurdsson and colleagues[54] described PCa cases from known Icelandic HBOC families each caused by the *BRCA2* 999del5 mutation. Of the 12 patients with PCa that were available for genetic testing, 9 of the men inherited the *BRCA2* 999del5 allele and the remaining 3 men did not carry the allele. Interesting, all 9 mutation carriers died of PCa compared with only 1 of the noncarriers, suggesting that *BRCA2* mutation status correlates with a poorer prognosis from the disease. In a larger study of 527 Icelandic men with PCa, including 30 men who were carriers of the *BRCA2* 999del5 allele, carriers were shown to have a significantly earlier age at diagnosis, more advanced tumor stage and grade, and shorter survival time.[55] After adjusting for year of diagnosis and birth, mutation carriers were also shown to be at increased risk of dying of PCa, and this association remained after adjusting for stage and grade. The role of *BRCA1* and *BRCA2* in clinically aggressive PCa has been strengthened from studies of both men known to carry *BRCA1/2* germline mutations and also men discovered to have *BRCA1/2* germline mutations through clinical studies of metastatic PCa tissue.[35,56,57]

LYNCH SYNDROME FAMILIES

In addition to colorectal cancer, there are several cancers that occur with increased frequency in individuals carrying a pathogenic germline mutation in a Lynch syndrome (LS)–associated mismatch repair (MMR) gene (most commonly *MLH1*, *MSH2*, *MSH6*, and *PMS2*). These LS-associated cancers occur in the endometrium, ovary, stomach, small bowel, and ureter, but data supporting an LS-PCa correlation have been conflicting. In 2014, Raymond and colleagues, Han and colleagues[58,59] reported an overall HR for PCa of 1.99 (95% CI, 1.34–4.59; *P* = .0038) across 2 large familial LS cancer registries, whereas an independent meta-analysis identified a risk increase of 2.28-fold (95% CI, 2.32–6.67) for men with MMR mutations in LS families. Interestingly, PCa tumors sequenced from individuals with LS carry classic microsatellite instability signatures, an uncommon observation in PCa.[60] In light of this new information, there is general consensus among experts that men harboring MMR mutations are at an increased risk for PCa, but the magnitude of the risk increase is not fully defined.

USE OF SINGLE GENE POLYMORPHISMS IN RISK ASSESSMENT

To date, more than 160 inherited PCa risk–associated SNPs have been identified through genome-wide association studies (GWASs).[61] Because of stringent criteria used for declaring statistically significant risk SNPs, including multiple-stage study design, large sample size of cases and controls, and a minimum requirement of $P < 5 \times 10E\text{-}8$ to account for multiple testing, most of these risk SNPs can be replicated in independent study populations. Compared with rare monogenic mutations, SNPs are more common, and each has a modest individual effect on PCa risk. However, SNPs have a stronger cumulative effect that can be measured by a polygenic risk score.

VARIOUS POLYGENIC RISK SCORE METHODS

Polygenic risk score is a generic term for statistical methods that measure the cumulative effect of multiple risk-associated SNPs. Several polygenic risk score methods have been commonly used in the last 10 years, including a direct risk allele count, an OR-weighted risk allele count (often specifically referred to as polygenic risk score), or an OR-weighted and population-standardization method, typically termed GRS.[62] A common feature of these methods is that they are based on well-established risk-associated SNPs.

Recently, a novel polygenic risk score method based on millions of SNPs in the genome (not limited to the well-established risk-associated SNPs), called genome-wide polygenic score (GPS), was proposed.[63–65] In addition, a polygenic hazard score that is based on a set of SNPs that are associated with age at diagnosis of aggressive PCa has also been developed.[66]

Except for the weaker performance of the direct risk allele count method, which does not take the effect (OR) of risk allele into account, the performance of other polygenic risk score methods in risk stratification is similar. Specifically, the performance and percentile of polygenic risk score and GRS is exactly the same if the same SNPs and OR of risk alleles are used.[62] The only difference is that GRS is population standardized and can be interpreted as RR to the general population regardless of numbers of SNPs used in the calculation (therefore, the mean GRS in the population is always 1). In contrast, the values of polygenic risk score increase with the number of SNPs used in the calculation. Although many more SNPs are used in the GPS, its performance is similar to GRS,[64,67] likely because most of the risk stratification signals in GPS come from well-established risk-associated SNPs that have already been accounted for in GRS.

POLYGENIC RISK SCORE FOR PROSTATE CANCER RISK

Since the first demonstration of the cumulative effect of the first 5 established risk-associated SNPs on PCa risk in 2008 by our research group,[68] published studies to date consistently show associations between polygenic risk score and PCa risk, including those from large case-control studies,[61,69] retrospective analysis of prospective studies,[70,71] prostate biopsy cohorts,[72,73] and population-based prospective studies.[74] A dose-response association between higher percentile of polygenic risk scores and higher PCa risk is observed in all published studies. For example, using a large prospective cohort derived from the UK Biobank, where 208,685 PCa diagnosis–free participants at recruitment were followed via the UK cancer and death registries, we found that a GRS based on 130 known risk-associated SNPs significantly predicted risk and mortality for PCa.[75] Men in higher GRS deciles had significantly higher PCa incidence and PCa mortality, both *P* trend less than .001. Furthermore, a head-to-head comparison showed that GRS was more informative for stratifying inherited PCa risk than family history and RPMs. In addition, this study revealed that the association between GRS and

PCa incidence was independent of family history and RPMs and can therefore complement family history and RPMs for inherited risk assessment. Although family history and RPMs identified 11% of men at higher PCa risk, adding GRS (>1.5) identified an additional 15% of men at higher PCa risk with comparable PCa incidence and mortality.

Higher polygenic risk scores are also consistently associated with an earlier age of PCa diagnosis.[66,76,77] Based on a retrospective analysis of The Reduction by Dutasteride of Prostate Cancer Events (REDUCE) chemoprevention trial, men in higher GRS risk groups (based on 110 known PCa risk-associated SNPs) were shown to have worse PCa diagnosis–free survival compared with the entire cohort (P trend <.0001).[76]

POLYGENIC RISK SCORE FOR DIFFERENTIATING AGGRESSIVENESS OF PROSTATE CANCER

Despite the consistent finding that polygenic risk score can effectively stratify disease risk, its association with disease is inconsistent and generally negative.[78–81] For example, in a study of 5895 surgically treated PCa cases in which each tumor was uniformly graded and staged using the same protocol, there were no statistically significant differences (P>.05) in risk allele frequencies between patients with more aggressive or less aggressive disease for 18 of the 20 reported PCa risk–associated SNPs.[78] In another recently published study on European men from the Prostate Cancer Prevention Trial (PCPT) (N = 2434) and the Selenium and Vitamin E Cancer Prevention Trial (SELECT) (N = 4885), a higher polygenic score based on 98 known risk-associated SNPs was associated with PCa risk in both trials but did not predict other outcomes.[79] These studies suggest that almost all PCa risk–associated SNPs are not associated with aggressiveness and currently have minimal utility in predicting the risk for developing more or less aggressive forms of PCa.

Lack of association between polygenic risk score and aggressiveness of PCa in case-case studies is not contradictory to its association with PCa mortality found in case-control studies. Because of the association of polygenic risk score and PCa risk, more men with higher polygenic risk score are expected to develop PCa (both indolent and aggressive PCa) compared with men in the general population. However, once diagnosed with PCa, polygenic risk score does not differentiate which patients are more likely to die from the disease. This explanation is supported by data from the large prospective cohort derived from the UK Biobank, with 209,588 men at risk

for PCa. After approximately 10 years' follow-up, 10,203 (4.87%) men developed PCa, and 695 died of the disease. The mortality was 0.33% (695 out of 209,588) among men at risk for PCa, and the mortality ratio was 6.81% (695 out of 10,203) among men diagnosed with PCa. The PCa incidence rate was higher in men with high GRS defined as greater than or equal to 1.5 (3615 out of 37,445 = 9.65%) than low GRS defined as less than 1.5 (6558 out of 172,143 = 3.83%; P<.001). The PCa-specific mortality was also higher in men with high GRS (239 out of 37,445 = 0.64%) than low GRS (456 out of 172,143 = 0.26%; P<.001). However, there was no significant difference in mortality ratio between patients with PCa with high GRS (239 out of 3615 = 6.61%) and low GRS (456 out of 6558 = 6.92%; P = .58).[75]

POTENTIAL CLINICAL UTILITY OF POLYGENIC RISK SCORE

The consistent findings of associations for polygenic risk score with PCa risk and also early age of diagnosis provide a basis for its use in PCa risk stratification. Furthermore, because the associations of polygenic risk score with PCa risk and age at diagnosis are independent of family history and RPMs, polygenic risk score can be used to supplement family history and RPMs to better stratify inherited risk.[12] At present, recommendations for inherited PCa risk assessment from the US Preventive Services Task Force and the European Association of Urology rely primarily on family history only, whereas the NCCN also recommends incorporation of RPMs.[82–84] In the future, incorporation of information regarding inherited risk based on family history, RPMs, and GRS may be considered in the discussion of potential benefits and harms for baseline PSA screening at an early age.

Polygenic risk scores may be useful in the clinic to refine estimates of disease penetrance for carriers of RPMs. As mentioned above, several studies have shown significantly higher penetrance between high and low polygenic risk score among men with RPMs of BRCA2 and HOXB13.[21,33,85]

Inherited risk assessment may also have potential clinical utility in decision making of prostate biopsy. Results from the REDUCE study,[70] several prostate biopsy cohorts,[72,73] and a study of Finnish men with and without PCa[86] suggest polygenic risk scores provide added value compared with PSA levels to improve the detection rate of PCa.

In contrast, the clinical utility of polygenic risk scores in differentiating aggressive from indolent PCa and in predicting prognosis of PCa is currently unclear. However, encouraging preliminary findings are emerging on the use of polygenic risk scores for predicting tumor upgrading in 2 active surveillance (AS) cohorts, as discussed by Helfand and Xu.[87] The prognostic value of polygenic risk scores may be unique for use in AS and this observation awaits confirmation in additional studies.

IMPORTANT CONSIDERATIONS FOR IMPLEMENTING POLYGENIC RISK SCORE IN THE CLINIC

Based on the consistent association between polygenic risk score percentile and PCa risk,[61,66,68–77,88] polygenic risk scores have been proposed and recently adopted by several genetic testing companies to estimate an individual's risks for common diseases, including PCa. However, the important and consistent trend between percentiles of polygenic risk score and disease risk in study populations is not sufficient to support their clinical use for risk assessment at the individual patient level. There are 2 major considerations for this statement. First, although an informative risk measurement, the percentile of risk only ranks an individual's probability of disease risk within a population. It does not specify the quantity of risk, and individuals with the same percentile may have different quantities of risks for different diseases and in different populations. Second, percentiles per se are not commonly used in current clinical guidelines for risk assessment. Instead, absolute risk, such as lifetime risk, is routinely used in clinical guidelines. Lifetime risk is calculated from an individual's RR derived from various risk factors (including polygenic risk) and population-based incidence and mortality.

Another important factor for translating polygenic risk score is the need to develop race-specific scores. This factor is critical because the effect size (OR) and allele frequency of risk-associated SNPs differ among racial populations.[59,89] To date, most GWASs and polygenic risk scores were based on white populations. As such, the validity and calibration of polygenic risk score for other minority racial groups are not well developed. This status quo may exacerbate existing racial disparities in PCa care. Substantial efforts should be devoted to address this need in order to fully realize the potential of polygenic risk scores for use in the clinical management of PCa.

SUMMARY

PCa remains a leading cause of cancer death among American men. Genetic testing to assess mutational status of DRGs is a noninvasive, reproducible means of identifying men at increased risk of lethal disease at a time when cure is still possible. Unaffected carriers of DRG and *HOXB13* mutations should managed with earlier and more intensive disease screening, whereas DRG mutation carrier status in men diagnosed with PCa should be used in both surgical and systemic treatment decision making. Although the data supporting the role of *BRCA2* and *ATM* in aggressive PCa seem unequivocal, some data also exist to support a role for mutations in other DRGs, including *BRCA1*, *MSH2*, *PALB2*, *CHEK2*, and *NBN*, as risk factors for aggressive disease, but larger studies are needed before these genes become actionable in terms of clinical decision making. The use of polygenic risk score to stratify risk of PCa diagnosis is highly effective, inexpensive, and informative, but currently underused. Future studies should focus on combining family history, RPMs, and polygenic risk score to more accurately define PCa risk in unaffected men.

CLINICS CARE POINTS

- PCa has a strong inherited component and having a family history of clinically significant PCa or other cancers, such as breast, colon, ovarian, or pancreatic cancer, particularly when diagnosed at an early age, increases the risk of developing clinically significant PCa ∼ 1.5-fold to 3-fold.

- The NCCN recommends offering genetic testing to men who are diagnosed with high-risk or very-high-risk PCa and if the patient has a family history of *BRCA1* or *BRCA2* mutations, LS, or comes from a high-risk ancestry group such as the Ashkenazi Jewish.

- Pathogenic mutations in *BRCA2* and *ATM* are the most consistent and reproducible genetic risk factors for aggressive, potentially lethal PCa. *MSH2* mutations, although much less common, seem to be associated with high-risk disease as well. Because of their rarity, further studies are necessary to more fully determine the prognostic importance of mutations in *PALB2*, *NBN*, *CHEK2*, *BRCA1*, *HOXB13*, and most other putative PCa risk genes tested on most cancer gene panels. *HOXB13* G84E continues to be a reproducible and informative risk factor for all PCa risk.

- Polygenic risk scores determined using well-characterized common genetic factors are powerful and informative predictors of PCa risk in Americans of both European and African descent. However, there are important differences in the panel of SNPs that stratify risk most effectively in these 2 groups.

- Increased use of combined, ancestry-optimized polygenic risk score and genetic testing for BRCA2, ATM, and MSH2 should be strongly considered for inclusion in routine disease screening paradigms to optimize patient management in the era of precision medicine.

DISCLOSURE

The generous support from the Patrick C Walsh Hereditary Prostate Cancer program is gratefully acknowledged. This study was supported by grants from Department of Defense (W81XWH-16-1-0764, W81XWH-16-1-0765, and W81XWH-16-1-0766).

REFERENCES

1. Mucci LA, Hjelmborg JB, Harris JR, et al. Familial risk and heritability of cancer among twins in nordic countries. JAMA 2016;315(1):68–76.
2. NVSS - Mortality Data. Available at: https://www.cdc.gov/nchs/nvss/deaths.htm?CDC_AA_refVal=https%3A%2F%2Fwww.cdc.gov%2Fnchs%2Fdeaths.htm. Accessed October 23, 2020.
3. About Prostate Cancer. Available at: www.cancer.org/cancer/prostate-cancer/detection-diagnosis-staging/how-. Accessed October 23, 2020.
4. Pernar CH, Ebot EM, Wilson KM, et al. The epidemiology of prostate cancer. Cold Spring Harb Perspect Med 2018;8(12). https://doi.org/10.1101/cshperspect.a030361.
5. Sandhu GS, Andriole GL. Overdiagnosis of prostate cancer. J Natl Cancer Inst Monogr 2012;2012(45): 146–51.
6. Prostate cancer statistics | Cancer Research UK. Available at: https://www.cancerresearchuk.org/health-professional/cancer-statistics/statistics-by-cancer-type/prostate-cancer. Accessed October 23, 2020.
7. Kiviharju-af Hällström TM, Jäämaa S, Mönkkönen M, et al. Human prostate epithelium lacks Wee1A-mediated DNA damage-induced checkpoint enforcement. Proc Natl Acad Sci U S A 2007; 104(17):7211–6.
8. Woolf CM. An investigation of the familial aspects of carcinoma of the prostate. Cancer 1960;13:739–44.
9. Nelson Q, Agarwal N, Stephenson R, et al. A population-based analysis of clustering identifies a strong genetic contribution to lethal prostate cancer. Front Genet 2013;4:152.
10. Steinberg GD, Carter BS, Beaty TH, et al. Family history and the risk of prostate cancer. Prostate 1990; 17(4):337–47.
11. Carlsson S, Castle EP, Catalona WJ, et al. NCCN guidelines version 2.2020 prostate cancer early detection. Plymouth Meeting: National Comprehensive Cancer Network; 2020.
12. Xu J, Labbate CV, Isaacs WB, et al. Inherited risk assessment of prostate cancer: it takes three to do it right. Prostate Cancer Prostatic Dis 2020;23(1):59–61.
13. Cremers RG, Aben KK, van Oort IM, et al. The clinical phenotype of hereditary versus sporadic prostate cancer: HPC definition revisited. Prostate 2016;76(10):897–904.
14. Carter BS, Ewing CM, Ward WS, et al. Allelic loss of chromosomes 16q and 10q in human prostate cancer. Proc Natl Acad Sci U S A 1990;87(22):8751–5.
15. Hemminki K, Ji A, Försti A, et al. Concordance of survival in family members with prostate cancer. J Clin Oncol 2008;26(10):1705–9.
16. Lindström LS, Hall P, Hartman M, et al. Familial concordance in cancer survival: a Swedish population-based study. Lancet Oncol 2007;8(11):1001–6.
17. Albright FS, Stephenson RA, Agarwal N, et al. Relative risks for lethal prostate cancer based on complete family history of prostate cancer death. Prostate 2017;77(1):41–8.
18. Xu J, Dimitrov L, Chang BL, et al. A combined genomewide linkage scan of 1,233 families for prostate cancer-susceptibility genes conducted by the international consortium for prostate cancer genetics. Am J Hum Genet 2005;77(2):219–29.
19. Ewing CM, Ray AM, Lange EM, et al. Germline mutations in HOXB13 and prostate-cancer risk. N Engl J Med 2012;366(2):141–9.
20. Xu J, Lange EM, Lu L, et al. HOXB13 is a susceptibility gene for prostate cancer: results from the International Consortium for Prostate Cancer Genetics (ICPCG). Hum Genet 2013;132(1):5–14.
21. Karlsson R, Aly M, Clements M, et al. A population-based assessment of germline HOXB13 G84E mutation and prostate cancer risk. Eur Urol 2014; 65(1):169–76.
22. Laitinen VH, Wahlfors T, Saaristo L, et al. HOXB13 G84E mutation in Finland: population-based analysis of prostate, breast, and colorectal cancer risk. Cancer Epidemiol Biomarkers Prev 2013;22(3): 452–60.
23. Momozawa Y, Iwasaki Y, Hirata M, et al. Germline pathogenic variants in 7636 Japanese patients with prostate cancer and 12 366 controls. J Natl Cancer Inst 2020;112(4):369–76.
24. Lin X, Qu L, Chen Z, et al. A novel germline mutation in HOXB13 is associated with prostate cancer risk in Chinese men. Prostate 2013;73(2):169–75.
25. Bhanvadia RR, Van Opstall C, Brechka H, et al. MEIS1 and MEIS2 expression and prostate cancer

progression: a role for HOXB13 binding partners in metastatic disease. Clin Cancer Res 2018;24(15): 3668–80.

26. Johng D, Torga G, Ewing CM, et al. HOXB13 interaction with MEIS1 modifies proliferation and gene expression in prostate cancer. Prostate 2019;79(4): 414–24.

27. Marlin R, Créoff M, Merle S, et al. Mutation HOXB13 c.853delT in Martinican prostate cancer patients. Prostate 2020;80(6):463–70.

28. Landrum MJ, Lee JM, Benson M, et al. ClinVar: improving access to variant interpretations and supporting evidence. Nucleic Acids Res 2018;46(D1): D1062–7.

29. Economides KD, Capecchi MR. Hoxb13 is required for normal differentiation and secretory function of the ventral prostate. Development 2003;130(10): 2061–9.

30. Norris JD, Chang CY, Wittmann BM, et al. The homeodomain protein HOXB13 regulates the cellular response to androgens. Mol Cell 2009;36(3): 405–16.

31. Luo Z, Farnham PJ. Genome-wide analysis of HOXC4 and HOXC6 regulated genes and binding sites in prostate cancer cells. PLoS One 2020;15(2). https://doi.org/10.1371/journal.pone.0228590.

32. Nyberg T, Govindasami K, Leslie G, et al. Homeobox B13 G84E mutation and prostate cancer risk. Eur Urol 2019;75:834–45.

33. Kote-Jarai Z, Mikropoulos C, Leongamornlert DA, et al. Prevalence of the HOXB13 G84E germline mutation in British men and correlation with prostate cancer risk, tumour characteristics and clinical outcomes. Ann Oncol 2015;26(4):756–61.

34. Wei J, Shi Z, Na R, et al. Germline HOXB13 G84E mutation carriers and risk to twenty common types of cancer: results from the UK Biobank. Br J Cancer 2020; 123(9). https://doi.org/10.1038/s41416-020-01036-8.

35. Robinson D, Van Allen EM, Wu YM, et al. Integrative clinical genomics of advanced prostate cancer. Cell 2015;162(2):454.

36. Pritchard CC, Mateo J, Walsh MF, et al. Inherited DNA-repair gene mutations in men with metastatic prostate cancer. N Engl J Med 2016;375(5):443–53.

37. Na R, Zheng SL, Han M, et al. Germline mutations in ATM and BRCA1/2 distinguish risk for lethal and indolent prostate cancer and are associated with early age at death [figure presented]. Eur Urol 2017;71:740–7.

38. Carter HB, Helfand B, Mamawala M, et al. Germline mutations in ATM and BRCA1/2 are associated with grade reclassification in men on active surveillance for prostate cancer (figure presented.). Eur Urol 2019;75(5):743–9.

39. Wu Y, Yu H, Zheng SL, et al. A comprehensive evaluation of CHEK2 germline mutations in men with prostate cancer. Prostate 2018;78(8):607–15.

40. Wokołorczyk D, Kluźniak W, Huzarski T, et al. Mutations in ATM, NBN and BRCA2 predispose to aggressive prostate cancer in Poland. Int J Cancer 2020;147(10):2793–800.

41. Wu Y, Yu H, Li S, et al. Rare germline pathogenic mutations of DNA repair genes are most strongly associated with grade group 5 prostate cancer. Eur Urol Oncol 2020;3:224–30.

42. Schaid DJ, McDonnell SK, FitzGerald LM, et al. Two-stage study of familial prostate cancer by whole-exome sequencing and custom capture identifies 10 novel genes associated with the risk of prostate cancer. Eur Urol 2020. https://doi.org/10.1016/j.eururo.2020.07.038.

43. Mateo J, Carreira S, Sandhu S, et al. DNA-repair defects and olaparib in metastatic prostate cancer. N Engl J Med 2015;373(18):1697–708.

44. Hughley R, Karlic R, Joshi H, et al. Etiologic index — A case-only measure of BRCA1/2–associated cancer risk. N Engl J Med 2020;383(3):286–8.

45. Hoffman RM, Gilliland FD, Eley JW, et al. Racial and ethnic differences in advanced-stage prostate cancer: the prostate cancer outcomes study. J Natl Cancer Inst 2001;93(5):388–95.

46. Matejcic M, Patel Y, Lilyquist J, et al. Pathogenic variants in cancer predisposition genes and prostate cancer risk in men of African ancestry. JCO Precis Oncol 2020;4(4):32–43.

47. Miki Y, Swensen J, Shattuck-Eidens D, et al. A strong candidate for the breast and ovarian cancer susceptibility gene BRCA1. Science 1994;266:66–71.

48. Wooster R, Bignell G, Lancaster J, et al. Identification of the breast cancer susceptibility gene BRCA2. Nature 1995;378:789–91.

49. Thompson D, Easton DF. Cancer Incidence in BRCA1 mutation carriers. J Natl Cancer Inst 2002; 94(18):1358–65. Available at: http://www.ncbi.nlm.nih.gov/pubmed/12237281.

50. The Breast Cancer Linkage C. Cancer risks in BRCA2 mutation carriers. J Natl Cancer Inst 1999; 91(15):1310–6.

51. Wilkens EP, Freije D, Xu J, et al. No evidence for a role of BRCA1 or BRCA2 mutations in Ashkenazi Jewish families with hereditary prostate cancer. Prostate 1999;39(4):280–4.

52. Zuhlke KA, Madeoy JJ, Beebe-Dimmer J, et al. Truncating BRCA1 mutations are uncommon in a cohort of hereditary prostate cancer families with evidence of linkage to 17q markers. Clin Cancer Res 2004; 10(18 Pt 1):5975–80.

53. Thorlacius S, Olafsdottir G, Tryggvadottir L, et al. A single BRCA2 mutation in male and female breast cancer families from Iceland with varied cancer phenotypes. Nat Genet 1996;13:117–9.

54. Sigurdsson S, Thorlacius S, Tomasson J, et al. BRCA2 mutation in Icelandic prostate cancer patients. J Mol Med 1997;75(10):758–61.

55. Tryggvadottir L, Vidarsdottir L, Thorgeirsson T, et al. Prostate cancer progression and survival in BRCA2 mutation carriers. J Natl Cancer Inst 2007;99(12): 929–35.

56. Castro E, Goh C, Olmos D, et al. Germline BRCA mutations are associated with higher risk of nodal involvement, distant metastasis, and poor survival outcomes in prostate cancer. J Clin Oncol 2013; 31(14):1748–57.

57. Mateo J, Cheng HH, Beltran H, et al. Clinical outcome of prostate cancer patients with germline DNA repair mutations: retrospective analysis from an international study. Eur Urol 2018;73(5):687–93.

58. Raymond VM, Mukherjee B, Wang F, et al. Elevated risk of prostate cancer among men with Lynch syndrome. J Clin Oncol 2013;31(14):1713–8.

59. Han Y, Signorello LB, Strom SS, et al. Generalizability of established prostate cancer risk variants in men of African ancestry. Int J Cancer 2015; 136(5):1210–7.

60. Bauer CM, Ray AM, Halstead-Nussloch BA, et al. Hereditary prostate cancer as a feature of Lynch syndrome. Fam Cancer 2011;10(1):37–42.

61. Schumacher FR, Al Olama AA, Berndt SI, et al. Association analyses of more than 140,000 men identify 63 new prostate cancer susceptibility loci. Nat Genet 2018;50(7):928–36.

62. Conran CA, Na R, Chen H, et al. Population-standardized genetic risk score: the SNP-based method of choice for inherited risk assessment of prostate cancer. Asian J Androl 2016;18(4):520–4.

63. Vilhjalmsson BJ, Yang J, Finucane HK, et al. Modeling linkage disequilibrium increases accuracy of polygenic risk scores. Am J Hum Genet 2015; 97(4):576–92.

64. Khera AV, Chaffin M, Aragam KG, et al. Genome-wide polygenic scores for common diseases identify individuals with risk equivalent to monogenic mutations. Nat Genet 2018;50(9):1219–24.

65. Ge T, Chen CY, Ni Y, et al. Polygenic prediction via Bayesian regression and continuous shrinkage priors. Nat Commun 2019;10(1):1776.

66. Seibert TM, Fan CC, Wang Y, et al. Polygenic hazard score to guide screening for aggressive prostate cancer: development and validation in large scale cohorts. BMJ 2018;360:j5757.

67. Yu H, Shi Z, Wu Y, et al. Concept and benchmarks for assessing narrow-sense validity of genetic risk score values. Prostate 2019;79(10):1099–105.

68. Zheng SL, Sun J, Wiklund F, et al. Cumulative association of five genetic variants with prostate cancer. N Engl J Med 2008;358(9):910–9.

69. Hoffmann TJ, Van Den Eeden SK, Sakoda LC, et al. A large multiethnic genome-wide association study of prostate cancer identifies novel risk variants and substantial ethnic differences. Cancer Discov 2015;5(8):878–91.

70. Kader AK, Sun J, Reck BH, et al. Potential impact of adding genetic markers to clinical parameters in predicting prostate biopsy outcomes in men following an initial negative biopsy: findings from the REDUCE trial. Eur Urol 2012;62(6):953–61.

71. Chen H, Liu X, Brendler CB, et al. Adding genetic risk score to family history identifies twice as many high-risk men for prostate cancer: results from the prostate cancer prevention trial. Prostate 2016; 76(12):1120–9.

72. Ren S, Xu J, Zhou T, et al. Plateau effect of prostate cancer risk-associated SNPs in discriminating prostate biopsy outcomes. Prostate 2013;73(16): 1824–35.

73. Jiang H, Liu F, Wang Z, et al. Prediction of prostate cancer from prostate biopsy in Chinese men using a genetic score derived from 24 prostate cancer risk-associated SNPs. Prostate 2013;73(15):1651–9.

74. Gronberg H, Adolfsson J, Aly M, et al. Prostate cancer screening in men aged 50-69 years (STHLM3): a prospective population-based diagnostic study. Lancet Oncol 2015;16(16):1667–76.

75. Shi Z, Platz E, Wei J, et al. Performance of three inherited risk measures for predicting prostate cancer incidence and mortality: a population-based prospective analysis. Eur Urol 2021;79(3):419–26.

76. Na R, Labbate C, Yu H, et al. Single-nucleotide polymorphism-based genetic risk score and patient age at prostate cancer diagnosis. JAMA Netw Open 2019;2(12):e1918145.

77. Karunamuni RA, Huynh-Le MP, Fan CC, et al. African-specific improvement of a polygenic hazard score for age at diagnosis of prostate cancer. Int J Cancer 2020. https://doi.org/10.1002/ijc.33282.

78. Kader AK, Sun J, Isaacs SD, et al. Individual and cumulative effect of prostate cancer risk-associated variants on clinicopathologic variables in 5,895 prostate cancer patients. Prostate 2009;69(11): 1195–205.

79. Ahmed M, Goh C, Saunders E, et al. Germline genetic variation in prostate susceptibility does not predict outcomes in the chemoprevention trials PCPT and SELECT. Prostate Cancer Prostatic Dis 2020;23(2):333–42.

80. Helfand BT, Roehl KA, Cooper PR, et al. Associations of prostate cancer risk variants with disease aggressiveness: results of the NCI-SPORE Genetics Working Group analysis of 18,343 cases. Hum Genet 2015;134(4):439–50.

81. Pomerantz MM, Werner L, Xie W, et al. Association of prostate cancer risk Loci with disease aggressiveness and prostate cancer-specific mortality. Cancer Prev Res (Phila) 2011;4(5):719–28.

82. Force USPST, Grossman DC, Curry SJ, et al. Screening for prostate cancer: US preventive services task force recommendation statement. JAMA 2018;319(18):1901–13.

83. Mottet N, Bellmunt J, Bolla M, et al. EAU-ESTRO-SIOG guidelines on prostate cancer. part 1: screening, diagnosis, and local treatment with curative intent. Eur Urol 2017;71(4):618–29.

84. Mohler JL, Higano CS, Schaeffer EM, et al. Current recommendations for prostate cancer genetic testing: NCCN prostate guideline. Can J Urol 2019; 26(5 Suppl 2):34–7. Available at: https://www.ncbi.nlm.nih.gov/pubmed/31629426.

85. Lecarpentier J, Silvestri V, Kuchenbaecker KB, et al. Prediction of breast and prostate cancer risks in male BRCA1 and BRCA2 mutation carriers using polygenic risk scores. J Clin Oncol 2017;35(20): 2240–50.

86. Li-Sheng Chen S, Ching-Yuan Fann J, Sipeky C, et al. Risk prediction of prostate cancer with single nucleotide polymorphisms and prostate specific antigen. J Urol 2019;201(3):486–95.

87. Helfand BT, Xu J. Germline testing for prostate cancer prognosis: implications for active surveillance. Can J Urol 2019;26(5 Suppl 2):48–9.

88. Yu H, Shi Z, Lin X, et al. Broad- and narrow-sense validity performance of three polygenic risk score methods for prostate cancer risk assessment. Prostate 2020;80(1):83–7.

89. Du Z, Hopp H, Ingles SA, et al. A genome-wide association study of prostate cancer in Latinos. Int J Cancer 2020;146(7):1819–26.

Clinical Multigene Testing for Prostate Cancer

Tala Berro, MS, CGC[a,1], Elizabeth Barrett, MS[b,1], Saud H. AlDubayan, MD[a,b,]*

KEYWORDS

• Multigene panel testing • Prostate cancer • Germline genetic testing • Genetic counseling

KEY POINTS

- Germline genetic testing has ever-expanding diagnostic, prognostic, and therapeutic utility in prostate cancer.
- When indicated, germline genetic testing should be offered to prostate cancer patients in a timely manner because this information can change clinical management.
- Multigene panels are the most time-efficient and cost-effective way to evaluate the presence of a germline pathogenic variant in patients with prostate cancer.
- The choice of germline multigene panels to test prostate cancer patients should be dependent on a patient's overall clinical phenotype, disease status (primary vs metastatic), family history of cancer, response to current treatment regimen, and potential enrollment in clinical trials.
- The vast majority of PC patients who have undergone genetic analysis are of European ancestry, which severely limits the ability to generalize the findings of these studies to prostate cancer patients from other ancestral and ethnic groups.
- Pretest genetic and post-test genetic counseling will become increasingly important with the increased utilization of multigene panels that can uncover unexpected findings.

INTRODUCTION

Prostate cancer (PC) is the most common cancer in men.[1] It is estimated that more than 3 million men are living with PC in the United States,[2] with approximately 190,000 estimated new diagnoses annually.[3] On average, men have a 1 in 8 chance of developing PC at some point in their lifetime, and, despite having the highest 5-year survival rate of any cancer (approximately 98%), approximately 1 man in 41 still dies of PC.[4] This underscores the need to develop a more comprehensive molecular-based stratification framework that can identify patients with heritable forms of PC and inform decision making across various clinical settings.

Large twin studies have provided a better understanding of PC heritability, which describes the amount of variation in the PC risk across a population that can be explained by genetic variants.[5] In a study by Lichtenstein and colleagues[6] that leveraged twin registries across the Nordic countries, the PC heritability was estimated to be 42% (95% CI, 29%–50%), which is much higher than the heritability of other common cancers, such as breast (27%; 95% CI, 4%–41%) and colorectal (35%; 95% CI, 10%–48%) cancers in the same population. A more recent analysis of cancer heritability in more than 80,000 monozygotic and 123,000 dizygotic twins in the population-based registers of Denmark, Finland, Norway, and Sweden confirmed the substantially high heritability of PC and showed that 57% (95% CI, 51%–63%) of PC risk is attributed to inherited genetic factors.[7,8] Despite the high heritability of PC, case-control

[a] Division of Genetics, Brigham and Women's Hospital, EC Alumnae Hall, Suite 302, 41 Avenue Louis Pasteur, Boston, MA 02115, USA; [b] Department of Medical Oncology, Dana-Farber Cancer Institute, Harvard Medical School, 41 Avenue Louis Pasteur, Suite 303-0, Boston, MA 02115, USA
[1] These authors contributed equally to this work.
* Corresponding author. Dana-Farber Cancer Institute, 41 Avenue Louis Pasteur, Suite 303-01, Boston, MA 02115.
E-mail address: SAUD_ALDUBAYAN@DFCI.HARVARD.EDU
Twitter: @tala_berro (T.B.); @Liz13arrett (E.B.); @s_aldubayan (S.H.A.)

Urol Clin N Am 48 (2021) 297–309
https://doi.org/10.1016/j.ucl.2021.03.002
0094-0143/21/© 2021 Elsevier Inc. All rights reserved.

and family-based germline studies in PC so far have elucidated only some, but not all, of the low-penetrance, intermediate-penetrance, and high-penetrance genetic factors driving PC susceptibility.[9] For example, pathogenic metastatic germline variants in all known PC predisposition genes are present in only under 5% and 10% of primary and metastatic PC patients,[10] respectively, strongly suggesting the presence of yet to be discovered mendelian PC susceptibility genes.

Despite the relatively small percentage of PC patients with identifiable mendelian predisposition variants, clinical germline genetic testing, using multigene panels (MGPs), has become increasingly used to implement a more personalized clinical screening and management plan for PC patients. Diagnostically, germline pathogenic variants in the PC predisposition genes confer a substantial increase in the risk of developing PC and several other malignancies where gene-specific screening recommendations are available. Furthermore, germline analysis also can be expanded to other family members to identify asymptomatic carriers of pathogenic variants in whom cancer preventive measures can be lifesaving. In addition to characterizing cancer risk, germline testing can identify variants associated with a higher risk of metastatic disease and those that confer greater tumor sensitivity and overall survival benefit to targeted therapeutics, such as PARP (poly (Adenosine di-phosphate-ribose) polymerase) inhibitors (PARPi) and immune checkpoint blockades (ICBs).[10,11] Given the expanding diagnostic and therapeutic utility of germline testing in PC, the effort to maximally utilize germline genetic analysis at the point of care has culminated in a multidisciplinary, consensus-driven genetic implementation framework to guide clinical germline genetic testing in PC.[9]

This review explores the current landscape of MGP testing in PC with a focus on clinical experiences. Known and suspected predisposition genes for PC in clinical patient cohorts also are reviewed and the counseling implications for future providers looking to integrate this testing into their clinical care for patients with PC discussed.

GENES WITH ESTABLISHED OR POTENTIAL CLINICAL UTILITY IN PROSTATE CANCER

Several germline genetic variants have established or potential implications for the clinical management of PC through risk assessment or predictive utility for disease progression and therapeutic response. So far, BRCA2[12] and HOXB13[13] have been associated with the highest risk increase

for PC. Germline pathogenic variants in BRCA2 are, on average, associated with a 2-6 fold increased risk of PC, which translates to approximately 20%-60% lifetime risk of developing PC[12,14–22] (Table 1). Several studies also have demonstrated the association of the HOXB13 p.Gly84Glu (G84E) variant with a 3.5-times to 8.0-times higher risk of PC in general and a 6-fold higher risk of early-onset disease.[9,13,23–27] On the other hand, BRCA1[28] and the mismatch repair (MMR) genes[29,30] are more moderately penetrant risk alleles for PC, with an overall lifetime risk of approximately 20% to 40%[9,20,30–34] (see Table 1). In addition to these established PC predisposition genes, recently emerging evidence supports germline pathogenic alterations in other DNA repair genes, such as CHEK2,[35] ATM,[36] and NBN[37] (also known as NBS1) as mediators of PC susceptibility. For example, 2 founder pathogenic variants in CHEK2, c.1100delC (p.Thr367fs) and c.470T>C (p.Ile157Thr), have been shown to confer 3.29-fold and 1.80-fold increases, respectively, in the risk of PC.[35,38] Similarly, pathogenic germline ATM variant c.3161G (p.P1054R) and founder NBN variant c.657_661del (p.Lys219fs) have been shown to increase susceptibility to PC[36,37,39–41] (see Table 1). Additional studies still are needed, however, to further delineate the PC risk increase associated with each gene and if they are associated with a higher predisposition to an early-onset or a more aggressive form of the disease.

In addition to PC risk stratification and counseling, germline variants have prognostic and therapeutic predictive utility that can guide decision making in oncology settings. For example, pathogenic variants in BRCA2 (and potentially CHEK2) are independent prognostic indicators of a higher risk of disease progression and distant metastasis in PC[10,16,42–46] (see Table 1). Although germline pathogenic variants in other DNA repair genes have been proposed as having predictive utility in PC,[47] well-designed large-scale studies still are needed to explore the role of these germline events in PC tumorigenesis. Therapeutically, germline analysis of DNA repair pathways, namely the homologous recombination, MMR, and the Fanconi anemia pathways, also can inform treatment decisions in PC. For example, germline pathogenic alterations in BRCA1/2; the MMR genes, CHEK2, ATM, PALB2, and RAD51C/D; and the FANC gene family modulate PC tumorigenesis leading to DNA repair-deficient tumors that are sensitive to various therapeutic interventions[11,48–53] (see Table 1). Response to other systemic therapies besides PARPi, platinum-based chemotherapy, and ICBs also might be influenced

Table 1
Genes with established or emerging evidence for prostate cancer susceptibility

Gene	Evidence Level	Fold Increase in Prostate Cancer Risk	Lifetime Prostate Cancer Risk	Fold Increase in the Risk of Early-Onset Disease	Fold Increase in Risk of Metastatic Disease	Therapeutic Utility
BRCA2	+++	6	20%-60%	7.8 ($\leq$65 y of age)	18.6–26.7	PARPi PBC
BRCA1	+++	2.0–3.8	20%–40%	Not well defined	Not well defined	PARPi PBC
HOXB13	+++	3.5–8.0	30%–60%	6 ($\leq$55 y of age)	Not well defined	Not well defined
MSH2	+++	5.8	20%	Not well defined	Not well defined	ICB
MLH1	+++	1.7	Not well defined	Not well defined	Not well defined	ICB
MSH6	+++	1.3	Not well defined	Not well defined	Not well defined	ICB
PMS2	+++	Not well defined	Not well defined	Not well defined	Not well defined	ICB
CHEK2	++	1.80–3.29	25%–45%	Not well defined	4.7–7.86	Not well defined
ATM	++	2	Increased	Not well defined	Not well defined	PARPi PBC[b]
NBN	++	3–4[a]	Increased	Not well defined	Not well defined	Not well defined

+++, established; ++, emerging; mPC, metastatic prostate cancer; PBT, platinum-based chemotherapy.
[a] In Eastern European populations.
[b] Potential association, needs further study.

by germline variants in the DNA repair genes. As such, the presence of these pathogenic variants increasingly is becoming an eligibility requirement to enroll PC patients in clinical trials,[54] supporting the inclusion of DNA repair genes with less defined diagnostic utility in germline testing for men with PC considering clinical trials.[11,55,56]

Collectively, germline variants in several DNA repair genes have established diagnostic and predictive utility in PC, highlighting the importance of germline genetic testing in this patient population. Universal testing of metastatic PC patients already has been recommended by the National Comprehensive Cancer Network guidelines and endorsed by an expert consensus.[9] Germline genetic testing in PC should utilize an MGP approach that prioritizes established and suspected PC susceptibility genes as well as genes that can inform disease prognosis and treatment approach in PC.

LANDSCAPE OF AVAILABLE CLINICAL MULTIGENE PANELS FOR PROSTATE CANCER

Clinical germline genetic testing has evolved significantly over the past 2 decades, from stepwise single-gene testing to MGPs and even exome sequencing. As such, clinical germline testing has become an increasingly useful tool in the clinical management of PC patients.[57] Single-gene or limited gene testing first was used to identify germline variants in patients with personal and family histories highly suspicious for hereditary cancer syndromes, such as Lynch syndrome or hereditary breast and ovarian cancer.[58] The general paradigm of this approach consisted of an initial phase of testing for some of the commonly mutated genes, such as BRCA1 and BRCA2, and, if negative, testing sequentially for additional gene(s) as indicated.[58] This kind of testing is time-consuming and costly and lacks the comprehensive coverage achieved by MGP testing. Following the invention of next-generation massively parallel sequencing in 2005 and the 2013 court ruling against gene patenting, it became more feasible to sequence multiple genes at once in focused gene panels. These factors made MPG testing more affordable and time-efficient and enabled clinicians to cast a wider net, which increases testing yield compared with single-gene or limited gene testing.[59] Additionally, exome sequencing also has begun to be offered by clinical laboratories in the United States and has been shown to have a relatively high diagnostic utility and potentially be more cost-efficient for patients who remain undiagnosed after initial testing using the MGP approach.[60] The lack of proved higher diagnostic yield and cost-effectiveness, however, compared with phenotype-focused MGPs as well as insufficient standardization regarding informed consent, data sharing, and results management remain barriers to the implementation of exome sequencing as a first-tier clinical diagnostic test in cancer patients.[61] In summary, MGP testing is the most common first-tier clinical diagnostic test utilized in germline cancer genetics, being both more time-efficient and affordable than single-gene testing and more focused than exome sequencing.

The number of clinical PC-specific MGPs available in the United States grew from 3 in 2017[56,62] to at least 13 panels that can be ordered as of October 2020. On average, 12 genes were included in these panels (ranging from 5 to 16) (**Fig. 1**A). Although all MGPs included *BRCA1* and *BRCA2,* which are established PC susceptibility genes, 15% of MGPs did not test the DNA MMR genes or *HOXB13*, which also are established PC predisposition genes (**Fig. 1**B). Similarly, although all MGPs included *NBN* and *TP53*, which have limited or no clinical utility in PC, only 50% of these panels included canonical DNA repair genes, such as *PALB2* and *RAD51D*, where germline pathogenic variants can substantially influence treatment decision making. Overall, the MGPs currently available are variable, and although most include the established PC susceptibility genes, a significant fraction of these MGPs do not test *HOXB13*, the DNA MMR genes, and other DNA repair genes that have established or potential clinical implications in PC, underscoring the importance of choosing the most suitable MGP

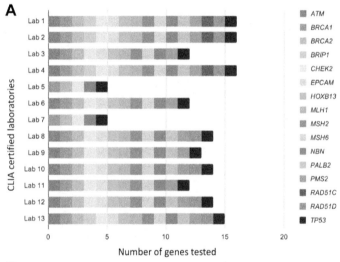

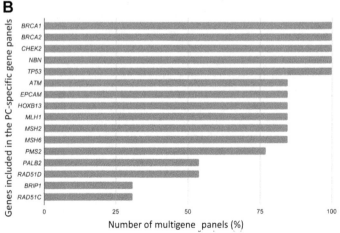

Fig. 1. Germline MGPs clinically available to test PC patients. (*A*) As of October 2020, a total of 13 germline MGPs were offered by Clinical Laboratory Improvement Amendments-certified laboratories in the United States to test PC patients. Although most of these MGPs included 12 to 16 genes, some panels included as few as 5 genes. (*B*) Of the established PC susceptibility genes, only *BRCA1* and *BRCA2* consistently were included in all the clinical PC-specific MGPs, whereas *HOXB13* and the DNA MMR genes were included in most but not all the panels. Furthermore, other DNA repair genes with established prognostic or therapeutic predictive utility in PC were tested only occasionally in these clinically oriented panels, highlighting an area for potential improvement.

based on a patient's overall phenotype, disease status (primary vs metastatic), presence of a positive family history of cancer, and response to the current treatment regimen.

GENETICALLY CHARACTERIZED CLINICAL PROSTATE CANCER COHORTS
Clinical Characteristics of the Tested Prostate Cancer Patients

Despite the high prevalence of PC, there remain few published clinical PC cohorts who underwent germline genetic analysis for cancer risk assessment at the point of care. The first of these clinical PC cohorts was reported by Giri and colleagues[63] and described the germline molecular findings in 200 men, 125 patients with PC and 75 cancer-free patients, who are at a high risk of PC. Of this cohort, 11 (5.5%; 95% CI, 3.0%–9.9%) patients were found to have pathogenic germline variants in the cancer predisposition genes, 63.6% of which involved 1 of the DNA repair genes. Subsequently, 3 larger clinical PC cohorts were described by Nicolosi and colleagues,[64] Pritzlaff and colleagues,[65] and Na and colleagues,[46] which collectively evaluated a total of 4406 PC patients. To better understand the landscape of germline genetic variation in PC, the clinical, histologic, and molecular findings of these 3 large clinical PC patient cohorts are systematically reviewed.

Nicolosi and colleagues[64] described the germline genetic findings in 3607 PC patients who underwent germline genetic analysis between 2013 and 2018. Ages of patients at testing ranged from less than 50 years old to greater than 90 years old, with 43% of the PC patients having a positive family history of PC. Although Gleason score was unknown for 57% of the tested PC patients, 38% of PC patients with a reported score had a Gleason score between 7 and 10 whereas the remaining patients had a Gleason score between 3 and 6 (**Fig. 2**A). Importantly, PC patients in the study by Nicolosi and colleagues[64] underwent an MGP approach with a variable number of genes (2–80 genes), with 62% of orders having a minimum of 14 genes tested, which included *ATM*, *BRCA1*, *BRCA2*, *CHEK2*, *EPCAM*, *HOXB13*, *MLH1*, *MSH2*, *MSH6*, *NBN*, *PMS2*, *TP53*, *RAD51D*, and *PALB2*.

The second clinical PC cohort was reported by Pritzlaff and colleagues[65] and described the germline genetic findings in 1878 PC patients who underwent genetic analysis between 2012 and 2017. The median age at testing was 66 years, with most individuals (92.4%) having a family history of cancer, 50.6% with a family

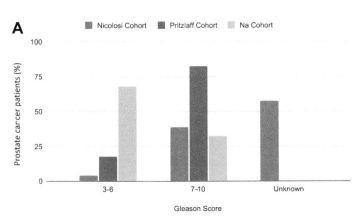

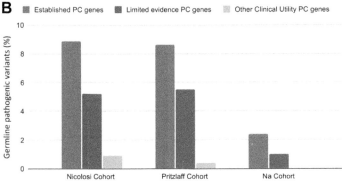

Fig. 2. Clinical and molecular characteristics of clinical PC cohorts. (*A*) Although most of the PC patients reported in the study of Pritzlaff and colleagues[65] had a Gleason score of 7 or more, only a small fraction of the clinical PC cohorts reported by Nicolosi and colleagues[64] and Na and colleagues[46] had a high Gleason score, underscoring the heterogeneity of the PC patients described in these studies. (*B*) Prevalence of germline pathogenic variants in genes with established or emerging clinical utility in PC.

history of PC specifically. The Gleason score was known for all PC patients in this study, with 82.3% of the patients having a Gleason score higher than 7 (see **Fig. 2**A). The high rates of positive family history of cancer and a Gleason score of over 7 in this study group underscore the high-risk nature of this clinical cohort. The PC patients in the Pritzlaff and colleagues[65] study also were tested using a variable expanded MGP testing approach, which included up to 67 cancer susceptibility genes.

Lastly, the study by Na and colleagues[46] described the molecular findings of clinical MGP analysis in 799 PC patients, 313 with lethal PC disease and 486 patients with localized PC. The median age at diagnosis was 62 years for patients with lethal PC and 65 years for patients with localized PC. The Gleason score was known for all PC patients in this study, with the majority (67.9%) having a score under 7 (see **Fig. 2**A). This study included PC patients with African ancestry and Chinese ancestry, making up 14.9% and 8.3% of the total participants, respectively. Although PC patients studied by Na and colleagues[46] underwent exome sequencing or a next-generation sequencing panel of 222 cancer-related genes, the study described only pathogenic variants found in BRCA1, BRCA2, and ATM.

Molecular Findings: Pathogenic Results of Known Significance

Although each of these studies investigated cancer predisposition genes using large MGPs or a clinical exome, the genes with known clinical utility in PC remain limited. Collectively, the prevalence of germline pathogenic variants in the established PC genes (BRCA1, BRCA2, MMR genes, and HOXB13) were 8.85%, 8.6%, and 2.38% in the Nicolosi and colleagues,[64] Pritzlaff and colleagues,[65] and Na and colleagues[46] cohorts, respectively (**Fig. 2**B; **Table 2**), underscoring the relatively small fraction of PC patients who received a clear informative result for PC risk assessment. When genes with emerging evidence as mediators of PC susceptibility (CHEK2, ATM, and NBN) were considered, however, the diagnostic yield of germline testing for cancer risk assessment at the point of care increased by 5.23%, 5.5%, and 1% in the Nicolosi and colleagues,[64] Pritzlaff and colleagues,[65] and Na and colleagues[46] studies, respectively (see **Fig. 2**B and **Table 2**). The relatively low diagnostic yield

Table 2
Frequency of germline pathogenic variants in genes with established or emerging clinical utility in clinical prostate cancer cohorts studied by Nicolosi and colleagues,[64] Pritzlaff and colleagues,[65] and Na and colleagues[46]

Genes	Count of Patients with a Pathogenic Finding in the Nicolosi and Colleagues[64] Cohort (%)	Count of Patients with a Pathogenic Finding in the Pritzlaff and Colleagues[65] Cohort (%)	Count of Patients with a Pathogenic Finding in the Na and Colleagues[46] Cohort (%)[a]
BRCA1	43 (1.25)	10 (0.8)	4 (0.5)
BRCA2	164 (4.74)	56 (3.8)	15 (1.88)
HOXB13	30 (1.12)	8 (1.2)	
MLH1	2 (0.06)	2 (0.1)	
MSH2	23 (0.69)	11 (1.2)	
MSH6	15 (0.45)	5 (0.8)	
PMS2	18 (0.54)	7 (0.6)	
CHEK2	95 (2.88)	38 (2.5)	
ATM	65 (2.03)	37 (2.7)	8 (1)
NBN	10 (0.32)	4 (0.3)	
PALB2	17 (0.56)	7 (0.4)	
BRIP1	7 (0.28)	0	
RAD51C	5 (0.21)	0	
RAD51D	4 (0.15)	0	

[a] Only BRCA1, BRCA2, and ATM were reported in the study of Na and colleagues.[46]

reported by Na and colleagues,[46] however, is related to the fact that this study examined only 3 cancer genes, BRCA1, BRCA2, and ATM. Beyond cancer risk assessment, the frequency of germline pathogenic variants in other genes with potential therapeutic utility for PC (PALB2, RAD51C, RAD51D, FANCA, and other Fanconi anemia genes) were 0.92% and 0.4% in the Nicolosi and colleagues[64] and Pritzlaff and colleagues[65] cohorts, respectively (see **Fig. 2**B and **Table 2**).

Intriguingly, PC patients in these clinical cohorts had relatively high prevalence of germline pathogenic variants in BRCA2 (4.74%, 3.8%, and 1.88% for Niclosi and colleagues,[64] Pritzlaff and colleagues,[65] and Na and colleagues,[46] respectively) and CHEK2 (2.88% and 2.5% for Niclosi and colleagues[64] and Pritzlaff and colleagues,[65] respectively), which were more similar to the prevalence of these germline alterations in the metastatic PC cohort than the primary PC cohort reported by Pritchard and colleagues[10] (primary PC: 0.2% and 0.4% for BRCA2 and CHEK2, respectively; and metastatic PC: 5.35% and 1.87% for BRCA2 and CHEK2, respectively) (**Fig. 3**A; see **Table 2**). These observations highlight the high-risk and advanced disease nature of the patients within these clinical PC cohorts, where early detection of germline pathogenic

variants can be therapeutically beneficial. Furthermore, the high-risk nature of the reported clinical PC cohorts limits the generalizability of the germline molecular findings in these studies and is an important consideration when offering germline testing to PC patients with low-risk features.

Molecular Findings: Pathogenic Results of Unknown Significance

In addition to identifying pathogenic variants in the genes with known clinical utility in PC, the studies by Nicolosi and colleagues[64] and Pritzlaff and colleagues[65] tested an expanded set of genes, most of which have unknown clinical significance to the clinical phenotype under assessment (ie, PC). For example, a total of 4.93% of PC patients in the Nicolosi and colleagues[64] study received a result for pathogenic variants in a gene with unknown clinical utility in PC. Similarly, Pritzlaff and colleagues[65] reported that 6.7% of PC patients in their cohort had 1 or more pathogenic variants of unknown clinical relevance in PC. Variable gene sets, however, were used in the study by Pritzlaff and colleagues,[65] so the true prevalence of germline pathogenic variants in cancer genes with unknown clinical relevance in PC might differ from the calculated frequency. Although these findings may shed light on the prevalence of these gene alterations in PC patients, the lack of an ancestry-matched

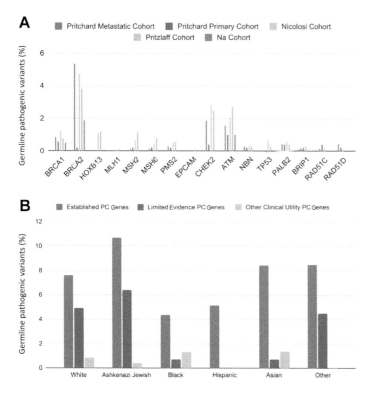

Fig. 3. Prevalence of germline pathogenic variants in PC patients sequenced at the point of care. (A) The prevalence of germline PC variants in the clinically tested cohorts was more similar to the prevalence of these germline alterations in the metastatic PC cohort reported by Pritchard and colleagues[10] than the primary PC cohort of The Genome Cancer Atlas, underscoring the high-risk nature of these cohorts. (B) The molecular diagnostic yield of germline analysis was variable across various ancestral groups, which is a critical consideration when evaluating PC patients from one of these understudied populations.

control cohort to account for the baseline frequency of these alterations in the general population makes it difficult to make firm conclusions on the clinical and biological relevance of these pathogenic germline variants in PC. For example, the frequency of pathogenic variants in *APC* and *MUTYH* in the study by Nicolosi and colleagues[64] were relatively high, at 1.28% and 2.37%, respectively. Pathogenic variants in these genes, however, also are relatively prevalent in the general population, with the frequency of the common Ashkenazi Jewish *APC* founder variant (c.3920T>A, p.Ile1307Lys) 6% to 12%[66] and the frequency of an individual having a heterozygous pathogenic *MUTYH* variant 1% to 2% in the general northern European, Australian, and US populations.[67] As such, large case-control studies of PC patients and genetically matched cancer-free individuals are needed to dissect the biological relevance of these germline pathogenic variants in PC.

Limitations and Heterogeneity of Cohorts

Given that 190,000 new diagnoses of PC have been estimated to take place in 2020,[3] the described clinical cohorts constitute only a small amount of the possible data on PC. These data are limited further by the lack of comprehensive reporting of relevant clinical characteristics, such as disease stage and grade, therapeutic interventions, and disease outcomes, that could provide valuable insight into additional germline genetic determinants with prognostic or therapeutic predictive utility in PC. For example, it has been shown that 25% of requisition forms from clinical genetic testing laboratories lacked the clinical information relevant to interpret the genetic results.[68] This raises the difficulty of parsing out whether patients tested for PC genes have localized PC, metastatic PC, or lethal PC, and additionally whether or not they have a family history of PC or cancer in general.

A further limitation of these data, and genetic data in general, is the substantial heterogeneity of the tested cohorts. For example, although 67.9% of PC patients in the study by Na and colleagues[46] had a Gleason score under 7%, 82.3% of the PC patients studied by Pritzlaff and colleagues[65] had a Gleason score higher than 7 (see **Fig. 2**A). Furthermore, 2 of the 3 studies were spearheaded by commercial genetic testing companies, which brings the challenge that these tests have been ordered by providers in many different clinical settings and are not uniform in their ordering practices.

Lack of Representation in Ancestral Groups

Across all the clinical PC cohorts, 72.8% of PC patients who have undergone genetic analysis are of European ancestry (**Table 3**), which severely limits the ability to generalize the findings of these studies to PC patients from other ancestral and ethnic groups. This lack of data from non-European

Table 3
Prevalence of germline pathogenic variants in patients with prostate cancer across various ancestral groups

Ancestral Group	Total (%)	Count of Patients with a Pathogenic Result in the Established Prostate Cancer Predisposition Genes (%)	Count of Patients with a Pathogenic Result in Genes with Limited Evidence for Prostate Cancer Susceptibility (%)	Count of Patients with a Pathogenic Result in Genes with Other Clinical Utility in Prostate Cancer (%)	Count of Patients with a Pathogenic Result in all Genes Relevant to Prostate Cancer (%)	Count of Patients with a Pathogenic Result in any Cancer Susceptibility Gene (%)
White	3207 (72.8)	219 (6.8)	138 (4.3)	22 (0.7)	379 (11.8)	483 (15.06)
Ashkenazi Jewish	234 (5.3)	22 (9.4)	25 (6.4)	1 (0.4)	38 (16.23)	52 (22.22)
Black	346 (7.8)	13 (3.7)	4 (1.1)	3 (0.9)	20 (5.8)	24 (6.94)
Hispanic	78 (1.8)	4 (5.1)	0	0	4 (5.1)	5 (6.41)
Asian	140 (3.2)	10 (7.1)	3 (2.1)	1 (0.7)	14 (10.0)	15 (10.71)
Other	401 (9.1)	33 (8.2)	18 (4.5)	1 (0.2)	52 (12.9)	67 (16.71)
All	4406 (100)	301 (6.8)	178 (4.0)	28 (0.6)	507 (11.5)	646 (14.66)

communities further perpetuates an already existing disparity and poor disease outcome in PC.[69,70] These limitations of paucity of clinical data and diverse populations are important to consider, as these clinical PC cohorts are described further.

When stratifying the results by ancestral groups studied in the Nicolosi and colleagues[64] and Na and colleagues[46] cohorts, the frequency rates of pathogenic variants in the established PC genes for individuals with European ancestry and Ashkenazi Jewish ancestry are 6.8% and 9.4%, respectively (see **Table 3**). These frequencies are juxtaposed with lower prevalence rates in individuals with black/African ancestry of 3.7% and Hispanic ancestry of 5.1%. The frequency rate of pathogenic variants in the established PC risk genes in PC patients of the Asian ancestry was 7.1%, which is closer to the prevalence of these germline variants in PC patients from the European and Ashkenazi Jewish ancestries (see **Table 3**). This variability in the molecular diagnostic yield of germline analysis also is seen for genes with emerging evidence for PC susceptibility, all PC relevant genes, and all tested cancer genes (**Fig. 3**B). Collectively, these results underscore the need for increased representation for African and Hispanic ancestral groups to further identify ancestry-specific genetic variants that may lead to additional clinical benefit for PC patients from these understudied populations.

GENETIC COUNSELING IMPLICATIONS AND CHALLENGES

In order to further understanding of the utility of germline molecular analysis in PC improve, more patients need to have clinical testing at the point of care. Should uptake of genetic testing increase, it will affect the genetic counselors directly, who likely will be the providers involved in post-test counseling of these patients. Given this, some genetic counseling implications and anticipated challenges for this patient population are highlighted. As noted in **Table 3**, there were 646 (14.66%) patients included in the clinical PC cohorts who were found to have a pathogenic variant in a gene that confers a significant increase in the risk of developing one or more cancers. These findings require counseling patients regarding genetic variants with increased cancer risk that may not correlate with their personal or family history of cancer.[58] In a meta-analysis of studies on distress and anxiety of patients undergoing germline genetic testing, it was shown that patients tend to have emotional distress at the time of receiving results. This anxiety, however, appears to subside soon after for those with negative or inconclusive results.[71] Furthermore, the appropriate

screening modalities for patients with pathogenic variants not related to their phenotype are unclear, which has been noted to be a concern.[72] Additionally, although the clinical cohorts described received panel testing, exome testing increasingly is becoming utilized in the clinical space and presents a possible challenge of returning incidental or secondary findings.[73] In this case, incidental or secondary findings refer to variants that are associated with a condition other than PC, such as cardiomyopathy. Another counseling difficulty that may arise when testing a higher volume of PC patients is the presence of variants of uncertain significance (VUSs). In the study by Nicolosi and colleagues,[64] there were 941 VUS findings detected across 3607 patients,[64] whereas 35% of the participants in the study by Giri and colleagues[9] were found to have at least 1 VUS.[63] Other studies similarly have shown that approximately 44% of tested patients received 1 or more VUS findings when undergoing germline genetic testing for indications related to cancer.[58] The return of VUS findings may lead to increased screening for patients who may not be clinically indicated for such interventions,[74] thereby contributing to unnecessary medical costs and stress. In cases of patients found to have a pathogenic variant, genetic counselors may have to facilitate cascade testing for at-risk family members in order to ensure proper access to early detection and screening. These considerations highlight the importance of appropriate post-test genetic counseling to better explain the impact of off-phenotypic-target and incidental findings, VUSs, and cascade testing to patients.

In addition to the need for appropriate post-test counseling, providers must navigate health insurance policies when ordering genetic testing for cancer risk. This can prove challenging, as a review of the insurance landscape for MGP testing found substantial variations in how payers cover these tests.[75] Furthermore, insurance coverage influences not only if people pursue genetic testing[76] but also how they pay for genetic testing. Namely, some individuals may choose to pay for genetic testing out-of-pocket because genetic testing results can affect insurance coverage. Although the passage of the Genetic Information Nondiscrimination Act[77] in 2008 prevents genetic test results from affecting coverage of health insurance, life insurance and long-term disability insurance coverage still may be affected.[78] Understanding and discussing the impact of insurance coverage on genetic testing and vice versa increasingly are expected of genetic counselors and other clinical providers ordering germline genetic analysis[78,79] and may be important especially for cascade testing of asymptomatic at-risk family members.

In conclusion, understanding and communicating the intricacies of insurance coverage have the potential to increase access to genetic testing, which is necessary for increasing clinical germline genetic testing in PC patients.

Lastly, there was a nontrivial time lag between establishing the diagnosis of PC and performing germline genetic testing at the point of care. As observed in the Nicolosi and colleagues[64] study, the mean age at testing was 67 years whereas the mean age at diagnosis was 60 years. This highlights the importance of timing for initiating germline testing. The observed lag in genetic testing could be due to many barriers, but one to highlight is that geneticists and genetic counselors are in high demand.[80] Such challenges can be mitigated by adopting additional models for genetic consultation and counseling, which can include printed handouts, recorded video clips, and telemedicine services. There is an overall need to identify and address barriers better, in order to perform germline testing in oncology settings in a timely manner.

FUTURE DIRECTIONS

Moving forward, there are relevant and pertinent ways to continue to better understand the inherited genetics behind PC susceptibility and tumorigenesis. A key need continues to be increased representation of non-European PC patients in clinical and molecular studies, because this will increase understanding of the ancestry-specific genetic drivers for PC and better elucidate the true frequencies of pathogenic cancer variants in these populations. One possible direction is to increase the amount of diversity and representation within research investigators and collaborators, because it has been shown that participants have a preference for research studies that include research staff who share the same cultural background.[81] In addition, larger clinical cohorts still are necessary to further refine the prevalence of germline alterations in PC patients with different clinical characteristics. To do this, however, genetic testing needs to be more accessible, which can be achieved by implementing germline testing at the point of care by nongenetic providers or by adopting better mechanisms, such as telemedicine, to facilitate genetic testing for PC patients. Another way is through patient-partnered research, where clinical samples can be obtained directly from PC patients for genetic sequencing and analysis.[82] Such efforts can accelerate discoveries and bypass common barriers in provider-driven research studies. To continue learning the genetic drivers and mechanisms behind PC, it also would be prudent to turn to new modalities, such as RNA sequencing and long-read sequencing, which may provide useful insight into the germline determinants of cancer risk and disease outcomes that may escape detection using current standard analysis approaches.

SUMMARY

Despite the high prevalence and heritability of PC, the number of PC patients studied remains low and with limited diversity, highlighting the need for increased germline genetic testing in this patient population. Overall, clinical germline genetic testing in PC should utilize an MGP approach that prioritizes established and suspected PC susceptibility genes as well as genes that can inform disease prognosis and treatment approach in PC. A review of large published clinical PC cohorts shows that up to 15% of PC patients have clinically informative results following comprehensive germline genetic testing, a figure that may be higher when considering the limitations and heterogeneity of these studies. In addition to being the most cost-effective and time-efficient type of testing, a majority of MGPs that currently are available include genes with established diagnostic or therapeutic utility in PC. Accordingly, it is crucial to offer appropriate MGP testing to PC patients in a timely manner following diagnosis to inform clinical decisions related to screening, treatment interventions, and familial genetic testing. Lastly, as the uptake of genetic testing increases, genetic counseling services will be increasingly crucial for post-test counseling regarding unexpected and uncertain results as well as cascade testing.

CLINICS CARE POINTS

- If indicated, germline genetic testing or genetics referral should be initiated promptly for PC patients shortly after diagnosis to maximally inform clinical decision making.
- Depending on ancestry, approximately 10% to 16% of PC patients have 1 or more germline pathogenic variants that can inform cancer risk stratification or therapeutic interventions.
- MGPs are best suited for patients with PC because they routinely include established PC risk genes.
- Genetic counseling, especially after testing, can be utilized for PC patients to facilitate discussion of incidental findings, VUSs, and cascade testing.

DISCLOSURE

Research support for this work was generously provided by the Department of Defense (W81XWH-21-1-0084, PC200150, SHA) and Prostate Cancer Foundation (18YOUN02, SHA).

REFERENCES

1. Rawla P. Epidemiology of prostate cancer. World J Oncol 2019;10(2):63–89.
2. Institute NC. Cancer stat facts: prostate cancer 2014. Available at: https://seer.cancer.gov/statfacts/html/prost.html.
3. Siegel RL, Miller KD, Jemal A. Cancer statistics, 2020. CA Cancer J Clin 2020;70(1):7–30.
4. Society AC. Cancer facts and figures 2020.
5. Tenesa A, Haley CS. The heritability of human disease: estimation, uses and abuses. Nat Rev Genet 2013;14(2):139–49.
6. Lichtenstein P, Holm NV, Verkasalo PK, et al. Environmental and heritable factors in the causation of cancer—analyses of cohorts of twins from Sweden, Denmark, and Finland. N Engl J Med 2000;343(2):78–85.
7. Mucci LA, Hjelmborg JB, Harris JR, et al. Familial risk and heritability of cancer among Twins in Nordic Countries. JAMA 2016;315(1):68–76.
8. Hjelmborg JB, Scheike T, Holst K, et al. The heritability of prostate cancer in the Nordic Twin Study of Cancer. Cancer Epidemiol Biomarkers Prev 2014;23(11):2303–10.
9. Giri VN, Knudsen KE, Kelly WK, et al. Implementation of germline testing for prostate cancer: philadelphia prostate cancer consensus conference 2019. J Clin Oncol 2020. JCO2000046.
10. Pritchard CC, Mateo J, Walsh MF, et al. Inherited DNA-repair gene mutations in men with metastatic prostate cancer. N Engl J Med 2016;375(5):443–53.
11. Mateo J, Carreira S, Sandhu S, et al. DNA-repair defects and olaparib in metastatic prostate cancer. N Engl J Med 2015;373(18):1697–708.
12. Kote-Jarai Z, Leongamornlert D, Saunders E, et al. BRCA2 is a moderate penetrance gene contributing to young-onset prostate cancer: implications for genetic testing in prostate cancer patients. Br J Cancer 2011;105(8):1230–4.
13. Ewing CM, Ray AM, Lange EM, et al. Germline mutations in HOXB13 and prostate-cancer risk. N Engl J Med 2012;366(2):141–9.
14. Mersch J, Jackson MA, Park M, et al. Cancers associated with BRCA1 and BRCA2 mutations other than breast and ovarian. Cancer 2015;121:269–75.
15. Van Asperen CJ, Brohet RM, Meijers-Heijboer EJ, et al. Cancer risks in BRCA2 families: estimates for sites other than breast and ovary. J Med Genet 2005;42(9):711–9.
16. Gallagher DJ, Gaudet MM, Pal P, et al. Germline BRCA mutations denote a clinicopathologic subset of prostate cancer. Clin Cancer Res 2010;16(7):2115–21.
17. Moran A, O'Hara C, Khan S, et al. Risk of cancer other than breast or ovarian in individuals with BRCA1 and BRCA2 mutations. Fam Cancer 2012;11(2):235–42.
18. Roed Nielsen H, Petersen J, Therkildsen C, et al. Increased risk of male cancer and identification of a potential prostate cancer cluster region in BRCA2. Acta Oncol 2016;55(1):38–44.
19. Agalliu I, Karlins E, Kwon EM, et al. Rare germline mutations in the BRCA2 gene are associated with early-onset prostate cancer. Br J Cancer 2007;97(6):826–31.
20. Nyberg T, Frost D, Barrowdale D, et al. Prostate cancer risks for male BRCA1 and BRCA2 mutation carriers: a prospective cohort study. Eur Urol 2020;77(1):24–35.
21. Consortium BCL. Cancer risks in BRCA2 mutation carriers. J Natl Cancer Inst 1999;91(15):1310–6.
22. Kirchhoff T, Kauff ND, Mitra N, et al. BRCA mutations and risk of prostate cancer in Ashkenazi Jews. Clin Cancer Res 2004;10(9):2918–21.
23. Breyer JP, Avritt TG, McReynolds KM, et al. Confirmation of the HOXB13 G84E germline mutation in familial prostate cancer. Cancer Epidemiol Biomarkers Prev 2012;21(8):1348–53.
24. Karlsson R, Aly M, Clements M, et al. A population-based assessment of germline HOXB13 G84E mutation and prostate cancer risk. Eur Urol 2014;65(1):169–76.
25. Kote-Jarai Z, Mikropoulos C, Leongamornlert DA, et al. Prevalence of the HOXB13 G84E germline mutation in British men and correlation with prostate cancer risk, tumour characteristics and clinical outcomes. Ann Oncol 2015;26(4):756–61.
26. Xu J, Lange EM, Lu L, et al. HOXB13 is a susceptibility gene for prostate cancer: results from the International Consortium for Prostate Cancer Genetics (ICPCG). Hum Genet 2013;132(1):5–14.
27. Hoffmann TJ, Sakoda LC, Shen L, et al. Imputation of the rare HOXB13 G84E mutation and cancer risk in a large population-based cohort. PLoS Genet 2015;11(1):e1004930.
28. Leongamornlert D, Mahmud N, Tymrakiewicz M, et al. Germline BRCA1 mutations increase prostate cancer risk. Br J Cancer 2012;106(10):1697–701.
29. Grindedal EM, Møller P, Eeles R, et al. Germ-line mutations in mismatch repair genes associated with prostate cancer. Cancer Epidemiol Biomarkers Prev 2009;18(9):2460–7.
30. Raymond VM, Mukherjee B, Wang F, et al. Elevated risk of prostate cancer among men with Lynch syndrome. J Clin Oncol 2013;31(14):1713–8.
31. Bauer CM, Ray AM, Halstead-Nussloch BA, et al. Hereditary prostate cancer as a feature of Lynch syndrome. Fam Cancer 2011;10(1):37–42.

32. Ryan S, Jenkins MA, Win AK. Risk of prostate cancer in Lynch syndrome: a systematic review and meta-analysis. Cancer Epidemiol Biomarkers Prev 2014; 23(3):437–49.

33. Rosty C, Walsh MD, Lindor NM, et al. High prevalence of mismatch repair deficiency in prostate cancers diagnosed in mismatch repair gene mutation carriers from the colon cancer family registry. Fam Cancer 2014;13(4):573–82.

34. Thompson D, Easton DF, Breast Cancer Linkage Consortium. Cancer incidence in BRCA1 mutation carriers. J Natl Cancer Inst 2002;94(18):1358–65.

35. Wang Y, Dai B, Ye D. CHEK2 mutation and risk of prostate cancer: a systematic review and meta-analysis. Int J Clin Exp Med 2015;8(9):15708.

36. Meyer A, Wilhelm B, Dörk T, et al. ATM missense variant P1054R predisposes to prostate cancer. Radiother Oncol 2007;83(3):283–8.

37. Cybulski C, Wokołorczyk D, Kluźniak W, et al. An inherited NBN mutation is associated with poor prognosis prostate cancer. Br J Cancer 2013;108(2):461–8.

38. Hale V, Weischer M, Park JY. CHEK2 (*) 1100delC Mutation and Risk of Prostate Cancer. Prostate Cancer 2014;2014:294575.

39. Cybulski C, Górski B, Debniak T, et al. NBS1 is a prostate cancer susceptibility gene. Cancer Res 2004;64(4):1215–9.

40. Rusak B, Kluźniak W, Wokołorczykv D, et al. Inherited NBN mutations and prostate cancer risk and survival. Cancer Res Treat 2019;51(3):1180–7.

41. Angèle S, Falconer A, Edwards SM, et al. ATM polymorphisms as risk factors for prostate cancer development. Br J Cancer 2004;91(4):783–7.

42. Wu Y, Yu H, Zheng SL, et al. A comprehensive evaluation of CHEK2 germline mutations in men with prostate cancer. Prostate 2018;78(8):607–15.

43. Akbari MR, Wallis CJD, Toi A, et al. The impact of a BRCA2 mutation on mortality from screen-detected prostate cancer. Br J Cancer 2014; 111(6):1238–40.

44. Tryggvadóttir L, Vidarsdóttir L, Thorgeirsson T, et al. Prostate cancer progression and survival in BRCA2 mutation carriers. J Natl Cancer Inst 2007;99(12): 929–35.

45. Thorne H, Willems AJ, Niedermayr E, et al. Decreased prostate cancer-specific survival of men with BRCA2 mutations from multiple breast cancer families. Cancer Prev Res 2011;4(7):1002–10.

46. Na R, Zheng SL, Han M, et al. Germline Mutations in ATM and BRCA1/2 distinguish risk for lethal and indolent prostate cancer and are associated with early age at death. Eur Urol 2017;71(5):740–7.

47. Leongamornlert D, Saunders E, Dadaev T, et al. Frequent germline deleterious mutations in DNA repair genes in familial prostate cancer cases are associated with advanced disease. Br J Cancer 2014;110(6):1663–72.

48. Jeggo PA, Pearl LH, Carr AM. DNA repair, genome stability and cancer: a historical perspective. Nat Rev Cancer 2016;16(1):35–42.

49. Ratta R, Guida A, Scotté F, et al. PARP inhibitors as a new therapeutic option in metastatic prostate cancer: a systematic review. Prostate Cancer Prostatic Dis 2020. https://doi.org/10.1038/s41391-020-0233-3.

50. Mateo J, Porta N, Bianchini D, et al. Olaparib in patients with metastatic castration-resistant prostate cancer with DNA repair gene aberrations (TOPARP-B): a multicentre, open-label, randomised, phase 2 trial. Lancet Oncol 2020;21(1):162–74.

51. Pomerantz MM, Spisák S, Jia L, et al. The association between germline BRCA2 variants and sensitivity to platinum-based chemotherapy among men with metastatic prostate cancer. Cancer 2017; 123(18):3532–9.

52. Le DT, Durham JN, Smith KN, et al. Mismatch repair deficiency predicts response of solid tumors to PD-1 blockade. Science 2017;357(6349):409–13.

53. Abida W, Cheng ML, Armenia J, et al. Analysis of the prevalence of microsatellite instability in prostate cancer and response to immune checkpoint blockade. JAMA Oncol 2019;5(4):471–8.

54. Carlo MI, Giri VN, Paller CJ, et al. Evolving intersection between inherited cancer genetics and therapeutic clinical trials in prostate cancer: a white paper from the Germline Genetics Working Group of the Prostate Cancer Clinical Trials Consortium. JCO Precision Oncol 2018;2:1–14.

55. Gillessen S, Attard G, Beer TM, et al. Management of patients with advanced prostate cancer: the report of the advanced prostate cancer consensus conference APCCC 2017. Eur Urol 2018;73(2): 178–211.

56. Giri VN, Knudsen KE, Kelly WK, et al. Role of genetic testing for inherited prostate cancer risk: Philadelphia prostate cancer consensus conference 2017. J Clin Oncol 2018;36(4):414–24.

57. AlDubayan SH. Leveraging clinical tumor-profiling programs to achieve comprehensive germline-inclusive precision cancer medicine. JCO Precision Oncol 2019;(3):1–3.

58. Lynce F, Isaacs C. How far do we go with genetic evaluation? gene, panel, and tumor testing. Am Soc Clin Oncol Educ Book 2016;35:e72–8.

59. Susswein LR, Marshall ML, Nusbaum R, et al. Pathogenic and likely pathogenic variant prevalence among the first 10,000 patients referred for next-generation cancer panel testing. Genet Med 2016; 18(8):823–32.

60. Xue Y, Ankala A, Wilcox WR, et al. Solving the molecular diagnostic testing conundrum for Mendelian disorders in the era of next-generation sequencing: single-gene, gene panel, or exome/genome sequencing. Genet Med 2015;17(6):444–51.

61. Jamal SM, Yu J-H, Chong JX, et al. Practices and policies of clinical exome sequencing providers: analysis and implications. Am J Med Genet A 2013;161A(5):935–50.

62. AlDubayan SH. Considerations of multigene test findings among men with prostate cancer - knowns and unknowns. Can J Urol 2019;26(5 Suppl 2):14–6.

63. Giri VN, Obeid E, Gross L, et al. Inherited mutations in men undergoing multigene panel testing for prostate cancer: emerging implications for personalized prostate cancer genetic evaluation. JCO Precision Oncol 2017;(1):1–17.

64. Nicolosi P, Ledet E, Yang S, et al. Prevalence of germline variants in prostate cancer and implications for current genetic testing guidelines. JAMA Oncol 2019;5(4):523–8.

65. Pritzlaff M, Tian Y, Reineke P, et al. Diagnosing hereditary cancer predisposition in men with prostate cancer. Genet Med 2020. https://doi.org/10.1038/s41436-020-0830-5.

66. Cox DM, Nelson KL, Clytone M, et al. Hereditary cancer screening: case reports and review of literature on ten Ashkenazi Jewish founder mutations. Mol Genet Genomic Med 2018;6(6):1236–42.

67. Nielsen M, Infante E, Brand R. MUTYH polyposis. In: Adam MP, Ardinger HH, Pagon RA, et al, editors. GeneReviews®. Seattle: University of Washington; 2012.

68. Lubin IM, Caggana M, Constantin C, et al. Ordering molecular genetic tests and reporting results: practices in laboratory and clinical settings. J Mol Diagn 2008;10(5):459–68.

69. Bentley AR, Callier S, Rotimi CN. Diversity and inclusion in genomic research: why the uneven progress? J Community Genet 2017;8(4):255–66.

70. Mills MC, Rahal C. A scientometric review of genome-wide association studies. Commun Biol 2019;2:9.

71. Hamilton JG, Lobel M, Moyer A. Emotional distress following genetic testing for hereditary breast and ovarian cancer: a meta-analytic review. Health Psychol 2009;28(4):510.

72. Stanislaw C, Xue Y, Wilcox WR. Genetic evaluation and testing for hereditary forms of cancer in the era of next-generation sequencing. Cancer Biol Med 2016;13(1):55–67.

73. Manolio TA, Chisholm RL, Ozenberger B, et al. Implementing genomic medicine in the clinic: the future is here. Genet Med 2013;15(4):258–67.

74. Okur V, Chung WK. The impact of hereditary cancer gene panels on clinical care and lessons learned. Cold Spring Harb Mol Case Stud 2017;3(6).

75. Lu CY, Loomer S, Ceccarelli R, et al. Insurance coverage policies for pharmacogenomic and multigene testing for cancer. J Pers Med 2018;8(2).

76. Roberts MC, Kurian AW, Petkov VI. Uptake of the 21-gene assay among women with node-positive, hormone receptor-positive breast cancer. J Natl Compr Canc Netw 2019;17(6):662–8.

77. The Genetic Information Nondiscrimination Act of 2008. Available at: https://www.eeoc.gov/statutes/genetic-information-nondiscrimination-act-2008. Accessed October 15, 2020.

78. Prince AER, Roche MI. Genetic information, nondiscrimination, and privacy protections in genetic counseling practice. J Genet Couns 2014;23(6):891–902.

79. Wagner C, Murphy L, Harkenrider J, et al. Genesurance counseling: patient perspectives. J Genet Couns 2018;27(4):814–22.

80. Penon-Portmann M, Chang J, Cheng M, et al. Genetics workforce: distribution of genetics services and challenges to health care in California. Genet Med 2020;22(1):227–31.

81. George S, Duran N, Norris K. A systematic review of barriers and facilitators to minority research participation among African Americans, Latinos, Asian Americans, and Pacific Islanders. Am J Public Health 2014;104(2):e16–31.

82. Metastatic prostate cancer project. Available at: https://mpcproject.org/count-me-in. Accessed September 30, 2020.

Genetic Testing Guidelines and Education of Health Care Providers Involved in Prostate Cancer Care

James Ryan Mark, MD[a], Carey McDougall, LCGC[b,c], Veda N. Giri, MD[a,b,c],*

KEYWORDS

• Germline testing • Prostate cancer • Genetic education • Precision medicine

KEY POINTS

- Prostate cancer (PCA) germline testing is now necessary to determine candidacy for targeted therapy in the metastatic setting and screening approaches and will likely inform management of localized disease in the future, impacting urology and oncology practices.
- Implementation of PCA germline testing requires working knowledge of National Comprehensive Cancer Network (NCCN) guidelines, considerations of pretest and posttest informed consent and recommendations, testing options, hereditary cancer risks and impact on families, and insight into the field of genetic counseling.
- NCCN guidelines for PCA germline testing are regularly updated, and therefore, providers need to maintain knowledge of revised guidelines.
- Many educational resources are available for providers to gain formal or informal training and knowledge of principles and practice of germline testing for PCA.

INTRODUCTION

Germline testing for prostate cancer (PCA) has become a central part of PCA care.[1,2] Current National Comprehensive Cancer Network (NCCN) guidelines recommend germline testing for all men with metastatic PCA because of the role in determining candidacy for targeted therapies such as PARP inhibitors or immune checkpoint therapy.[1–4] Furthermore, NCCN guidelines define germline testing criteria for men with early-stage PCA based on pathologic and disease features and family history. For unaffected men interested in cancer risk assessment, germline testing is based primarily on family history.[3,4] Germline testing is therefore becoming an integral part of

PCA care across multiple disciplines, including medical oncology, urology, radiation oncology, and primary care. Germline testing is a complex process involving pretest genetic counseling or informed consent, optimal genetic testing, intake of family history, and disclosure of genetic test results and recommendations relevant to men and their families.[1] Given that germline testing is increasing in PCA care, referral of all men to genetic counseling is not a sustainable model because of the increasing demand for genetic counseling.[1,5,6] As such, health care providers are increasingly faced with ordering germline testing in their practices or determining how to refer to genetic counseling, which requires working knowledge of germline testing and practice

a Department of Urology, Thomas Jefferson University, Philadelphia, PA, USA; b Cancer Risk Assessment and Clinical Cancer Genetics, Department of Medical Oncology, Sidney Kimmel Cancer Center, Thomas Jefferson University, Philadelphia, PA, USA; c Cancer Risk Assessment and Clinical Cancer Genetics, Department of Cancer Biology, Sidney Kimmel Cancer Center, Thomas Jefferson University, Philadelphia, PA, USA
* Corresponding author. Medical Oncology, Cancer Biology, Urology, Cancer Risk Assessment and Clinical Cancer Genetics, 1025 Walnut Street, Suite 1015, Philadelphia, PA 19107.
E-mail address: Veda.Giri@jefferson.edu

Urol Clin N Am 48 (2021) 311–322
https://doi.org/10.1016/j.ucl.2021.03.003

considerations for responsible delivery of germline testing to men.

Here, the authors provide a brief overview of key aspects of germline testing in the pretest and posttest scenarios, current NCCN guidelines addressing germline testing and management for PCA, differences in germline and somatic testing in PCA care, and implementation elements for practice. They also highlight educational resources for formal learning of key aspects of germline testing.

GENETICS KNOWLEDGE AND PRACTICE CHALLENGES FOR UROLOGISTS

The role of germline testing in urology practice is increasing and is primarily indicated to inform PCA screening strategies and identify hereditary cancer syndromes at this time.[1,3,4,7] Specifically, men with BRCA2 mutations are recommended to start PSA screening starting at age 40 and to consider annual versus semiannual screening because of emerging data stating that men with BRCA2 mutations are diagnosed at a younger age and had more clinically significant disease.[4,7,8] There are also early data in the setting of early-stage, low-risk PCA regarding upgrading of biopsies among men on active surveillance.[9] Men with BRCA2 mutations were found to have greater rates of upgrading of biopsies while on active surveillance, which deserves validation studies.[9] Germline testing also uncovers hereditary cancer syndromes, such as hereditary breast and ovarian cancer associated with BRCA1 and BRCA2 mutations or Lynch syndrome associated with mutations in multiple DNA mismatch repair genes.[10] Therefore, germline testing not only impacts men regarding PCA treatment and screening but also may inform additional cancer risks for men and their families, which urologists need to understand and address.

Despite the growing clinical relevance of germline testing in PCA screening and treatment, significant knowledge and practice challenges exist to widespread implementation in the urology clinic. One study of 132 urologists in the United States reported lower knowledge of germline testing indications.[11] When presented with hypothetical case scenarios where germline testing is indicated, many respondents indicated they would not offer genetic counseling or testing; 2% of respondents answered questions consistent with current NCCN guidelines regarding germline testing and 4% reported any formal education in genetics. Roughly 25% of urologists reported feeling unqualified to answer questions regarding the genetics of inheritable PCA. Younger age ($P = 0.03$), academic practice ($P = .04$), and

specialization in PCA oncology ($P = .007$) were significantly associated with performing or referring for germline testing.[11]

A survey of 52 large urology groups in the United States indicated practice challenges to implementing PCA germline testing.[12] Reimbursement concerns, time constraints preventing complete documentation of family history into the electronic medical record, and a fear of medicolegal liability were major barriers to genetic testing and counseling by urologists.[12] In addition to administrative hurdles, practicing urologists may not have adequate working knowledge of genetic testing and pretest informed consent to provide these services.[1,11]

GENETICS KNOWLEDGE AND PRACTICE CHALLENGES FOR ONCOLOGISTS

The rapid emergence of precision medicine is now a major driver for PCA germline testing.[1,2] In 2020, the Food and Drug Administration (FDA) approved olaparib and rucaparib for men with metastatic, castration-resistant PCA (mCRPC) with specific DNA repair gene mutations after progression on standard lines of therapy owing to improved clinical responses among men with specific DNA repair gene mutations, such as in BRCA1 and BRCA2.[13,14] The FDA has also approved pembrolizumab for patients with mismatch repair deficiency or microsatellite instability who have progressed on prior therapies, which can also impact a subset of men with PCA.[15] Therefore, germline testing for men with mCRPC is now critical to identify germline mutations to inform therapy options, which is predicted to impact a major subset of men with mCRPC because 12% to 15% have been reported to carry germline mutations in DNA repair genes.[16,17]

Literature regarding practice patterns and barriers among oncologists is also emerging relevant to PCA germline testing. One study surveying 26 primarily academic oncologists reported that 62% consider testing all metastatic PCA patients, whereas 11% consider testing all patients with high-risk localized disease.[18] Five key barriers to widespread implementation of germline testing for patients with PCA included delayed or limited access to genetic counseling, no insurance coverage, lack of effective clinical workflows, insufficient educational materials, and clinical time and space constraints.[18] Thus, knowledge gaps and practice challenges need to be urgently addressed in oncology practices given that germline testing for men with metastatic PCA is a major indication for germline testing.[3,4]

NATIONAL COMPREHENSIVE CANCER NETWORK GUIDELINES FOR PROSTATE CANCER GERMLINE TESTING

The NCCN addresses germline testing indications for men with PCA or at risk for PCA in multiple guidelines: the NCCN Genetic/Familial High-Risk Assessment: Breast, Ovarian Pancreatic (version 2.2021) guideline and the NCCN Prostate Cancer (version 2.2021) guideline (**Table 1**).[3,4] NCCN guidelines are regularly updated, and so urologists and oncologists need to stay up-to-date regarding new and revised germline testing indications. The current guidelines are concordant regarding PCA germline testing of men meeting any of the following criteria: metastatic PCA; Ashkenazi Jewish ancestry; intraductal/cribriform histology; very-high-risk disease (T3b-T4 or primary Gleason pattern 5 or >4 Scores with grade group 4 or 5); high-risk disease (T3a or grade group 4 or 5 or PSA >20).[3,4] There are differences regarding germline testing criteria based on family history. NCCN Guidelines Genetic/Familial High-Risk Assessment: Breast, Ovarian, and Pancreatic (version 2.2021) states to consider genetic testing for men with PCA with (1) ≥1 close blood relative diagnosed with breast cancer ≤ age 50, pancreatic, ovarian, or metastatic, intraductal/cribriform

PCA at any age; or (2) ≥2 close blood relatives with either breast cancer or PCA at any age.[4] The NCCN Prostate Cancer (version 2.2021) guideline states to consider family history as follows: (1) PCA family history: brother, father, or multiple family members diagnosed with PCA at less than 60 or died of PCA (grade groups 2–5); or (2) ≥3 cancers on the same side of the family (especially if diagnosed ≤50): bile duct, breast, colorectal, endometrial, gastric, kidney, melanoma, ovarian, pancreatic, prostate (grade groups 2–5), small bowel, or urothelial.[3] These complex guidelines can cause confusion in clinical practice and require ongoing education and attention to practice needs.

DIFFERENCES IN GENETIC TESTING STRATEGIES

One area that providers need to understand is the differences in "genetic testing" that encompass germline and somatic testing strategies (**Table 2**). Germline testing is performed to identify inherited genetic pathogenic variants (or mutations) that may predispose an individual to cancers and may now increasingly inform targeted therapies.[1,2,10] Germline testing involves testing blood or saliva specimens to assess for inherited genetic

Table 1
Current prostate cancer germline testing guidelines

NCCN Guidelines Genetic/Familial High-Risk Assessment: Breast, Ovarian, and Pancreatic (version 2.2021) *and* NCCN Guidelines Prostate Cancer Version (2.2021)

- Metastatic prostate cancer
- Ashkenazi Jewish ancestry
- Intraductal/cribriform histology
- Very high risk: T3P-T4 or primary Gleason pattern 5 or >4 cores with grade group 4 or 5
- High risk: T3a or grade group 4 or 5 or PSA >20

NCCN Guidelines Genetic/Familial High-Risk Assessment: Breast, Ovarian, and Pancreatic Version 1.2021	NCCN Guidelines Prostate Cancer Version 4.2019
- ≥1 close blood relative diagnosed with breast cancer ≤ age 50, pancreatic, ovarian, or metastatic, intraductal/cribriform prostate cancer at any age - ≥2 close blood relatives with either breast or prostate cancer at any age	- Prostate cancer family history: brother, father, or multiple family members diagnosed with prostate cancer at <60 y or died from prostate cancer (grade groups 2–5) - ≥3 cancers on the same side of the family (especially if diagnosed <=50): bile duct, breast, colorectal, endometrial, gastric, kidney, melanoma, ovarian, pancreatic, prostate (grade groups 2–5), small bowel, or urothelial

Note: Guidelines as of 10/18/2020.

Table 2
Comparison of genetic tests involved in prostate cancer care

Features	Germline Testing	Tumor Next-Generation Sequencing	Molecular Genomic Tests
Example tests/ laboratory tests	Invitae, Ambry Genetics, Myriad Genetics, GeneDx, Color	Foundation Medicine, Caris Life Sciences	Decipher, OncotypeDX, Prolaris, ConfirmMDx
Specimen	Blood or saliva	Tumor or circuiting tumor cells	Tumor or prostate specimen
Testing capacity	2–80+ genes	250+ genes	—
Testing capability	Full sequencing, deletion and duplication testing, rearrangement testing, single-site testing if known mutation in a family	Sequencing or hot-spot testing for targetable mutations	RNA expression or epigenetic assay
Information for metastatic disease treatment	++ (if mutations found in genes tested)	+++	—
Information for nonmetastatic disease management	+ (emerging for active surveillance)	—	+++
Information for prostate cancer screening discussions	++ (*BRCA2* specifically)	—	ConfirmMDx for rebiopsy
Hereditary cancer information	+++	+ (needs confirmatory germline testing)	—
NCCN criteria for testing	+++	—	++
Insurance coverage	+++ (insurance needs to be checked)	++ (insurance needs to be checked)	+++

mutations. Testing may involve as few as 2 genes (such as *BRCA1* and *BRCA2*) or up to 80 genes or more with comprehensive panel testing.[1] Ways to proceed with this testing is through guidelines-based panels, PCA-specific panels, comprehensive panels, or reflex panels where initial testing of a smaller set of genes is followed by expanded testing.[1] The testing capability involves full sequencing, deletion and duplication testing, rearrangement testing, and single-site testing if there is a known mutation in a patient's family. The classic purpose of testing was to identify individuals at risk for cancers to inform cancer screening and risk reduction measures.[10] Over recent years, the indication for germline testing has evolved to include identifying patients with cancer for targeted therapies.[1,2,6] For example, testing men with metastatic PCA is a clear indication for testing by NCCN guidelines to inform precision therapy, such as for PARP inhibitors, and identify hereditary cancer syndromes.[3,4]

Somatic next-generation sequencing (NGS) is a central part of oncologic care across multiple tumor types, including PCA. Somatic NGS testing involves sequencing of tumors or, increasingly, circulating tumor cells, to identify targetable mutations (see **Table 2**).[19] Testing capability can include 200 to 300+ genes and typically involves assessing for hot-spot regions for therapeutic targets. Approximately 3% to 12% of patients with tumor mutations have been reported to carry actionable germline mutations,[20] and therefore, providers need to have growing knowledge of patients to refer for genetic counseling and confirmatory germline testing. Mutations may be identified from tumor testing that may fit with the patient's clinical scenario or be discordant with the patient's personal or family history features. Mutations in specific highly penetrant genes to consider referring for confirmatory germline testing include *BRCA1*, *BRCA2*, *MLH1*, *MSH2*, *MSH6*, *PMS2*, *CHEK2*, and *ATM*, among others.[4] It is important to consult with a genetics professional to discuss which patients should be referred for genetic counseling based on tumor NGS results.

Urology practice has long entailed tumor or tissue-based analyses among men with PCA or those undergoing repeat biopsies to inform management (see **Table 2**). These tests evaluate messenger RNA expression or epigenetic profiles to determine risk of PCA recurrence or relapse to inform postprostatectomy treatment with radiation or need for repeat biopsies.[3] These tests do not provide information on hereditary cancer risk or chance of carrying a germline mutation among men with PCA or at risk for PCA.

IMPLEMENTATION OF GERMLINE TESTING FOR PATIENTS WITH PROSTATE CANCER

At the present time, many thousands of men with PCA on active treatment, PCA survivors, or men at risk for PCA will meet criteria for germline testing.[3,4] As such, urologists and oncologists need to consider strategies to address the germline testing needs of these patients. Central to this practice need is for providers to have a deeper understanding of the genetic counseling and informed consent process to inform areas of genetic education needed and how best to address elements of counseling and testing in practice. Because the increasing patient population in need of germline testing is rapidly outweighing genetic counseling availability,[13] urologists and oncologists need to have working knowledge of the field of genetic counseling, appropriate pretest informed consent, genetic results interpretation, hereditary cancer recommendations, and cascade testing to make informed practice decisions for streamlined collaboration with genetic counseling.[1,6] Later discussion describes the classic process of pretest genetic counseling and posttest counseling. Genetic counseling specific to men with PCA or at risk for PCA is covered in the article by Hyatt and colleagues[21] in this issue and has also been addressed more in-depth by others.[1,21]

Pretest Genetic Counseling

Pretest genetic counseling is done before ordering genetic testing in order to facilitate informed decision making. This process includes the necessary elements of informed consent for genetic testing.[1] During pretest genetic counseling, a genetic counselor will evaluate a patient's goals for testing (such as treatment decision making or risk assessment) to create a mutually agreed on plan for the session, obtain a personal medical and surgical history as well as a family history, educate about genetics and inheritance, identify the best relative to pursue genetic testing in the family (particularly for risk assessment), discuss appropriate genetic testing options and the possible types of genetic test results, and address privacy and psychosocial issues.[1,21,22] The genetic counselor will also discuss insurance coverage, cost of genetic testing, and genetic discrimination laws with the patient. Obtaining a thorough medical and family history is essential for pretest genetic counseling, as this helps to determine whether an individual meets criteria for genetic testing and to establish a differential diagnosis, allowing for discussion of appropriate genetic testing options.[1,21–23] In terms of medical history, a focus is placed on cancer diagnoses and treatments as well as cancer screening history or risk-reduction measures. Reported information surrounding medical, surgical, and family history is confirmed with pathology reports and medical records whenever possible to ensure accuracy. A large portion of the pretest genetic counseling session involves obtaining a comprehensive family history. Using standard pedigree nomenclature, a 3-generation medical pedigree is drawn to create a visual representation of the family history.[22,24] Information obtained about relatives includes cancer diagnoses, including age at diagnosis as well as relevant cancer screenings, risk-reducing surgeries, and genetic testing results. For hereditary PCA referrals, it is important to ask targeted family history questions, such as family history of metastatic PCA or whether any relatives died of PCA.[1,3,4,21,22] It is also important to inquire about ethnicity, particularly Ashkenazi Jewish ancestry, as these patients have higher rates of *BRCA* mutations.[3,4] With this information, the genetic counselor can discuss appropriate genetic testing and medical management options. In addition, information for family members about genetic counseling, genetic testing, and cancer screenings will be discussed.[25,26] There are known limitations of family history information. Many patients have limited family history information, such as for patients who are adopted, estranged from their relatives, or have a small family structure. Cancer diagnoses may not be openly discussed in families and therefore may not be known to patients; this may mask a hereditary cancer syndrome in a family history. Therefore, this needs to be taken into consideration when analyzing a pedigree.[27] Additional considerations in family history interpretation include variable expressivity of cancers or reduced cancer penetrance.[25]

Suspicion for hereditary cancer syndrome arises when there are multiple relatives with similar or related cancers, cancer diagnoses at young ages, and individuals who have bilateral or multiple primary cancers.[27] Criteria for PCA germline testing are described above and are shown in **Table 1**.

The purpose, benefits, and limitations of genetic testing are thoroughly reviewed during pretest genetic counseling. This pretest genetic counseling includes discussion of implications of the different type of genetic test results, positive, negative, and variant of uncertain significance (VUS). The genetic counselor also helps identify the best relative in the family to pursue genetic testing. It is most informative to initiate genetic testing in a family member who has had a cancer diagnosis.[25] Individuals without a personal cancer history can pursue genetic testing, but results are often considered inconclusive unless there is a known pathogenic mutation in the family.[25] Genetic testing options are also discussed, such as a PCA-focused panel, more expanded cancer panel as well as the availability of genes with emerging evidence for PCA.

The Genetic Information Non-Discrimination Act (GINA) is an important law to discuss, as many patients have concerns about their genetic test results being used against them. This law, enacted in 2008, provides some protections surrounding genetic discrimination in the areas of health insurance and employment.[25,28] Specifically, health insurance companies cannot use genetic information to determine eligibility or premiums. Employers cannot make decisions about hiring, firing, pay, or promotions based on genetic test results. GINA does not apply to health insurance through the US military, Veterans Administration, Indian Health Service, or Federal Employees Health Benefits plan, or employers with less than 15 employees. Additional limitations to GINA are that it does not protect life, disability, and long-term care insurance companies from discriminating on the basis of genetic information. Some states have laws that build on the protections in GINA.[28]

Posttest Genetic Counseling

Posttest genetic counseling consists of the genetic counselor reviewing the genetic testing results in detail with the patient. Cancer risks and medical management guidelines, when available, are discussed. Appropriate high-risk referrals are also facilitated to further discuss high-risk cancer screenings.[1,29]

Genetic results are classified into 5 major categories as established by the American College of Medical Genetics and Genomics.[30] The 5 categories of variant classification are pathogenic, likely pathogenic, uncertain significance, likely benign, and benign.[30] These classifications are grouped into 3 main result types for clinical disclosure: positive, negative, and VUS.

A positive test result means that a pathogenic or likely pathogenic variant was identified in one of the genes on the genetic testing panel. If a germline mutation is identified, appropriate high-risk cancer screening and risk-reduction options are recommended for the patient and implications for current cancer treatment, such as eligibility for PARP inhibitors.[1,6,13,14,27] Identifying a germline mutation can also uncover additional cancer risks, beyond PCA risk, and risks for other medical conditions. Implications for at-risk relatives are also discussed. Cascade testing of family members can then be pursued in order for relatives to be informed of their cancer risks and to implement appropriate medical management interventions as necessary.[27] Genetic counselors may provide a family letter to help patients convey this information to their at-risk relatives.

A negative test result means that no clinically significant variants or VUS was identified in any of the genes on the genetic testing panel. Most often this is considered an "inconclusive" result because other genetic regions or genes account for cancer risk or development, which were not tested. Cancer screening and medical management are based on personal and family history. If there is a known pathogenic variant in a family and a relative does not carry this mutation, that individual is considered to be a true negative. Patients with negative results may have cancer risks that are closer to the general population risk.[25]

A VUS means that a genetic variation was identified, but it is currently unknown whether this variant is related to increased cancer risk. Medical management and cancer screening recommendations are typically based on personal and family history. VUS results can be particularly difficult for patients to have an accurate understanding of, highlighting the importance of thorough posttest genetic counseling.[31] Over time, a VUS result may be reclassified as pathogenic, likely pathogenic, benign, or likely benign, as the genetic testing laboratory obtains additional evidence about the specific variant. These reclassifications are typically reported by the genetic testing laboratory to the genetic counselor or ordering provider. It is therefore important for ordering providers to understand the genetic testing laboratory's variant reclassification process and for the patient to keep in contact with their ordering provider.[25] Reclassification of VUS to pathogenic/likely pathogenic can also occur in rare instances.[32] It is also important that providers understand the limitations to genetic testing, including technological limitations to identify mutations, laboratory testing techniques (full sequencing with deletion/duplication testing vs targeted testing), variant reclassification programs, and family studies for assisting in classifying variants.[25]

In general, it has also been shown that pretest and posttest genetic counseling reduces negative outcomes, such as psychosocial effects, misunderstanding of genetic test results, inappropriate medical management, and unnecessary genetic testing,[26,31,33] although further research in male populations is needed.

GERMLINE TESTING EDUCATIONAL APPROACHES

Given the complexity of germline testing, urologists and oncologists need to consider how best to enhance education regarding germline testing principles and practice. The Philadelphia Prostate Cancer Consensus Conference 2019 endorsed specific priority topics for provider education with a high level of agreement.[1] These topics included genetic counseling principles, understanding types of results (mutation, VUS, negative), GINA law and other laws that address discrimination, hereditary cancer syndromes and additional cancer risks that may be uncovered, genetic testing panel options along with pros and limitations, understanding of insurance and out-of-pocket costs for genetic testing, genetic data privacy consideration, and cascade testing.[1]

Recent publications have described in detail how practices may consider implementing germline testing for PCA.[1,21] Overall, these strategies include (1) identification of a local or remote genetic counseling service to address the needs of referrals; (2) defining if all men with PCA meeting testing criteria will be referred to genetic counseling or a subset based on specific criteria (those with mutations, those with complex family history, those with psychosocial issues, those who prefer to see a genetic counselor); (3) determining if the practice and providers have adequate working knowledge to perform pretest informed consent for germline testing and insights into genetic testing ordering options at quality laboratories; (4) development of workflows for comprehensive family history collection whether in the provider practice or in the genetics practice to deliver full recommendations at disclosure; (5) considering if telegenetics services suit the patient and practice needs; (6) considering tools to help with identifying men who meet germline testing criteria; (7) determining if there is a working knowledge base of NCCN cancer risk, screening, and management guidelines across cancer types and hereditary syndromes; (8) developing pathways to address the needs of men and their families.[1,21]

To successfully and responsibly implement germline testing in practice, working knowledge of the principles of germline testing, genetic counseling, NCCN guidelines for testing and management, and management of hereditary cancer syndromes is needed. Multiple professional societies have educational resources for providers on these topics to facilitate responsible implementation of germline testing in practice (**Table 3**). Overall, these resources cover most of the pretest informed elements endorsed by the 2019 Philadelphia Prostate Cancer Consensus Conference, including purpose of germline testing, knowledge and identification of hereditary cancer syndromes, appropriate family history collection, multigene panel testing options and considerations, types of genetic results and implications for management, range of cancer risks that may be identified by genetic mutations, GINA law, potential cost of testing and possible insurance challenges, cascade testing for mutation carriers or further familial genetic testing based on family history, and data sharing and data privacy.[1] Some of these resources are cost-free, whereas others are for members of these professional societies with or without a fee. A certification in cancer genetic risk assessment is available through City of Hope Comprehensive Cancer Center, which is an approximate year-long remote-learning course with engagement needed throughout and with a cost associated for the course (see **Table 3**). However, this course offers complete learning regarding all elements of germline testing across cancer types, including PCA. Multiple additional tools and opportunities to gain knowledge regarding germline testing for PCA will become available in the future. For example, Thomas Jefferson University is developing a Web-based tool (Helix) for providers to rapidly identify men with PCA who meet genetic testing criteria to refer for genetic counseling and genetic testing. The tool also includes brief educational modules regarding basic elements of genetic counseling and genetic testing.

DISCUSSION

Urologists and oncologists are now having to consider how to gain knowledge of PCA germline testing and develop practice strategies to responsibly implement germline testing for their patients because germline testing is a new standard of care for PCA.[3,4] Given this fact, some of the challenges that arise include remaining up-to-date on NCCN guidelines, developing a knowledge base

Table 3
Germline testing educational resources relevant to urology and oncology

Organization	Description of Resources	Contact Links
City of Hope Comprehensive Cancer Center	Intensive course in genomic cancer risk assessment: approximately 1-y remote learning course with certification delivered after completion; fee required. Reviews fundamentals of hereditary cancer risk, genetic counseling, genetic testing, cancer risk management, and emerging precision therapies	https://www.ccgcop.org/home
American Society of Clinical Oncology eLearning	Cancer genetics: 10-module toolkit reviews the genetic basis of cancer and the role of genetics and genomics in precision oncology; reviews hereditary cancer genetics, risk assessment, diagnosis, and treatment of several hereditary cancers and syndromes; covers genetic and genomic testing technologies, interpretation of genetics and genomics test results, genetics and genomics counseling, and informed consent for genetic testing. Includes hereditary prostate cancer module	https://elearning.asco.org/coursecollection/genetics-and-genomics
National Cancer Institute (PDQ) Summaries	Cancer genetics: provides detailed summaries of hereditary cancer syndromes, cancer genetic testing covering multiple cancer types, and genetic basis of cancer risk and treatment with synthesis of new research. Entire section devoted to genetics of prostate cancer	https://www.cancer.gov/publications/pdq/information-summaries/genetics https://www.cancer.gov/tvpes/prostate/hp/prostate-genetics-pdq

(continued on next page)

Table 3
(continued)

Organization	Description of Resources	Contact Links
National Comprehensive Cancer Network	Prostate cancer germline testing guidelines: includes germline testing criteria for prostate cancer and several other cancers. Also includes impact of genetic test results and family history on cancer screening, treatment, and risk reduction. NCCN guidelines that include germline testing for prostate cancer are • Genetic/familial high-risk assessment: breast, ovarian, and pancreatic (version 2.2021) • Prostate cancer (version 2.2021) • Prostate cancer early detection (2.2020)	https://www.nccn.orx/
American Urologic Association: AUA University	Evolving role of the urologist in metastatic and castration-resistant prostate cancer: a guidelines and case-based discussion—2020: describes the emerging role of prostate cancer germline testing, genes of top priority, and role in treatment, management, and screening	https://auau.auanet.org/
Harvard HMX Fundamentals: genetics	3-mo online class. Requires 3–6 h of course work per week. Includes basic concepts in genetics as well as cancer genetics and precision medicine	https://onlinelearning.hms. harvard.edu/hmx/courses/ hmx- genetics/
2019 Philadelphia Prostate Cancer Consensus: implementation of genetic testing for inherited prostate cancer	Multidisciplinary consensus statement reviewing and proposing models for implementing germline testing for prostate cancer. Reviews basic elements of genetic counseling and genetic testing. Provides a model for addressing these elements in practice. Additional articles and media presentation links provided	https://ascopubs.org/doi/full/ 10.1200/jc0.20.00046 https://grandroundsinurology. com/implementation-of-germ line-testing-for-prostate-cancer-philadelphia-prostate-cancer-consensus-conference-2019/ https://www.medpagetoday. com/reading-room/asco/ non-prostate-genitourinary-cancer/89231
National Society of Genetic Counselors	Cancer predisposition evaluation practice resource	https://www.nsgc.org/
	Webinars and online education courses for various areas of genetic counseling, including hereditary cancer	
	Locate local genetic counseling services	

(continued on next page)

Table 3
(*continued*)

Organization	Description of Resources	Contact Links
American College of Medical Genetics and Genomics	A practice guideline from the American College of Medical Genetics and Genomics and the National Society of Genetic Counselors: referral indications for cancer predisposition	https://www.acmg.net/ACMG/Medical-Genetics-Practice-Resources/Practice-Guidelines.aspx
GeneReviews	A point-of-care resource for health care providers for inherited conditions	https://www.ncbi.nlm.nih.gov/books/NBK1116/
UpToDate	Provides summaries of genetic risk and management of prostate cancer based on genetic factors	https://www.uptodate.com/contents/genetic-risk-factors-for-prostate-cancer

of hereditary cancer syndromes and NCCN guidelines regarding germline testing and management, and building collaborative models with genetic counseling to address the variety of needs of men with PCA, men at risk for PCA, and their families. Key gaps that currently exist include lack of genetic data and clinical challenges of germline testing for African American men, reimbursement for telehealth and telephone counseling, which is needed now increasingly in the pandemic and postpandemic era, virtual genetics boards to engage with experts regarding the complexities of germline testing from case-based discussion, streamlined insurance coverage, increased advocacy and public awareness of germline testing for PCA, and need to engage primary care providers in this process.[1] Further research and practice models are needed to address these gaps.

SUMMARY

Germline testing for PCA is central to PCA care, and urologists and oncologists now need to include dedicated learning of germline testing principles and practice to maintain a high level of care for their patients. Proactive collaboration of urology and oncology with genetic counseling is a top priority in practice to address patient and family needs. Core curricula for urology, oncology, and genetic counseling students and trainees need to include principles and practice of germline testing for PCA to make ongoing advances in this era of precision medicine.

CLINICS CARE POINTS

- Germline testing for prostate cancer is now a new standard of care, requiring that urologists and oncologists develop dedicated educational and practice strategies of the principles and practice of this field.

- Key elements to gain working knowledge of germline testing include understanding National Comprehensive Cancer Network germline testing guidelines, appropriate pretest informed consent, impact on precision treatment, management, and screening, hereditary cancer implications, germline testing results and impact on care, and implications for families.

- Urologists and oncologists need to proactively develop collaborative approaches for their patients with prostate cancer or at risk for prostate cancer to address the various clinical and psychosocial needs of men and their families regarding prostate cancer germline testing.

DISCLOSURE

The authors have no relevant disclosures to this article.

REFERENCES

1. Giri VN, Knudsen KE, Kelly WK, et al. Implementation of germline testing for prostate cancer: Philadelphia

prostate cancer consensus conference 2019. J Clin Oncol 2020. https://doi.org/10.1200/JCO.20.00046.

2. Cheng HH, Sokolova AO, Schaeffer EM, et al. Germline and somatic mutations in prostate cancer for the clinician. J Natl Compr Canc Netw 2019;17(5):515–21.

3. National Comprehensive Cancer Network Clinical Guidelines in Oncology (NCCN Guidelines): prostate cancer (version 2.2021). Available at: NCCN.org. Accessed August 4, 2020.

4. National Comprehensive Cancer Network Clinical Guidelines in Oncology (NCCN Guideline): Genetic/Familial High-Risk Assessment: Breast, Ovarian, and Pancreatic (version 2.2021). Available at: NCCN.org. Accessed August 4, 2020.

5. Abacan M, Alsubaie L, Barlow-Stewart K, et al. The global state of the genetic counseling profession. Eur J Hum Genet 2019;27:183–97.

6. Giri VN, Hyatt C, Gomella LG. Germline testing for men with prostate cancer: navigating an expanding new world of genetic evaluation for precision therapy and precision management. J Clin Oncol 2019.

7. National Comprehensive Cancer Network Clinical Guidelines in Oncology (NCCN Guidelines): prostate cancer early detection (version 2.2020). Available at: NCCN.org. Accessed August 29, 2020.

8. Page EC, Bancroft EK, Brook MN, et al. Interim results from the IMPACT study: evidence for prostate-specific antigen screening in BRCA2 mutation carriers. Eur Urol 2019;76(6):831–42.

9. Carter HB, Helfand B, Mamawala M, et al. Germline mutations in ATM and BRCA1/2 are associated with grade reclassification in men on active surveillance for prostate cancer. Eur Urol 2019;75(5):743–9.

10. Genetics of prostate cancer (PDQ®)–health professional version. National Cancer Institute. Available at: www.cancer.gov. Accessed August 29, 2020.

11. Loeb S, Byrne N, Walter D, et al. Knowledge and practice regarding prostate cancer germline testing among urologists: gaps to address for optimal implementation. Cancer Treat Res Commun 2020. https://doi.org/10.1016/j.ctarc.2020.100212.

12. Concepcion RS. Germline testing for prostate cancer: community urology perspective. Can J Urol 2019;26:50–1.

13. Abida W, Patnaik A, Campbell D, et al. Rucaparib in men with metastatic castration-resistant prostate cancer harboring a BRCA1 or BRCA2 gene alteration [published online ahead of print, 2020 Aug 14]. J Clin Oncol 2020;JCO2001035.

14. de Bono J, Mateo J, Fizazi K, et al. Olaparib for metastatic castration-resistant prostate cancer. N Engl J Med 2020;382:2091–102.

15. Le DT, Durham JN, Smith KN, et al. Mismatch repair deficiency predicts response of solid tumors to PD-1 blockade. Science 2017;357(6349):409–13.

16. Pritchard CC, Mateo J, Walsh MF, et al. Inherited DNA-repair gene mutations in men with metastatic prostate cancer. N Engl J Med 2016;375(5):443–53.

17. Nicolosi P, Ledet E, Yang S, et al. Prevalence of germline variants in prostate cancer and implications for current genetic testing guidelines. JAMA Oncol 2019;5(4):523–8.

18. Paller CJ, Antonarakis ES, Beer TM, et al. Germline genetic testing in advanced prostate cancer; practices and barriers: survey results from the germline genetics working group of the prostate cancer clinical trials consortium. Clin Genitourin Cancer 2019;17(4):275–82.e1.

19. Berger MF, Mardis ER. The emerging clinical relevance of genomics in cancer medicine. Nat Rev Clin Oncol 2018;15(6):353–65.

20. Mandelker D, Zhang L. The emerging significance of secondary germline testing in cancer genomics. J Pathol 2018;244(5):610–5.

21. Szymaniak BM, Facchini LA, Giri VN, et al. Practical considerations and challenges for germline genetic testing in patients with prostate cancer: recommendations from the Germline Genetics Working Group of the PCCTC. JCO Oncol Pract 2020;OP2000431.

22. Hyatt C, Russo J, McDougall C. Genetic counseling perspective of engagement with urology and primary care. Can J Urol 2019;26(5 Suppl 2):52–3.

23. Hampel H, Grubs RE, Walton CS, et al. Genetic counseling practice analysis. J Genet Couns 2009;18:205–16.

24. Bennett RL, Steinhaus French K, Resta RG, et al. Standardized human pedigree nomenclature: update and assessment of the recommendations of the National Society of Genetic Counselors. J Genet Couns 2008;17:424–33.

25. Uhlmann WR, Schuette JL, Yashar B. A guide to genetic counseling. 2nd edition. Hoboken, NJ: Wiley-Blackwell; 2009.

26. Hampel H, Bennett RL, Buchanan A, et al. A practice guideline from the American College of Medical Genetics and Genomics and the National Society of Genetic Counselors: referral indications for cancer predisposition assessment. Genet Med 2015;17(1):70–87.

27. Riley BD, Culver JO, Skrzynia C, et al. Essential elements of genetic cancer risk assessment, counseling, and testing: updated recommendations of the National Society of Genetic Counselors. J Genet Couns 2012;21:151–61.

28. Genetic information Nondiscrimination Act of 2008: Pub.L. 110-233, 122 Stat. 881.

29. Giri VN, Obeid E, Gross L, et al. Inherited mutations in males undergoing multigene panel testing for PCA – emerging implications for personalized prostate cancer genetic evaluation. J Clin Oncol Precision Oncol 2017. https://doi.org/10.1200/PO.16.00039.

30. Richards S, Aziz N, Bale S, et al. Standards and guidelines for the interpretation of sequence variants: a joint consensus recommendation of the American College of Medical Genetics and Genomics and the Association for Molecular Pathology. Genet Med 2015;17(5):405–24. https://doi.org/10.1038/gim.2015.30.

31. Giri VN, Obeid E, Hegarty SE, et al. Understanding of multigene test results among males undergoing germline testing for inherited prostate cancer: implications for genetic counseling. Prostate 2018; 78:879–88.

32. Mersch J, Brown AN, Pirzadeh-Miller S, et al. Prevalence of variant reclassification following hereditary cancer genetic testing. JAMA 2018;320(12): 1266–74.

33. Bensend TA, Veach PM, Niendorf KB. What's the harm? Genetic counselor perceptions of adverse effects of genetics service provision by non-genetics professionals. J Genet Couns 2014; 23(1):48–63.

Genetic Counseling for Men with Prostate Cancer

Colette Hyatt, MS, CGC[a],*, Carey McDougall, MS, LCGC[b],
Susan Miller-Samuel, MSN, RN, AGN-BC[b], Jessica Russo, MS, LCGC[b]

KEYWORDS

- Genetic counseling • Prostate cancer • Genetic testing • Genetic counselor
- Hereditary prostate cancer

KEY POINTS

- Genetic testing is an important aspect of patient care in urology clinics for men with prostate cancer and/or patients with a family history of prostate cancer.
- Genetic counseling is an important component of genetic testing for prostate cancer.
- It is important to provide informed consent before genetic testing to allow the patient to make an autonomous decision regarding genetics testing.
- To help ensure informed consent before undergoing genetic testing for inherited risk of prostate cancer, it is important for the patients and/or their families to have genetic counseling.

INTRODUCTION TO GENETIC COUNSELING

As somatic and germline genetic testing continues to play an increasing role in oncology precision medicine, the need for genetic counseling by informed providers increases.[1] Germline genetic testing has become particularly important for patients with prostate cancer because of the possible therapeutic implications and high rate of detectable germline mutations. Germline mutation positivity may affect men's future cancer risk and treatment decisions, and may also have implications for their family members. This article reviews genetic counseling and how it relates to genetic testing in hereditary prostate cancer.

Overview of Genetic Counseling

In order to understand genetic counseling, it is important to have some historical perspective. As genetics knowledge made its way from the bench to clinical practice, genetic counseling emerged to meet a need for patient education and psychological support in what was the brave new world of twentieth century genetics. It was

in 1947 that the geneticist Dr Sheldon Clark Reed was the first to use the term genetic counseling.[2] In 1947, Dr Reed was chosen to be the Director of the Dight Institute for Human Genetics at the University of Minnesota. This appointment was during a time when medical geneticists were attempting to separate themselves from the eugenics movement. During his time at the Dight Institute, he learned about not only the medical implications of genetics but also the psychological aspects. He was the first to suggest the term genetic counseling to describe the process of providing medical information and psychological support to patients.[2] In the 1970s, genetic counseling emerged as a bona fide profession to help meet the needs of people considering genetic testing so they could obtain the correct information necessary to understand what genetic testing was and how it could affect them and their families, and to understand and manage psychologically their genetic test results.

Although genetic counseling initially existed in the reproductive and pediatric specialties, it has greatly expanded over time to meet the

[a] Familial Cancer Program, The University of Vermont Medical Center, Main Campus, East Pavilion, Level 2, 111 Colchester Avenue, Burlington, VT 05401, USA; [b] Sidney Kimmel Cancer Center, Clinical Cancer Genetics, 1100 Walnut Street, Suite 602, Philadelphia, PA 19107, USA
* Corresponding author.
E-mail address: Colette.Hyatt@uvmhealth.org

Urol Clin N Am 48 (2021) 323–337
https://doi.org/10.1016/j.ucl.2021.03.004

needs of new medical advances and the patients that opt to use them. Specifically, there has been an expansion in the role of genetic counseling in adult-onset diseases and specifically in oncology. For genetic counselors, this means an evolving role in patient care, including providing information related to risk assessment for complex disorders, chemoprevention, targeted drug therapy, cancer screenings, and prophylactic surgery.[3]

Definition of genetic counseling

The National Society of Genetic Counseling (NSGC) definition of genetic counseling states that "genetic counseling is the process of helping people understand and adapt to the medical, psychological, and familial implications of the genetic contributions to disease."[4] This process integrates:

1. Interpretation of family and medical histories to assess the chance of disease occurrence or recurrence.
2. Education about inheritance, testing, management, prevention, resources, and research.
3. Counseling to promote informed choices and adaptation to the risk or condition.

Most genetic counseling services are now provided by a board-certified genetic counselor that has completed, at minimum, a master's-level education program related to genetics and/or genetic counseling. Other qualified genetic counseling professionals include physicians and PhDs with advanced training in genetic counseling, and master's-prepared advanced practice nurses with advanced training and board certification in genetics.[3]

Along with collecting thorough personal and family history, a genetic counseling professional provides accurate, current information including the risks, benefits, and limitations of genetic testing, so that individuals can make informed decisions about whether to proceed with genetic testing. Also in the realm of the genetics professional is to help individuals to psychologically and operationally managing their genetic test results, whether positive or negative. Genetic counselors facilitate referrals to clinicians that specialize in certain high-risk aspects of individualized patient care. Thorough written summaries including current medical management and risk-reduction options for the patients and their family members are provided to the patients and their participating clinicians by the genetic counselor.

When positive genetic test results occur, the genetics counselor can facilitate cascade genetic testing in the family, or help the family find a qualified genetics provider in their geographic area.

At its core, genetic counseling strives to facilitate a trusting, collaborative relationship between counselor and patient that affords the patients unconditional positive regard and the control to make their own choices about genetic testing.[3] After participating in a genetic counseling session, some patients opt to go forward with testing, and others return later after they have had some time to digest what was discussed during counseling. Some need to first get their insurance situation settled. Others may opt to never proceed with genetic testing. The key element lies with the informed decision making and understanding of the patient. Patients should be in control of their own decisions, and confidently have been provided the correct understandable information, and nonjudgmental psychological support to reach those decisions.[3]

CANCER GENETIC COUNSELING SESSION

Traditionally, a genetic counseling session involves a pretest counseling session and then a posttest counseling session, if genetic testing was ordered. The components of pretest and posttest genetic counseling are outlined next.

Pretest genetic counseling

Pretest genetic counseling is done as a part of the cancer risk assessment before ordering genetic testing in order to facilitate informed decision making (see **Table 2**). This process should include evaluating the patient's needs; obtaining a comprehensive family, medical, and surgical history; creating a differential diagnosis; identifying the best relative to pursue genetic testing; educating about the basics of genetics and inheritance; discussing which genetic testing would be best and the possible types of genetic test results; and addressing privacy and psychosocial issues.[5,6] The genetic counselor also discusses insurance coverage and cost of genetic testing with the patient during this process. Pretest counseling has been shown to reduce negative outcomes such as psychosocial effects, misunderstanding of genetic test results, inappropriate medical management, and unnecessary genetic testing.[7,8]

At the beginning of a genetic counseling session, the genetic counselor sets an outline for the session together with the patient. Through contracting, the genetic counselor elicits the patient's goals for the session, often beginning by asking why the patient has come for genetic counseling.[3] This approach helps to establish rapport, identify specific questions and psychosocial concerns, and elicit the patient's expectations, thereby allowing the genetic counselor to tailor the session to meet the patient's goals.[3,9] Through this process, the genetic counselor and patient establish an agreed-on plan for the session.[3]

Once contracting is completed, a medical and family history are obtained, followed by a discussion of the necessary elements for optimal informed consent.[6,9] An essential part of pretest genetic counseling is discussing the purpose, benefits, and limitations of genetic testing. This process includes discussion of what it would mean to find a germline mutation with regard to implications for the patient and the patient's family. The genetic counselor also helps identify the best relative in the family to pursue genetic testing, because testing is most informative when pursued by a relative who has had a cancer diagnosis. Unaffected individuals can undergo genetic counseling but, in the absence of a known familial mutation, the results are often considered inconclusive. If applicable, testing options, such as a prostate cancer–focused panel compared with a more expanded cancer panel, are also discussed as well as the different types of test results that are possible, including positive, negative, and variant of uncertain significance (VUS).

It is common for individuals to overestimate their personal cancer risks. This possibility has been shown in many cancer genetics studies across various cancer types, including prostate cancer.[3,10,11] Effective genetic counseling does not cause increased risk perception and can result in a decrease in perceived cancer risk.[10,12] Perceived cancer risk has been shown to correlate with whether patients follow through on cancer screening and risk-reduction recommendations as well as psychosocial concerns.[13,14] Therefore, genetic counselors should address any discrepancy between a patient's perceived cancer risk and the actual cancer risk.

Importance of family history and pedigree

Obtaining a thorough family history is an integral part of the cancer genetic counseling session. This history allows genetic counselors to establish a differential diagnosis, perform a risk assessment, and make recommendations for genetic testing and medical management as well as to provide information for family members about genetic counseling, genetic testing, and cancer screening recommendations.[3,7] A comprehensive family history is obtained by creating a 3-generation medical pedigree, which is a visual representation of a patient's family history using standard pedigree

nomenclature.[5,15] The genetic counselor asks questions about all first-degree, second-degree, and third-degree relatives regarding cancer diagnoses, including age at diagnosis as well as relevant cancer screening, risk-reducing surgeries, and genetic testing results. In the evaluation of men for inherited prostate cancer risk, it is important to ask targeted family history questions in terms of prostate cancer history, including whether any relatives had metastatic prostate cancer or died of prostate cancer.[6] In addition, it is important to obtain information regarding ethnicity, particularly Ashkenazi Jewish ancestry, and consanguinity. This information is typically obtained during the pretest genetic counseling session before the risk assessment and counseling.[3] Through this process, a genetic counselor may learn about a patient's family and social relationships, which can assist in addressing a patient's psychosocial needs.[3]

The process of obtaining a detailed family history can present several challenges. It can take a significant amount of time to complete a thorough family history with a patient, which can be a limiting factor in many primary care and specialists' offices. Genetic counselors typically spend 60 to 90 minutes on each new patient appointment, allowing for adequate time to take a detailed family history.[5] Limited family history information, such as for patients who are adopted, estranged from their relatives, or have a small family structure, can also present a challenge in cancer genetic counseling. These factors may cause it to seem that there is a low risk for a hereditary cancer syndrome in a family and therefore need to be taken into consideration when analyzing a pedigree.[16] It is common for there to be inaccuracies in the information provided to the genetic counselor by the patient. Therefore, when possible, it is important for family history information to be confirmed with medical records.

The family history is an important tool to determine whether an individual meets criteria for genetic testing, establish a differential diagnosis, and discuss appropriate genetic testing options. Taken together, this information also assists genetic counselors in making referrals to appropriate specialists to further discuss high-risk cancer screenings. Factors that may indicate a hereditary cancer syndrome include many relatives with similar or related cancers, early-onset cancers, individuals with multiple primary or bilateral cancers, and the diagnosis of a rare cancer type.[16] Family history criteria for germline prostate cancer genetic testing include men with 1 first-degree relative or 2 or more male relatives diagnosed with prostate cancer before 60 years of age, who died of prostate cancer, or who had metastatic prostate cancer, as well as a family history of cancers associated with hereditary breast and ovarian cancer syndrome (HBOCS) or Lynch syndrome.[6] Additional considerations in family history interpretation include variable expressivity, reduced penetrance, and an extensive negative family history.

Posttest genetic counseling

In a posttest genetic counseling appointment, a genetic counselor thoroughly reviews genetic testing results with the patient and discusses cancer risk and associated management guidelines in the context of the patient's personal and family history.[3] At this time, referral to high-risk providers may also be discussed. In order to optimize management options for evaluation and medical care, results should be communicated in a timely manner.

Results of genetic testing do not always provide a clear answer. Most genetic variants are classified using the standards and guidelines established by the American College of Medical Genetics; however, available technology and methodology vary between laboratories.[17] Variants are classified using the following 5 tiers: benign, likely benign, VUS, likely pathogenic, and pathogenic.[18] When these findings are discussed with a patient, they are conveyed as either negative, positive, or uncertain results.

A negative result means that neither a clinically significant variant nor a VUS was detected in the genes that were analyzed.[3] For patients with a known highly penetrant mutation in the family, this can mean that the patient's risk of developing associated cancers is decreased and closer to the risk seen in the general population. These individuals are known as true negatives because they do not carry the pathogenic variant causing the cancer risks in their families. However, most do not have a known familial pathogenic mutation that explains their personal and/or family histories. For these individuals, a thorough risk assessment in the context of a negative test result is discussed. Screening and medical management guidelines discussion should be based on personal and family history. For all patients, it is imperative to discuss the limitations of genetic testing. These limitations can include technological limitations of the laboratory, limitations in genetic knowledge and technology, and not testing the best candidate in the family.

A positive genetic testing result means that a pathogenic or likely pathogenic variant was detected in one of the genes tested. A positive result can be emotional for the patient.[3] It is important to thoroughly discuss associated cancer risks and next steps in a way that the patient understands. Sometimes this can take multiple appointments to ensure that the patient has had time to think through the initial information and is comfortable discussing the next steps. Next steps will depend on what gene the pathogenic or likely pathogenic variant was detected in, and they may include high-risk screening for prostate and other cancer risks depending on the specific gene mutation and notifying family members of their risk. In some cases, this involves surgery for the patient or family members for risk reduction. To identify other family members that may be at risk, testing for an identified pathogenic variant must then extend to relatives in a process known as cascade testing. Cascade testing can identify at risk relatives as well as true-negatives, allowing appropriate family members to undergo high-risk screening.[1,5]

An uncertain result or VUS means that, at the time of interpretation, there was not sufficient evidence to determine whether the variant was positive or negative. Although VUSs are reported to patients in their genetic test results, they usually have no implications for management at the time of reporting.[3] VUSs are followed over time by genetic testing laboratories for evidence in support of pathogenicity and are reclassified as either pathogenic or benign. A 2018 study including more than 1 million genetic test results showed that, in a span of 10 years, 7.7% of VUS results detected in testing were reclassified, of which 91.2% were downgraded from a VUS to benign or likely benign. Although extremely rare, reclassification can also occur in variants previously thought to be pathogenic or benign.[19] Given the eventual reclassification of these variants, all patients that have had genetic testing should keep in contact with their genetics programs or other ordering providers to be aware of any reclassifications. It is also important for the ordering provider to know how the ordering laboratory treats VUSs. Some genetic testing laboratories regularly evaluate VUS results and make ordering providers aware of any future reclassifications, but not every laboratory has this policy in place.

Multigene testing has increased the complexity of the typical results discussion. In particular, understanding of VUS results on cancer risk can be difficult for patients. With multigene panel testing becoming the standard of care, rates of VUS results have increased.[17,20] A research study on 109 men with prostate cancer undergoing genetic testing showed a discordance of reported genetic testing results with actual reported results. This discordance was specifically true for those with a VUS.[21] This finding highlights the importance of an in-depth discussion of results regardless of the type of result obtained.

Past research has consistently reported no long-term adverse psychological outcomes for the most individuals undergoing testing and receiving results.[22] However, this understanding may not apply to family members being tested in cascade testing. A study of 297 families of Lynch syndrome probands measured genetic testing–related distress, depressive symptoms, and cancer worries in relation to the amount of time passed since the proband was tested and found to carry a mutation. The study found that cascade genetic testing significantly increased test-related stress and cancer worry as time increased between testing of the proband and other family members. This finding was specifically true for individuals in the same generation as the proband.[23]

BRIEF REVIEW OF HEREDITARY CANCER SYNDROMES WITH PROSTATE CANCER RISK WITH GENETIC COUNSELING IMPLICATIONS

There are multiple genes related to hereditary prostate cancer risk. Some risk levels are better understood than others as this area continues to advance. The following information is based on current knowledge and is likely to evolve over time (**Table 1**).

Hereditary breast and ovarian cancer syndrome

Perhaps best recognized for increased risk of female breast cancer and ovarian/fallopian tube cancers, the BRCA1 and BRCA2 germline mutations characteristic of hereditary breast and ovarian cancer syndrome (HBOCS) are also associated with an increased risk for prostate cancer, more so with BRCA2 positivity.[24–26] BRCA1 and BRCA2 are tumor suppressor genes associated with overall genomic stability.

Although the BRCA1-associated prostate cancer risk is less well quantified, men with BRCA2 germline positivity have an approximate 20% to 60% lifetime risk for developing prostate cancer.[27,28] These prostate cancers are often associated with more aggressive disease, including a Gleason score of greater than or equal to 7.[29]

Women with a pathogenic BRCA2 variant have approximately a 40% to 85% lifetime risk of breast cancer. The lifetime risk for ovarian, fallopian tube, or peritoneal cancer is 17% to 27%.[30–32] In addition, individuals affected with HBOCS have increased risks for melanoma, male breast cancer, and pancreatic cancer.[33] Appropriate high-risk referrals should be facilitated. Autosomal recessive biallelic pathogenic variants in the BRCA genes are associated with Fanconi anemia.[34–36]

BRCA2 mutations are associated with a particularly severe form of Fanconi anemia type D1 (FA-D1), which is characterized by bone marrow failure, short stature, abnormal skin pigmentation, developmental delay, and malformations of the thumbs and skeletal and central nervous systems. Risks of leukemia and early-onset solid tumors are significantly increased, with up to a 97% risk of malignancy by 5 years of age.[34]

It was previously thought that inherited biallelic germline positivity for BRCA1 was an embryonic lethal event. However, survival of inherited biallelic BRCA1 positivity is possible, and those incidents need to be recognized because these individuals may be destined for a different type of Fanconi anemia (Fanconi anemia, complementation group S [FANCS]).[35,36]

HOXB13-related Cancer Risks

The G84E variant in the HOXB13 gene is associated with increased risk of prostate cancer and also an earlier age of onset of prostate cancer.[37,38] Inheritance is autosomal dominant. Studies have shown the lifetime risk of prostate cancer to be up to 33%.[39]

Lynch syndrome (hereditary nonpolyposis colorectal cancer)

An increased risk for prostate cancer has been documented in multiple studies of men with Lynch syndrome. Estimates range from an approximately 2-fold to 5-fold increase in risk, or up to 30% depending on the affected Lynch syndrome gene.[6,40,41,42,43,44]

Lynch syndrome is a hereditary cancer syndrome that occurs when 1 or more of 5 mismatch repair (MMR) genes (MLH1, MSH2, MSH6, PMS2, EPCAM) has a germline mutation. An indication for this may be found when on immunohistochemistry (IHC) a pathologist finds that 1 or more of the mismatch repair genes is not expressed in a person's tumor.

Men and women with Lynch syndrome have a high risk of developing colorectal cancer, often at younger ages than are seen in the general population.[45] Women with Lynch syndrome also have a high risk for developing endometrial cancer and an increased risk for ovarian cancer.[45]

Patients with Lynch syndrome also have an increased risk of developing a wide variety of other Lynch syndrome–associated cancers, including prostate gastric, small bowel, urinary tract, hepatobiliary tract, brain (usually glioblastoma), sebaceous gland, and pancreatic.[45,46]

Table 1
Autosomal dominant and autosomal recessive characteristics of hereditary prostate cancer genes

Hereditary Prostate Cancer Genes	AD (Monoallelic) Mutation	Increased Cancer Risk and AD Inheritance	AR (Biallelic) Mutation	Risks Related to AR Inheritance
ATM	ATM-related disorders	Prostate, male and female breast, pancreatic	AT	• Ataxia, usually before age 5. Balance problems chorea, myoclonus, neuropathy[81] • Slurred speech and oculomotor apraxia • Telangiectasia, in the eyes and on the surface of the skin • Increased risk of cancer, particularly leukemia and lymphoma • Very sensitive to radiation exposure, including medical x-rays • Life expectancy varies greatly, but affected individuals typically live into early adulthood
BRCA1	HBOCS	Prostate, male and female breast, ovarian/fallopian tube, pancreatic, melanoma	Fanconi anemia (FANCS)	• Developmental delay apparent from infancy, short stature, microcephaly, and coarse dysmorphic features[82] • Laboratory studies show defective DNA repair and increased chromosomal breakage during stress • Some patients have radial ray anomalies, anemia, and increased risk of cancer; patients often have a family history of cancer in family members who have heterozygous mutations
BRCA2	HBOCS	Prostate, male and female breast, ovarian/fallopian tube, pancreatic, melanoma	Fanconi anemia (FA-D1)	• Risks of leukemia and early-onset solid tumors are increased with up to a 97% risk of malignancy by 5 y of age[83] • Short stature, abnormal skin pigmentation, skeletal malformations of the upper and lower limbs, microcephaly, and ophthalmic and genitourinary tract anomalies • Progressive bone marrow failure with pancytopenia typically presents in the first decade, often initially with thrombocytopenia or leukopenia

(continued on next page)

Hereditary Prostate Cancer Genes	AD (Monoallelic) Mutation	Increased Cancer Risk and AD Inheritance	AR (Biallelic) Mutation	Risks Related to AR Inheritance
Table 1 *(continued)*				
CHEK2	CHEK2-related disorders	Prostate, male and female breast, thyroid, CRC	—	—
HOXB13	Hereditary prostate cancer	Prostate	—	—
MLH1, MSH2, MSH6, PMS2, EPCAM	Lynch Syndrome	CRC, prostate, endometrial, ovarian, gastric, small bowel, urinary tract, hepatobiliary tract, brain, sebaceous gland, pancreatic	CMMR-D	• CMMR-D is a rare childhood cancer predisposition syndrome with hematologic malignances, brain/central nervous system tumors, colorectal tumors, and multiple intestinal polyps and other malignancies, including embryonic tumors and rhabdomyosarcoma[46,84] • Many patients show signs reminiscent of neurofibromatosis type I, particularly multiple café au lait macules

Abbreviations: AD, autosomal dominant; AR, autosomal recessive; AT, ataxia telangiectasia; CMMR-D, constitutional mismatch repair deficiency; CRC, colorectal cancer; FANCS, Fanconi anemia, complementation group S; HBOCS, Hereditary Breast and Ovarian Cancer Syndrome; LS, Lynch syndrome.

It is recommended that patients with a diagnosis of Lynch syndrome be managed by a multidisciplinary team with expertise in medical genetics and the care of patients with this condition. Appropriate high-risk clinician referrals should be facilitated. In rare instances, an individual may inherit mutations in both copies of a Lynch syndrome gene, leading to the autosomal recessive condition constitutional mismatch repair deficiency syndrome (CMMR-D).[47] Individuals with CMMR-D often have significant complications in childhood, including colorectal polyposis and a high risk for colorectal, small bowel, brain, and hematologic cancers.[47] The children of Lynch syndrome mutation carriers are at risk of inheriting CMMR-D if the other parent is also a carrier of a Lynch syndrome mutation.

ATM-ASSOCIATED CANCER RISKS

Women who are heterozygous ATM mutation carriers have an increased risk of breast cancer. Men have an increased risk of prostate cancer. Men and women have an increased risk of pancreatic cancer. For men with prostate cancer, ATM genetic mutations are associated with more aggressive prostate cancer.[48,49] Individuals who are homozygous for ATM genetic mutations have an autosomal recessive disorder known as ataxia telangiectasia (AT).[50] AT is a neurodegenerative disorder that causes extreme sensitivity to radiation, increased risk of cancer, early-onset ataxia, and immunodeficiency.[50]

GENES WITH EMERGING EVIDENCE FOR PROSTATE CANCER RISK (*CHEK2, NBN, BRIP1*)

There are genes that have early and emerging evidence for association with hereditary prostate cancer risk. These genes include *CHEK2*, *NBN*, and *BRIP1*.[51–54] *CHEK2* is a tumor suppressor gene that is associated with increased risk of breast and colon cancer. There are inconsistent data regarding heterozygous NBN genetic mutations and female breast cancer risk. People who are carriers for NBN genetic mutations have a risk of having a child with Nijmegen breakage syndrome. Genetic mutations in *BRIP1* are associated with increased risk of ovarian cancer. *BRIP1* is also associated with Fanconi anemia complementation group J (FANCJ).

REPRODUCTIVE DECISION MAKING AND GENETIC TESTING FOR INHERITED PROSTATE CANCER

An important part of the genetic counseling process for patients and their families is to understand reproductive implications for themselves and/or their families. As discussed earlier, some of the genes associated with inherited prostate cancer can also be inherited autosomal recessively and this has implications for discussion of reproductive risks for the patient and/or the families.[34-36,47,50] Parents concerned about the possibility of passing on a monoallelic or biallelic genetic mutations to a future child should discuss options for preconception genetic testing and assisted reproduction techniques, such as preimplantation genetic testing with a qualified provider. It is important to counsel patients about the possibility of an autosomal recessive condition in their offspring, and the importance of discussing this with their close family members that are of reproductive age. This discussion should be thoroughly documented in notes shared with the patient and in the patient's medical record.

PSYCHOSOCIAL CONCERNS FOR GENETIC COUNSELING IN MEN

Past literature regarding genetic testing communication and psychosocial implications associated with the cancer predispositions discussed earlier focused almost exclusively on women. This focus was likely attributable to more women receiving genetic testing given the higher level of cancer risk and more medical management options available for women.[55] Although women may be more likely to undergo genetic testing for such genes, research has shown that genetic testing uptake between men and women is similar. Distress following positive genetic testing results is also thought to be similar for men and women, indicating that individuals with a positive result generally show more distress than those that are negative, regardless of gender.[56]

However, prostate cancer genetic testing uniquely focuses on testing men, and many other psychosocial and counseling concerns may differ. From past studies that include both men and women disseminating information about BRCA risk, it seemed that women were often the "point person" in the family and men tended to restrict communication of test results to immediate family members such as spouses, children, and siblings. Specifically, it seemed that men were most concerned about their obligation to share information with their children and grandchildren, rather than other family members.[57] More recent studies show that communication of BRCA-related cancer risk in the family is not gendered and men may take a more active role as disseminators of familial genetic information as well as support providers, and even co-decision makers, than was previously thought. However, although men are taking over more communication roles in the family, many men are neglecting focusing on how they were managing their own risks in consideration of helping their children and close female relatives manage their risks. This finding may indicate a need to educate men about their own risk management in the context of a family-centered approach, especially given their interest in obtaining this information for other family members. These studies also highlighted a need for better education for providers regarding identification of at-risk men as well as a strong desire from patients to participate in support groups where they can connect with other men.[57,58]

CLINICAL IMPLICATIONS
Germline genetic testing

Germline genetic testing is important for men that have a personal and/or family history of prostate cancer.[1] There can be therapeutic implications for men with a personal history of prostate cancer that are found to carry mutations in certain genes. Also, information regarding genetic mutations can provide patients with information to share with family members regarding their cancer risks and the patient's future cancer risk. For men without a personal history of prostate cancer but with a family history of cancer, this information can help inform cancer screening and also provide guidance for other family members. Given the potential impact on therapeutic and cancer risk information, it is important that patients and their families receive the proper genetic counseling and the correct genetic test.

Precision medicine

Germline genetic testing is very important for treatment implications for men with prostate cancer, regardless of family history and age of diagnosis. Approximately 15% to 17% of men with prostate cancer have been shown to have germline mutations.[25,59] For men with metastatic prostate cancer, approximately 12% have a germline mutation.[60]

Metastatic prostate cancer

Germline genetic testing is important for treatment implications for men with metastatic prostate cancer. Research has shown benefits for platinum-based chemotherapy in those with metastatic CRPC and BRCA mutations. In addition, poly-(ADP-ribose) polymerase (PARP) inhibitors have shown responses for men with germline or somatic mutations in *BRCA1*, *BRCA2*, and *ATM*. There have been 2 approvals by the US Food and Drug Administration for use of PARP inhibitors rucaparib and olaparib in the treatment of prostate cancer.[61] Men with loss of DNA mismatch repair or who have Lynch syndrome can be candidates for immune checkpoint inhibitor immunotherapy.[62]

Potential role in active surveillance discussions

Active surveillance is the situation when favorable-risk prostate cancer is actively monitored but treatment is delayed with the understanding that if, based on results from active surveillance, the cancer progresses, treatment will be initiated. Advantages are that men will avoid or delay possible unnecessary side effects of therapy. A significant disadvantage in pursuing this would be missing the window of opportunity for potential cure. Genetic testing results have the potential to be helpful in these discussions when men are making decisions on active surveillance, such as men with *BRCA2* mutations, where prostate cancers can be more aggressive.[49,63] There are also early data with *ATM* mutation carriers.[49]

Implications for screening decisions

Men with *BRCA2* mutations tend to have earlier onset of prostate cancer and it tends to be more aggressive.[49,63] Men with *BRCA2* genetic mutations should consider starting prostate-specific antigen screening at age 40 years, or 10 years younger than the youngest prostate cancer diagnosis in the family.[6] This plan can also be considered with other gene mutations associated with inherited prostate cancer risk.[6]

Somatic testing

Somatic genetic testing is an important piece of care for prostate cancer.[64] Patients and providers need to understand the difference between somatic and germline genetic testing for understanding of meaning for current treatments, future cancer risk for the patient, and implications for family members. Germline genetic testing evaluates genetic mutations in DNA that a patient was born with, whereas tumor testing evaluates acquired mutations in the tumor.

Most mutations detected in tumor testing are of somatic origin (the mutation occurred within the formation of the tumor and was not inherited). However, germline mutations can also be uncovered in tumor testing; various studies have reported rates of 3% to 17.5% of patients with tumor testing having germline mutations depending on patient population and specific genes studied.[64–67] It is important during the counseling process that patients understand that tumor testing may uncover germline mutations and thus have hereditary cancer implications.[68,69] Genetic variants that are suspected to be of germline origin from tumor testing need to have confirmatory germline testing. Tumor genetic testing results can help with discussion of platinum chemotherapy and PARP inhibitor therapy.[64] Genetic mutations in tumor tissue may change over time; therefore, this testing might need to be repeated at different stages of the cancer.[64] However, germline mutations do not change over time.

NEW TECHNOLOGIES

As need for genetic counseling for men with prostate cancer increases, it is important to consider alternative delivery models and the use of technologies such as videos and chatbots. These options have the potential to improve access to genetic counselors, facilitate timely genetic testing, and also allow more effective use of genetic counselor time, leading to more tailored counseling sessions.[6,25,70] It has been recommended that additional strategies, such as the incorporation of videos, be used to provide pretest informed consent for men undergoing genetic testing for inherited prostate cancer.[6]

Chatbots are an artificial-intelligence tool that simulate conversation and can be used to gather information before a genetic counseling session, provide pretest genetic education, and assist providers with posttest care coordination.[70] In addition, chatbots can be used to inform relatives of patients with positive genetic testing results to aid in cascade testing.[70]

Studies have shown that patients are willing to incorporate these technologies into their care.[68] However, additional research is needed in order to ensure that these tools provide patients with an adequate understanding and that individual needs are met.[25] In addition, it will be important that these are thoughtfully integrated into cancer genetic counseling models to allow optimal use.[1,25] With increased clinical utility of genetic testing in the setting of prostate cancer, the demand for genetic counseling is increasing.[1] For this reason, more non–genetics providers are ordering their own genetic testing. It is important for providers who order their own genetic testing to either collaborate with their local genetics teams or use some of these new technologies to aid in providing informed consent to their patients before genetic testing is done and to ensure appropriate genetic testing is ordered.

ETHICAL/LEGAL CONCERNS WITH GENETIC COUNSELING AND PROSTATE CANCER
Nondirectiveness and genetic counseling

Nondirectiveness has historically been considered an essential element of the genetic counseling session.[3,71] Nondirectiveness is when information is presented without leaning toward a particular choice.[3] This approach aims to provide patients with balanced information in order to promote patient autonomy and informed decision making.[3,71,72] Over time, however, the field has moved away from nondirectiveness while still prioritizing patient autonomy.[72] In the emerging area of precision medicine, in which genetic variations are used to direct a more personalized treatment plan, there is a move away from the nondirectiveness approach to genetic counseling.[71–74] It is therefore vital for genetic counselors to balance bioethical principles and, in appropriate situations, provide active guidance to patients.[72]

Autonomy and informed consent

With increasing use and utility of germline genetic testing in the treatment of prostate cancer, it is important for health care providers involved in the care of patients to consider ethical implications for patients and their families. An important component of genetic counseling is informed consent, which allows the patients to have autonomy over choosing whether genetic testing is right for them.

If patients get true informed consent, then they can make an autonomous decision with regard to genetic testing. In order to get consent, the

Table 2
Topics to be covered in genetic counseling for prostate cancer germline testing

Elements of Informed Consent	Description
Purpose of germline testing	Precision therapy, early detection strategies, and/or to identify hereditary cancer syndrome/risk
Possibility of uncovering hereditary cancer syndromes	Depending on the test, it might uncover a hereditary cancer syndrome such as HBOCS and LS (see **Table 1**)
Panel options	Various multigene panels can be considered for genetic testing. Benefits and risks of each option should be discussed
Potential types of test results	Mutation (pathogenic/likely pathogenic variant). Variant of uncertain (unknown) significance and negative
Potential to uncover additional cancer risks	Multiple gene-specific cancer risks may be identified beyond prostate cancer risk that affects men and their families (see **Table 1**)
Potential out-of-pocket cost	Not all insurance plans cover genetic testing; some mandate referral to genetic counselor
GINA and other laws that address genetic discrimination	See **Box 1**, **Table 3** on GINA and genetic protections
Cascade testing/additional familial testing	Testing blood relatives for pathogenic variants or additional genetic testing by family history; worry and anxiety that may result from hereditary cancer testing; effect on family relationships
Data-sharing/data-selling policies of genetic laboratories	Each genetic testing laboratory may have unique data-sharing and data-selling policies that patients must be aware of
Privacy of genetic tests	Protection of genetic data from data breach or access by third parties

Abbreviation: GINA, Genetic Information Nondiscrimination Act.
Data From Giri VN, Knudsen KE, Kelly WK, et al. Implementation of Germline Testing for Prostate Cancer: Philadelphia Prostate Cancer Consensus Conference 2019. *J Clin Oncol.* 2020;38(24):2798-2811. https://doi.org/10.1200/JCO.20.00046

patients must be competent and understand what they are being told, be able to exercise judgment, be provided relevant information in a clear and understandable way, and be free to make decisions without coercion and outside influence.[75]

Autonomy is the principle that refers to the right of individuals to make health care decisions without interference from others and to make choices that best fit their beliefs and personal values.[76] For this to occur, individuals must understand the consequences of their choices without any interference or influence from others. Autonomy is both a negative (others should not influence choice) and positive obligation (need the proper information to make the choice).[76]

An important way to promote autonomous decision making is with genetic counseling. With help from a genetic counselor or health care provider with expertise in genetics, patients receive the appropriate pretest and posttest counseling and therefore are properly supported in making the right decisions for them.[3] To respect the autonomy of a patient, professionals in health care have an ethical obligation to disclose the right information to ensure that the patient understands, which helps promote adequate decision making.[3,75,76] This process is done successfully by the provider or genetic counselor knowing the social, emotional, and cultural experiences of the patient.[3]

Specifically for getting informed consent with genetic testing for prostate cancer, there are areas of importance that are important to cover before providing genetic testing (see **Table 2**). These areas include the purpose of the germline genetic testing, the chance of finding a hereditary cancer syndrome, the types of genetic testing results, the chance to discover other cancer risks, possibility of out-of-pocket costs for genetic testing, the Genetic Information Nondiscrimination Act (GINA) and other laws that address genetic discrimination (**Box 1** and discussed later), cascade testing, and additional familial testing.[6] Also to be considered are discussion of multigene panel genetic testing options, data-sharing and data-selling policies of genetic testing laboratories, and privacy with genetic testing.[6]

Concerns with Genetic Discrimination The Genetic Information Nondiscrimination Act

Patients and their families often have concerns about genetic discrimination, which is the misuse of genetic information.[3] For providers ordering genetic testing, it is important to be aware of where patients are protected legally and where protection is incomplete.

In 2008, GINA was enacted, which provided some protections for patients regarding their genetic information, which is their genetic testing results or family health history (see **Box 1**).[77] GINA states that it is illegal for health insurance companies to use genetic information to make decisions for a person's eligibility for health insurance or to determine how much the person will pay for health insurance. Also, GINA makes it illegal for employers to demand a genetic test be done and to use genetic information for any pay, firing, or hiring decisions.[77]

GINA has some large gaps, because it does not currently extend these nondiscrimination protections to life insurance, disability insurance, and long-term care insurance.[77] It also does not prevent health insurers from using this information to establish eligibility or premium rates once an individual afflicted with an inheritable disorder has started to show symptoms. GINA also does not

---

Box 1
Summary of Genetic Information Nondiscrimination Act of 2008 protections

What is covered:

- Health insurance
  - Illegal to use genetic information to make decisions on eligibility or determine cost for health insurance
- Employment
  - Cannot use genetic information for hiring, firing, or pay decisions
  - Cannot demand a genetic test be done

What is not covered:

- Does not apply to:
  - Individuals in the United States military who get their care through the Veterans' Administration[a]
  - Individuals with Indian Health Services[a]
  - Individuals with federal employee health benefits plans[a]
  - Does not prevent discrimination for eligibility or rates once symptoms show
- Does not include protections for life insurance, disability insurance, or long-term care insurance[b]

[a]These plans have protections in place similar to GINA.

[b]Some state laws have protections for genetic discrimination for life insurance, disability insurance, and long-term care insurance.

apply to individuals who have Indian Health Service, federal employees who have federal employee health benefits plans, and members of the United States military who get their care through the Veterans' Administration. There are protections in place with these groups that are like GINA. However, individuals with these types of health care insurance should speak with a case manager or supervisor at their insurance company to obtain a written iteration of that insurers genetic antidiscrimination policy to factor into decision making and avoid potential vulnerability in this area. With regard to employment, GINA also does not extend protection to employees of businesses with fewer than 15 employees. There are some state laws that have additional protections, and this can include protections with life insurance, disability insurance, and long-term care insurance.

Other protections for patients

The Americans with Disabilities Act (ADA) makes it illegal to discriminate in employment, public services, accommodations, and communications based on a disability (**Table 3**).[78,79] Discrimination based on genetic information is also protected by the ADA.[80] There are protections in place for individuals who have a preexisting condition or genetic disease from discrimination with the Health Insurance Portability and Accountability Act and the Affordable Care Act of 2010.

Table 3
Protections with regard to genetic discrimination

Law	What is Protected
GINA of 2008	Provides protections for misuse of genetic information with regard to health insurance and employment
ACA of 2010	Prevents health insurers from discriminating against patients because of preexisting conditions, including genetic conditions
ADA	Illegal for discrimination in employment, public services, accommodation, and communications based on disability
HIPAA	Protects individuals who have a genetic disease or a preexisting condition from discrimination

Abbreviations: ACA, Affordable Care Act; HIPAA, Health Insurance Portability and Accountability Act.

Genetic privacy

Privacy and confidentiality are important in any area of health care; however, there are unique considerations with regard to genetics and genetic testing.[3] Germline genetic testing provides information regarding the patient's risk and also the risk of family members. This information may be stigmatizing, which could put the patient and the family members at risk for discrimination in the workplace or procuring certain types of insurance.[75]

SUMMARY

Somatic and germline genetic testing has become relevant for the treatment of prostate cancer and for identifying hereditary cancer syndromes in affected men and their family members. Genetic counseling is an important component of genetic testing. It is important for treating clinicians to ensure that the patients receive the proper genetic counseling to allow informed decision making. Because of limited access to genetic counselors, alternative models have emerged to aid and even substitute components of the traditional model. However, it is important to ensure all aspects and implications of genetic testing are discussed with patients in both a pretest and posttest setting to facilitate and maintain positive regard and confidence between patient and clinician by avoiding discordant expectations and information when genetic testing is being considered.

CLINICS CARE POINTS

Genetic counseling for prostate cancer

- An important step for germline genetic testing for men with a personal and/or family history of prostate cancer and women with a family history of prostate cancer is genetic counseling.

- Genetic counseling helps maintain positive regard and confidence between patient and clinician by avoiding discordant expectations and information when genetic testing is being considered.

- It is essential to provide informed consent for the patient before undergoing germline genetic testing.

- Posttest genetic counseling includes discussing the implications of germline genetic testing results for the patient and family members and facilitating appropriate high-risk referrals.

- An important part of cascade testing of family members, if a germline genetic mutation is detected, is genetic counseling.
- Genetic counselors provide psychosocial support to patients throughout the genetic testing process.

DISCLOSURE

C. Hyatt was previously a consultant and held stock in GenomeSmart. The other authors have nothing to disclose.

REFERENCES

1. Giri VN, Hyatt C, Gomella LG. GT for men with prostate cancer: Navigating an expanding new world of genetic evaluation for precision therapy and precision management. J Clin Oncol 2019;37:1455–9.
2. Resta RG. The historical perspective: sheldon reed and 50 years of genetic counseling. J Genet Couns 1997;6:375–7.
3. Uhlmann WR, Schuette JL, Yashar B. A guide to genetic counseling. 2nd edition. Hoboken (NJ): Wiley-Blackwell; 2009.
4. Resta R, Biesecker BB, Bennett RL, et al. A new definition of genetic counseling: national society of genetic counselors' task force report. J Genet Counsel 2006;15:77–83.
5. Hyatt C, Russo J, McDougall C. Genetic counseling perspective of engagement with urology and primary care. Can J Urol 2019;26(5 Suppl 2):52–3.
6. Giri VN, Knudsen KE, Kelly WK, et al. Implementation of Germline Testing for Prostate Cancer: Philadelphia Prostate Cancer Consensus Conference 2019. J Clin Oncol 2020;38(24):2798–811.
7. Hampel H, Bennett RL, Buchanan A, et al. A practice guideline from the American College of Medical Genetics and Genomics and the National Society of Genetic Counselors: referral indications for cancer predisposition assessment. Genet Med 2015;17(1):70–87.
8. Bensend TA, Veach PM, Niendorf KB. What's the harm? Genetic counselor perceptions of adverse effects of genetics service provision by non-genetics professionals. J Genet Couns 2014;23(1):48–63.
9. Hampel H, Grubs RE, Walton CS, et al. Genetic counseling practice analysis. J Genet Couns 2009;18:205–16.
10. Bjorvatn C, Eide GE, Hanestad BR, et al. Risk perception, worry and satisfaction related to genetic counseling for hereditary cancer. J Genet Couns 2007;16(2):211–22.
11. Bratt O, Damber JE, Emanuelsson M, et al. Risk perception, screening practice and interest in genetic testing among unaffected men in families

with hereditary prostate cancer. Eur J Cancer 2000;36:235–41.
12. Culver JO, Brinkerhoff CD, Clague J, et al. Variants of uncertain significance in BRCA testing: Evaluation of surgical decisions, risk perception, and cancer distress. Clin Genet 2014;84(5):464–72.
13. Cicero G, DeLuca R, Dorangricchia P, et al. Risk perception and psychological distress in genetic counselling for hereditary breast and/or ovarian cancer. J Genet Couns 2017;26:999–1007.
14. Palmero EI, Campacci N, Schuler-Faccini L, et al. Cancer-related worry and risk perception in Brazilian individuals seeking genetic counseling for hereditary breast cancer. Genet Mol Biol 2020;43(2):1–7.
15. Bennett RL, Steinhaus French K, Resta RG, et al. Standardized human pedigree nomenclature: Update and assessment of the recommendations of the National Society of Genetic Counselors. J Genet Couns 2008;17:424–33.
16. Riley BD, Culver JO, Skrzynia C, et al. Essential elements of genetic cancer risk assessment, counseling, and testing: Updated recommendations of the National Society of Genetic Counselors. J Genet Couns 2012;21:151–61.
17. Balmaña J, Digiovanni L, Gaddam P, et al. Conflicting interpretation of genetic variants and cancer risk by commercial laboratories as assessed by the prospective registry of multiplex testing. J Clin Oncol 2016;34(34):4071–8.
18. Richards S, Aziz N, Bale S, et al. Standards and guidelines for the interpretation of sequence variants: a joint consensus recommendation of the American College of Medical Genetics and Genomics and the Association for Molecular Pathology. Genet Med 2015;17:405–23.
19. Mersch J, Brown N, Pirzadeh-Miller S, et al. Prevalence of variant reclassification following hereditary cancer genetic testing. JAMA 2018;320(12):1266–74.
20. Giri VN, Obeid E, Gross L, et al. Inherited Mutations in Males Undergoing Multigene Panel Testing for PCA – emerging implications for personalized prostate cancer genetic evaluation. J Clin Oncol 2017. https://doi.org/10.1200/PO.16.00039.
21. Giri VN, Obeid E, Hegarty SE, et al. Understanding of multigene test results among males undergoing germline testing for inherited prostate cancer: implications for genetic counseling. Prostate 2018;78:879–88.
22. Meiser B Psychological impact of genetic testing for cancer susceptibility: an update of the literature. Psychooncology 2005;14:1060–74.
23. Hadley DW, Ashida S, Jenkins JF, et al. Generation after generation: exploring the psychological impact of providing genetic services through a cascading approach. Genet Med 2010;12(12):808–15.

24. Castro E, Eeles RA. The role of BRCA1 and BRCA2 in prostate cancer. Asian J Androl 2012;14(3): 409–14. Available at: https://ncbi.nlm.nih.gov/pmc/articles/pmc3720154. Retrieved August 30, 2020.

25. Giri VN, Hegarty SE, Hyatt C, et al. Germline genetic testing for inherited prostate cancer in practice: Implications for genetic testing, precision therapy, and cascade testing. Prostate 2019;79(4):333–9. Available at: https://onlinelibrary.wiley.com/doi/full/10.1002/pros.23739. Retrieved August 30, 2020.

26. Friedenson B. BRCA1 and BRCA2 pathways and the risk of cancers other than breast or ovarian. MedGenMed 2005;7(2):60. Available at: https://ncbi.nlm.nih.gov/pmc/articles/pmc1681605. Retrieved August 30, 2020.

27. Nyberg T, Frost D, Barrowdale D, et al. Prostate Cancer Risks for Male BRCA1 and BRCA2 Mutation Carriers: A Prospective Cohort Study. Eur Urol 2020; 77(1):24–35.

28. Taneja SS. Re: Prostate Cancer Risks for Male BRCA1 and BRCA2 Mutation Carriers: A Prospective Cohort Study. J Urol 2020;203(3):463–4.

29. Castro E, Goh C, Olmos D, et al. Germline BRCA mutations are associated with higher risk of nodal involvement, distant metastasis, and poor survival outcomes in prostate cancer. J Clin Oncol 2013; 31(14):1748–57.

30. Struewing JP, Hartge P, Wacholder S, et al. The risk of cancer associated with specific mutations of BRCA1 and BRCA2 among Ashkenazi Jews. N Engl J Med 1997;336(20):1401–8.

31. Ford D, Easton DF, Stratton M, et al. Genetic heterogeneity and penetrance analysis of the BRCA1 and BRCA2 genes in breast cancer families. The Breast Cancer Linkage Consortium. Am J Hum Genet 1998; 62(3):676–89.

32. Kuchenbaecker KB, Hopper JL, Barnes DR, et al. Risks of Breast, Ovarian, and Contralateral Breast Cancer for BRCA1 and BRCA2 Mutation Carriers. JAMA 2017;317(23):2402–16.

33. Breast Cancer Linkage Consortium. Cancer risks in BRCA2 mutation carriers. J Natl Cancer Inst 1999; 91(15):1310–6.

34. Nalepa G, Clapp DW. Fanconi anaemia and cancer: an intricate relationship. Nat Rev Cancer 2018;18(3): 168–85.

35. Domchek SM, Tang J, Stopfer J, et al. Biallelic deleterious BRCA1 mutations in a woman with early-onset ovarian cancer. Cancer Discov 2013;3(4):399–405.

36. Sawyer SL, Tian L, Kähkönen M, et al. Biallelic mutations in BRCA1 cause a new Fanconi anemia subtype. Cancer Discov 2015;5(2):135–42.

37. Ewing CM, Ray AM, Lange EM, et al. Germline mutations in HOXB13 and prostate-cancer risk. N Engl J Med 2012;366(2):141–9.

38. Laitinen VH, Wahlfors T, Saaristo L, et al. HOXB13 G84E mutation in Finland: population-based analysis of prostate, breast, and colorectal cancer risk. Cancer Epidemiol Biomarkers Prev 2013; 22(3):452–60.

39. Karlsson R, Aly M, Clements M, et al. A population-based assessment of germline HOXB13 G84E mutation and prostate cancer risk. Eur Urol 2014; 65(1):169–76.

40. Bauer CM, Ray AM, Halstead-Nussloch BA, et al. Hereditary prostate cancer as a feature of Lynch Syndrome. Fam Cancer 2011;10(1):37–42. Available at: https://ncbi.nlm.nih.gov/pmc/articles/pmc3089958. Retrieved August 30, 2020.

41. Soravia C, Klift HM, Brundler M-A, et al. Prostate cancer is part of the hereditary non-polyposis colorectal cancer (HNPCC) tumor spectrum. Am J Med Genet A 2003;121(2):159–62. Available at: https://ncbi.nlm.nih.gov/pubmed/12910497. Retrieved August 30, 2020.

42. Shan A, Wick M, Persons D. Microsatellite instability in prostate cancer. Am J Hum Genet 1994;55. Available at: http://osti.gov/scitech/biblio/133573-microsatellite-instability-prostate-cancer. Retrieved August 30, 2020.

43. Duraturo F, Liccardo R, De Rosa M, et al. Genetics, diagnosis and treatment of Lynch syndrome: Old lessons and current challenges (Review). Oncol Lett 2019;17:3048–54.

44. Lynch H, Snyder C, Shaw T, et al. Milestones of Lynch syndrome: 1895–2015. Nat Rev Cancer 2015;15:181–94.

45. Jenkins MA, Baglietto L, Dowty JG, et al. Cancer risks for mismatch repair gene mutation carriers: a population-based early onset case-family study. Clin Gastroenterol Hepatol 2006;4(4):489–98.

46. Beebe-Dimmer JL, Kapron AL, Fraser AM, et al. Risk of prostate cancer associated with familial and hereditary cancer syndromes. J Clin Oncol 2020;38(16):1807–13.

47. Wimmer K, Kratz CP, Vasen HF, et al. Diagnostic criteria for constitutional mismatch repair deficiency syndrome: suggestions of the European consortium 'care for CMMRD' (C4CMMRD). J Med Genet 2014; 51(6):355–65.

48. Na R, Zheng SL, Han M, et al. Germline Mutations in ATM and BRCA1/2 distinguish risk for lethal and indolent prostate cancer and are associated with early age at death. Eur Urol 2017;71(5):740–7.

49. Carter HB, Helfand B, Mamawala M, et al. Germline Mutations in ATM and BRCA1/2 are associated with grade reclassification in men on active surveillance for prostate cancer. Eur Urol 2019;75(5):743–9.

50. Mavrou A, Tsangaris GT, Roma E, et al. The ATM gene and ataxia telangiectasia. Anticancer Res 2008;28(1B):401–5.

51. Seppälä EH, Ikonen T, Mononen N, et al. CHEK2 variants associate with hereditary prostate cancer. Br J Cancer 2003;89(10):1966–70.

52. Cybulski C, Gorski B, Debriak T, et al. NBS1 is a prostate cancer susceptibility gene. Cancer Res 2004;64(4):1215–9.

53. Kote-Jarai Z, Jugurnauth S, Mulholland S, et al. A recurrent truncating germline mutation in the BRIP1/FANCJ gene and susceptibility to prostate cancer. Br J Cancer 2009;100(2):426–30.

54. Giri VN, Obeid E, Gross L, et al: Inherited mutations in males undergoing multigene panel testing for prostate cancer: emerging implications for personalized prostate cancer genetic evaluation. JCO Precis Oncol 2017;10.1200/PO.16.00039

55. d'Agincourt-Canning L. Experiences of genetic risk: disclosure and the gendering of responsibility. Bioethics 2001;15:231–47.

56. Graves K, Gatammah R, Peshkin B, et al. BRCA1/2 genetic testing uptake and psychosocial outcomes in men. Fam Cancer 2011;1-:213–23.

57. Rauscher EA, Dean M, Campbell-Salome GM. "I Am Uncertain About What My Uncertainty Even Is": Men's Uncertainty and Information Management of Their BRCA-Related Cancer Risks. J Genet Couns 2018;27(6):1417–27.

58. Suttman A, Pilarski R, Agnese DM, et al. "Second-class status?" insight into communication patterns and common concerns among men with hereditary breast and ovarian cancer syndrome. J Genet Couns 2018;27(4):886–93.

59. Nicolosi P, Ledet E, Yang S, et al. Prevalence of germline variants in prostate cancer and implications for current genetic testing guidelines. JAMA Oncol 2019. https://doi.org/10.1001/jamaoncol.2018.6760.

60. Pritchard CC, Mateo J, Walsh MF, et al. Inherited DNA-repair gene mutations in men with metastatic prostate cancer. N Engl J Med 2016;375:443–53.

61. NCI Staff. 2020. Available at: https://www.cancer.gov/news-events/cancer-currents-blog/2020/fda-olaparib-rucaparib-prostate-cancer. Accessed October 2020.

62. Abida W, Cheng ML, Armenia J, et al. Analysis of the prevalence of microsatellite instability in prostate cancer and response to immune checkpoint blockade. JAMA Oncol 2019;5(4):471–8. Available at: https://jamanetwork.com/journals/jamaoncology/fullarticle/2718924?resultClick=1.

63. Edwards SM, Evans DG, Hope Q, et al. Prostate cancer in BRCA2 germline mutation carriers is associated with poorer prognosis. Br J Cancer 2010;103:918.

64. Cheng HH, Sokolova AO, Schaeffer EM, et al. Germline and Somatic Mutations in Prostate Cancer for the Clinician. J Natl Compr Cancer Netw 2019;17(5):515–21.

65. Mandelker D, Zhang L, Kemel Y, et al. Mutation Detection in Patients With Advanced Cancer by Universal Sequencing of Cancer-Related Genes in Tumor and Normal DNA vs Guideline-Based Germline Testing. JAMA 2017;318(9):825–35 [published correction appears in JAMA. 2018 Dec 11;320(22):2381].

66. Mandelker D, Zhang L. The emerging significance of secondary germline testing in cancer genomics. J Pathol 2018;244(5):610–5.

67. Schrader KA, Cheng DT, Joseph V, et al. Germline Variants in Targeted Tumor Sequencing Using Matched Normal DNA. JAMA Oncol 2016;2(1):104–11 [published correction appears in JAMA Oncol. 2016 Feb;2(2):279. Hyman, David [corrected to Hyman, David M]].

68. Robinson D, Van Allen EM, Wu YM, et al. Integrative clinical genomics of advanced prostate cancer. Cell 2015;161(5):1215–28.

69. Cancer Genome Atlas Research Network. The molecular taxonomy of primary prostate cancer. Cell 2015;163(4):1011–25.

70. Schmidlen T, Schwartz M, DiLoreto K, et al. Patient assessment of chatbots for the scalable delivery of genetic counseling. J Genet Couns 2019;28(6):1166–77.

71. Michie S, Bron F, Bobrow M, et al. Nondirectiveness in genetic counseling: An empirical study. Am J Hum Genet 1997;60:40–7.

72. Jamal L, Schupmann W, Berkman BE. An ethical framework for genetic counseling in the genomic era. J Genet Couns 2019;00:1–10.

73. Schupmann W, Jamal L, Berkman BE. Re-examining the ethics of genetic counseling in the genomic era. Bioethical Inq 2020;17(3):325–35.

74. Halbert CH, Harrison BW. Genetic counseling among minority populations in the era of precision medicine. Am J Hum Genet 2018;178(1):68–74.

75. Mundon R. Intervention and reflection: basic issues in medical ethics. 8th edition. Belmont (CA): Thomson Higher Education; 2008.

76. Beauchamp TL, Childress JF. Principles of biomedical ethics. 5th edition. New York: Oxford University Press; 2001.

77. Genetic Information Nondiscrimination Act of 2008: Pub.L. 110-233, 122 Stat. 881 (2008).

78. The health insurance portability and accountability Act (hipaa). Washington, DC: U.S. Dept. of Labor, Employee Benefits Security Administrations; 2004.

79. The Patient Protection and Affordable Care Act (PPACA). Pub. L. No. 111-148, 124 Stat. 119. (2010)

80. The Americans With Disabilities Act of 1990, Pub. L. No. 101-336, 2, 104 Stat. 328. (1991)

81. Genetics Home Reference. Ataxia-telangiectasia. Available at: https://ghr.nlm.nih.gov/condition/ataxia-telangiectasia. Accessed October 2020.

82. OMIM. Fanconi Anemia, complementation group S; FANCS. Available at: https://www.omim.org/entry/617883#2. Accessed October 2020.

83. NCBI. GTR: Genetic Testing Registry. Fanconi Anemia, complementation group D1. Available at: https://www.ncbi.nlm.nih.gov/gtr/conditions/C1838457/. Accessed October 2020.

84. OMIM. Mismatch Repair Cancer Syndrome; MMRCS. Available at: https://www.omim.org/entry/276300?search=CMMRD&highlight=%22cmmr%20d%22%20%22cmmr%7Cd%22%20%28cmmrd%7C%20%29%20cmmrd#2. Accessed October 2020.

Basic Science and Molecular Genetics of Prostate Cancer Aggressiveness

Matthew J. Schiewer, PhD[a,b],*, Karen E. Knudsen, MBA, PhD[c,d,e,f]

KEYWORDS

- Prostate cancer • Androgen receptor • Cellular plasticity • NEPC • DNA repair

KEY POINTS

- Prostate cancer development, progression, and aggressive behavior are often attributable to function of the androgen receptor.
- Tumor cell plasticity, neuroendocrine features, and loss of tumor suppressors lend aggressive behavior to prostate cancer cells.
- DNA repair defects have ramifications for prostate cancer cell behavior.

INTRODUCTION

Prostate cancer remains the most frequently diagnosed cancer in men in the United States, and is responsible for the second most cancer-related deaths in this group.[1] Although patients with organ-confined disease have a reasonable expectation of cure,[2] metastatic prostate cancer is largely incurable.[3] Despite this, there has been a decline in the morality rate caused by prostate cancer, which can be attributed to screening efforts,[4,5] appropriately aggressive management of primary disease,[6] and new therapeutic strategies for advanced disease.[7] Because prostate cancer cells are largely resistant to standard cytotoxic chemotherapy, and prostate cancer cells are heavily reliant on the androgen receptor (AR), androgen deprivation therapy (ADT) is first-line treatment of disseminated prostate cancer.[8] AR is targeted by pharmacologic means via administration of gonadotropin-releasing hormone (GnRH) agonists, which function to inhibit testicular androgen synthesis, thus limiting the available ligand for AR. ADT can be combined with direct AR antagonists (such as enzalutamide[9]), which function by reversibly binding to the ligand-binding domain of AR. It is likely that combined ADT and second-generation AR antagonists will become standard of care based on recent clinical trial findings that moving AR antagonist use to earlier disease history results in positive patient outcomes. Most patients respond positively to these treatments, for which the efficacy of AR-directed strategies is informed by PSA (prostate-specific antigen) quantification, given that the gene encoding PSA (*KLK3*) is stringently AR regulated. However, these therapeutic regimens are only transiently effective, because patients typically relapse within 24 to 36 months, and this relapse is often heralded by an increase in serum

[a] Department of Urology, Urology Research Laboratory, Thomas Jefferson University, Sidney Kimmel Cancer Center, 233 South 10th Street BLSB 804, Philadelphia, PA 19107, USA; [b] Department of Cancer Biology, Urology Research Laboratory, Thomas Jefferson University, Sidney Kimmel Cancer Center, 233 South 10th Street BLSB 804, Philadelphia, PA 19107, USA; [c] Department of Cancer Biology, Thomas Jefferson University, 233 South 10th Street BLSB 1050, Philadelphia, PA 19107, USA; [d] Department of Urology, Thomas Jefferson University, 233 South 10th Street BLSB 1050, Philadelphia, PA 19107, USA; [e] Department of Medical Oncology, Thomas Jefferson University, 233 South 10th Street BLSB 1050, Philadelphia, PA 19107, USA; [f] Department of Radiation Oncology, Thomas Jefferson University, 233 South 10th Street BLSB 1050, Philadelphia, PA 19107, USA
* Corresponding author. 233 South 10th Street BLSB 804, Philadelphia, PA 19107.
E-mail address: matthew.schiewer@jefferson.edu
Twitter: @MattSchiewer (M.J.S.); @SKCCDirector (K.E.K.)

Urol Clin N Am 48 (2021) 339–347
https://doi.org/10.1016/j.ucl.2021.04.004
0094-0143/21/© 2021 Elsevier Inc. All rights reserved.

PSA level, indicating that resurgent AR transcriptional activity has been reactivated despite continued therapeutic targeting. Castration-resistant prostate cancer (CRPC) is responsible for most prostate cancer–associated mortality[10–18]; although these tumors largely remain AR positive and AR responsive, a subset of cancers can transition to a less AR-dependent and/or neuroendocrine tumor type as a result of cellular plasticity.[19] CRPC-associated AR activity is induced by the selective pressure of the therapy itself, which leads to tumor cell evolution that allows aberrant activation of AR and is caused by nonredundant mechanisms that have been reviewed extensively elsewhere.[20] Regardless of the means by which AR is reactivated, the resultant CRPC-associated AR functions to induce cancer-associated phenotypes, including unchecked cell cycle progression.[21] Although management of advanced prostate cancer remains AR-centric, novel treatment strategies are forthcoming.[22] In addition, genetic testing in prostate cancer has recently gained increased traction,[23,24] and a recent consensus conference was held to discuss the implementation of genetic testing in prostate cancer.[25] This article delineates what has been published in the literature related to the basic science and molecular genetics of prostate cancer aggressiveness.

GERMLINE ALTERATIONS ASSOCIATED WITH PROSTATE CANCER AGGRESSIVENESS

Increased uptake of genetic testing is largely caused by the need for precision medicine in the management of prostate cancer,[26] such as use of poly(ADP)-ribose polymerase inhibitors (PARPi) in the context of homologous recombination (HR) deficiency.[27] Importantly, prostate cancer has been shown to be heritable in approximately 57% of cases,[28] 8% of metastatic CRPC tumors harbor actionable pathogenic germline alterations,[29] and most of the germline alterations found in prostate cancer are mutations in DNA repair genes.[30] Prevalence of germline DNA repair mutations is higher in metastatic prostate cancer than in primary disease, occurring in 11% to 33% of cases.[30,31] Although there are a number germline mutations associated with prostate cancer susceptibility (ATM, BRCA1, BRCA2, CHEK2, HOXB13, Lynch syndrome genes, NBN), only the DNA repair genes associated with susceptibility have been linked to prostate cancer aggressiveness (ATM, BRCA1, BRCA2, CHEK2, Lynch syndrome genes, NBN). In addition, although not linked to greater disease susceptibility, germline alterations in PALB2 have been linked to prostate

cancer aggressiveness. Interestingly, each of the DNA repair genes is less frequently mutated in the germline of African American men.[32]

ANDROGEN RECEPTOR PATHWAY

The AR signaling axis is critical for the development of the prostate, as well as tumorigenesis of most prostate cancers. In the context of normal prostate, AR function serves to regulate cellular differentiation and acts in an antiproliferative manner. The gene expression programs governed by AR become altered in tumorigenesis, and the function of AR becomes broadly proproliferative and prosurvival.[8] In prostate cells, testosterone is converted to the more potent AR ligand dihydrotestosterone by the activity of 5α-reductase. Canonically, AR is held inactive in the cytoplasm in complex with heat shock proteins/chaperones, and on ligand binding the N and C terminals of AR interact, and AR translocates to the nucleus through in an importin-α–dependent manner. AR dimerizes in the nucleus and subsequently binds to androgen response elements within the regulatory loci (promoters, but more often enhancers) or AR target genes. The function of AR on chromatin is to recruit basal transcriptional machinery and other cofactors, resulting in both activation and suppression of gene expression, depending on gene and biological contexts. **Fig. 1** provides a stylized depiction of the canonical AR pathway.[12,15,20,21,33] The transcriptional networks governed by AR function continue to be defined, but the major biological pathways under the control of AR include cancer cell proliferation and survival, DNA damage response, and secretion of proteases (such as PSA and TMPRSS2). Although tremendous effort was spent developing this elegant model for AR function, it is more complex and is the subject of ongoing study.

Means of targeting AR are in 2 basic categories: reduction/elimination of ligand (castration, GnRH-targeting drugs, abiraterone) or direct receptor antagonism (bicalutamide, enzalutamide, apalutamide, darolutamide, and so forth). Mechanisms that lead to therapeutic resistance include increased AR protein levels through gene amplification, altered protein stability, or deregulated gene expression[34]; gain-of-function mutation in AR, which can render antagonists less potent, or even push them to partial agonists[35]; other nuclear receptors, such as glucocorticoid receptor regulating AR-driven gene expression programs[36]; aberrant posttranslational modification of AR protein[15]; generation of so-called AR splice variants, which lack the ligand-binding domain and are constitutively active[37,38]; cofactor perturbation,

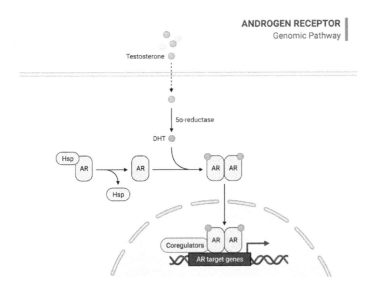

ANDROGEN RECEPTOR
Genomic Pathway

Fig. 1. The canonical AR pathway. (Created with BioRender.com.)

such as loss of corepressors or gain of coactivators[39]; and intracrine androgen synthesis, wherein tumor cells derange steroid metabolism to generate AR ligand,[40] which is targetable through use of abiraterone. These mechanisms are not mutually exclusive, and, irrespective of how tumor cells adapt to AR-directed therapy, the fact that most prostate cancer deaths occur after AR reactivation and CRPC development indicates the importance of AR in aggressive prostate cancer. Based on recent clinical trial data, addition of newer-generation AR antagonists with ADT will become commonplace, because using AR antagonists in combination with ADT has been shown to improve patient outcomes. As such, defining mechanisms of resistance to this combined modality will be of crucial importance.

LOSS OF KEY TUMOR SUPPRESSORS

Loss of specific tumor suppressors has been implicated in prostate cancer aggressiveness.

- The canonical function of the retinoblastoma (RB) tumor suppressor is to block the function of the E2F family of transcription factors, and RB sits at the interface of mitogenic signaling and cell cycle regulation.[41] *RB1* loss is common in small cell neuroendocrine prostate cancer.[42] A transcriptional signature of RB loss of function has been associated with poor clinical outcomes,[43] and model systems of RB loss in prostate cancer have shown:
  - Loss of RB increases E2F1-driven AR expression and leads to castration resistance.[44,45]
  - RB harbors tumor-suppressive functions distinct from cell cycle regulation that contribute to disease progression.[46]
- Combinatorial loss-of-function RB and p53 have also been modeled in prostate cancer, resulting in altered cellular plasticity, development of metastases, and resistance to AR-directed therapies.[47,48] The Transgenic Adenocarcinoma of the Mouse Prostate model results from SV40-dependent inactivation of p53 and RB and has been heavily used to study prostate cancer phenotypes, including aggressiveness.[49,50]
- The combined loss of *TP53*, *RB1*, and *PTEN* tumor suppressors is associated with increased risk of prostate cancer relapse and death from prostate cancer.[51]
- In addition, coloss of *RB1* and *BRCA2* in prostate cancer model systems leads to aggressive phenotypes, including resistance to castration, epithelial to mesenchymal transition (EMT), and increased invasive potential. Importantly, in human prostate cancer, this codeletion behaves aggressively.[52,53]

TUMOR CELL PLASTICITY

Lineage plasticity, mostly toward a neuroendocrine phenotype, confers aggressive behavior to prostate cancer.[54] Neuroendocrine prostate cancer (NEPC)[55–57] and aggressive-variant prostate cancer (AVPC)[58,59] are of increasing importance in the context of aggressive behavior of prostate cancer and are associated with loss of function of some of the tumor suppressors discussed earlier. Although de novo NEPC occurs infrequently, most instances of NEPC result from adaptation to AR-directed therapies. Critically, on development of treatment-induced NEPC, tumor cells no longer rely on AR signaling, rendering any AR-directed therapies largely ineffective. By this very nature, NEPC is considered aggressive. Although NEPC has been extensively reviewed elsewhere, the molecular features associated with NEPC include:

- Loss of luminal markers and suppressed AR expression and/or function.[56]
- Neuroendocrine markers, such as chromogranin A and synaptophysin.[56]
- Enrichment of gene expression programs associated with EMT, neuronal differentiation, stemlike, and developmental pathways.[56,60–62]
- TP53 and RB1 loss of function.[56]
- Increased expression of the oncogenic transcription factor N-Myc.[56,63]
- Derangement of epigenetic (such as EZH2[63] and DNA meythlation[64]), stem cell (such as SOX2), and lineage (such as placental PEG10[65,66]) factors.
- Importantly, NEPC is a potentially heterogenous phenotype, and there is a subset of prostate cancers that are both AR negative and also negative for markers of NEPC.[67]

Although there is overlap between NEPC and AVPC, AVPC harbors loss of 2 or more alterations in TP53, RB1, and PTEN and is defined by clinical phenotype, including being CRPC, sharing features of small cell prostate cancer, loss of AR signaling, and enrichment for a neural progenitor gene expression program.[58,59] By definition, both NEPC and AVPC are not responsive to AR-directed therapy, and, as such, developing means to target these aggressive prostate cancers is ongoing, and includes use of platinum-based and other chemotherapy as well as Aurora kinase inhibition[68] alone or in combination with PARPi.[69]

Other mechanisms that have been identified to result in cellular plasticity/aggressive behavior in prostate cancer models include (but are not limited to):

- c-MYC and AKT1 activation[70]
- SPINK1 upregulation through ADT[71]
- MUC1-C through MYC/BRN2, n-MYC, EZH2, and NEPC markers[72]
- Dysregulation of integrin signaling[73] and integrin modulation of small extracellular vesicles[74]
- Posttranscriptional regulation by microRNA-194[75]

- Acquired resistance to taxanes through NOTCH and Hedgehog signaling,[76] as well as GATA2-driven regulation of insulinlike growth factor 2[77]
- Deregulation of subunits of the SWI/SNF chromatin remodeling complex[78]

DNA REPAIR PATHWAYS

Part of the gene expression program governed by AR includes DNA repair genes, and alterations in DNA repair genes are associated with clinically aggressive prostate cancer.

- ATM is a kinase involved in DNA double-strand break repair, and germline mutations in ATM are associated with ataxia-telangiectasia. Germline mutation of ATM is associated with prostate cancer aggressiveness.[79–86] Although these data indicate that germline ATM alteration is implicated in more aggressive prostate cancer, it has been associated with improved outcomes in response to abiraterone or enzalutamide,[87] platinum-based chemotherapy,[88,89] and radium-223.[90,91] However, it has also been reported that there is no impact of ATM loss on outcomes after surgical intervention.[80] ATM mutations were thought to impart sensitivity to PARPi based early clinical data.[31] However, more recent trial data[92,93] indicate that this correlation is at the least controversial. In preclinical model systems, ATM activity has been associated with aggressive phenotypes through regulation of glucose uptake and glycolysis in the context of AKT hyperactivation,[94] and ATM loss has been associated with the Warburg effect.[95]
- BRCA1 and BRCA2 are tumor suppressor genes involved in homology-directed DNA damage repair, and germline mutations in these genes are responsible for hereditary breast and ovarian cancer syndromes. It is becoming increasingly appreciated that germline mutations in BRCA1/2 are associated with tumor types beyond breast and ovarian, including prostate.[96,97] Importantly, alterations in BRCA1/2 compromise high-fidelity HR, and cells with BRCA1/2 mutations are more reliant on error-prone DNA repair. Several studies have implicated germline BRCA1/2 mutation in aggressive behavior in prostate cancer.[86,98–106] Although it is apparent that BRCA1/2 mutations impart aggressiveness, not all BRCA2 mutations are equivalent,[107] and germline BRCA1 and BRCA2 mutations do not result in the same

level of risk or aggressiveness.[98,99,101–106] Similar to what has been seen with germline *ATM* mutations, *BRCA1/2* alterations have been associated with improved treatment response to platinum-based chemotherapy,[88,89,108] and poly(ADP)-ribose polymerase (PARP) inhibition,[31,109,110] with *BRCA2* mutation seeming to be better at selecting for PARPi responses.[110] However, it was recently determined that patients with advanced prostate cancer had positive responses to PARPi, irrespective of DNA repair gene status.[111] In preclinical models:

- Loss of *BRCA1/2* elicits sensitivity to PARPi.
- PARPi itself has been shown to reduce expression of DNA repair genes, including *BRCA2*.[112]
- Loss of BRCA2 in prostate cancer cells results in increased invasive potential through regulation of either c-kit[113] or matrix metalloproteinase-9.[114]
- Patient-derived xenografts from BRCA2 mutant tumors showed enrichment for intraductal histology, which is an aggressive subtype.[115,116]

SUMMARY

The preponderance of evidence shows AR functions to drive the basic biology of prostate cancer as well as aggressive phenotypes and disease progression. Given the importance of the AR in the natural history of prostate cancer, it is essential to note that there is significant crosstalk between AR and DNA damage repair proteins in prostate cancer.[117–120] It is hypothesized that targeting AR would reduce DNA repair gene expression, which should result in catastrophic loss of DNA repair capacity in carriers of DNA repair gene defects. However, the impact of germline *ATM* and *BRCA1/2* mutation on response to AR-directed therapy is controversial, ranging from reduced efficacy,[121] no difference,[122] to increased efficacy,[87] or having significance for sequence of treatment.[102] Furthermore, the impact of other DNA repair genes on response to AR-directed therapy remains underreported. Further prospective studies are needed to better understand the clinical impact of AR-DNA repair crosstalk, and how best to use this information to inform disease management.

The implications for tumor cell plasticity and loss of tumor suppressors on prostate cancer aggressiveness are clear based on the clinical data. However, defining the mechanisms by which plasticity/differentiation/NEPC drive aggressive behaviors remains an ongoing endeavor, and has the potential to unlock novel treatment strategies for aggressive prostate cancer.

In addition, alterations in DNA repair genes not only impart increased risk of developing prostate cancer but also are associated with more aggressive disease, defined variably as early age of onset, higher grade, shorter time to relapse, and metastases at diagnosis. Although the biology of these tumors associated with germline DNA repair defects may be associated with more aggressive behavior, that same biology may provide a means for better disease management through use of DNA damaging agents (such as platinum chemotherapy) or through targeting of DNA repair pathways (such as PARP inhibitors), as well as immune checkpoint inhibitors (in the case of mismatch repair deficiency). Although current approvals and recent clinical trial data are promising, further work will be needed to better understand the mechanisms by which germline DNA repair defects impart aggressive behavior to further improve outcomes.

DISCLOSURE

The authors report no conflicts relevant to this article. K.E. Knudsen reports the following unrelated disclosures for the last 3 years: research support from Celgene, Novartis, and CellCentric, and consultant/advisory relationships with CellCentric, Sanofi, Celgene, Janssen, and Genentech.

REFERENCES

1. Siegel RL, Miller KD, Jemal A. Cancer statistics, 2020. CA Cancer J Clin 2020;70:7–30.
2. Klein EA, Ciezki J, Kupelian PA, et al. Outcomes for intermediate risk prostate cancer: are there advantages for surgery, external radiation, or brachytherapy? Urol Oncol 2009;27:67–71.
3. Center MM, Jemal A, Lortet-Tieulent J, et al. International variation in prostate cancer incidence and mortality rates. Eur Urol 2012;61:1079–92.
4. Hugosson J, Roobol MJ, Månsson M, et al. A 16-yr Follow-up of the European Randomized study of Screening for Prostate Cancer. Eur Urol 2019;76:43–51.
5. Loeb S, Catalona WJ. Prostate-specific antigen screening: pro. Curr Opin Urol 2010;20:185–8.
6. Dahm P, Brasure M, Ester E, et al. in Therapies for clinically localized prostate cancer. Rockville (MD): 2020.
7. Teo MY, Rathkopf DE, Kantoff P. Treatment of advanced prostate cancer. Annu Rev Med 2019;70:479–99.
8. Chaturvedi AP, Dehm SM. Androgen receptor dependence. Adv Exp Med Biol 2019;1210:333–50.

9. Scher HI, Beer TM, Higano CS, et al. Antitumour activity of MDV3100 in castration-resistant prostate cancer: a phase 1-2 study. Lancet 2010;375:1437–46.

10. Chen Y, Sawyers CL, Scher HI. Targeting the androgen receptor pathway in prostate cancer. Curr Opin Pharmacol 2008;8:440–8.

11. Klotz L. Maximal androgen blockade for advanced prostate cancer. Best practice & research. Clin Endocrinol Metab 2008;22:331–40.

12. Knudsen KE, Scher HI. Starving the addiction: new opportunities for durable suppression of AR signaling in prostate cancer. Clin Cancer Res 2009;15:4792–8.

13. Loblaw DA, Virgo KS, Nam R, et al. Initial hormonal management of androgen-sensitive metastatic, recurrent, or progressive prostate cancer: 2006 update of an American Society of Clinical Oncology practice guideline. J Clin Oncol 2007;25:1596–605.

14. Taplin ME. Drug insight: role of the androgen receptor in the development and progression of prostate cancer. Nat Clin Pract Oncol 2007;4:236–44.

15. Yuan X, Balk SP. Mechanisms mediating androgen receptor reactivation after castration. Urol Oncol 2009;27:36–41.

16. Antonarakis ES, Armstrong AJ. Emerging therapeutic approaches in the management of metastatic castration-resistant prostate cancer. Prostate Cancer Prostatic Dis 2011;14:206–18.

17. Pezaro C, Attard G. Prostate cancer in 2011: redefining the therapeutic landscape for CRPC. Nat Rev Urol 2012;9:63–4.

18. Mukherji D, Eichholz A, De Bono JS. Management of metastatic castration-resistant prostate cancer: recent advances. Drugs 2012;72:1011–28.

19. Davies AH, Beltran H, Zoubeidi A. Cellular plasticity and the neuroendocrine phenotype in prostate cancer. Nat Rev Urol 2018;15:271–86.

20. Knudsen KE, Penning TM. Partners in crime: deregulation of AR activity and androgen synthesis in prostate cancer. Trends Endocrinol Metab 2010; 21:315–24.

21. Schiewer MJ, Augello MA, Knudsen KE. The AR dependent cell cycle: mechanisms and cancer relevance. Mol Cell Endocrinol 2012;352:34–45.

22. Marshall CH, Antonarakis ES. Emerging treatments for metastatic castration-resistant prostate cancer: Immunotherapy, PARP inhibitors, and PSMA-targeted approaches. Cancer Treat Res Commun 2020;23:100164.

23. Giri VN, Hyatt C, Gomella LG. Germline testing for men with prostate cancer: navigating an expanding new world of genetic evaluation for precision therapy and precision management. J Clin Oncol 2019;37:1455–9.

24. Cheng H, Powers J, Schaffer K, et al. Practical methods for integrating genetic testing into clinical practice for advanced prostate cancer. Am Soc Clin Oncol Educ Book 2018;38:372–81.

25. Giri VN, Knudsen KE, Kelly WK, et al. Implementation of germline testing for prostate cancer: philadelphia prostate cancer consensus conference 2019. J Clin Oncol 2020;38:2798–811.

26. Morgans AK, Szymaniak BM. Genetically-informed treatment for advanced and metastatic prostate cancer. Can J Urol 2019;26:54–6.

27. Antonarakis ES, Gomella LG, Petrylak DP. When and how to use PARP inhibitors in prostate cancer: a systematic review of the literature with an update on on-going trials. Eur Urol Oncol 2020; 3:594–611.

28. Mucci LA, Hjelmborg JB, Harris JR, et al. Familial risk and heritability of cancer among twins in nordic countries. JAMA 2016;315:68–76.

29. Robinson D, Van Allen EM, Wu YM, et al. Integrative clinical genomics of advanced prostate cancer. Cell 2015;162:454.

30. Pritchard CC, Mateo J, Walsh MF, et al. Inherited DNA-repair gene mutations in men with metastatic prostate cancer. N Engl J Med 2016;375: 443–53.

31. Mateo J, Carreira S, Sandhu S, et al. DNA-repair defects and olaparib in metastatic prostate cancer. N Engl J Med 2015;373:1697–708.

32. Sartor O, Yang S, Ledet E, et al. Inherited DNA-repair gene mutations in African American men with prostate cancer. Oncotarget 2020;11:440–2.

33. Estebanez-Perpina E, Bevan CL, McEwan IJ. Eighty years of targeting androgen receptor activity in prostate cancer: the fight goes on. Cancers (Basel) 2021;13:509.

34. Linja MJ, Savinainen KJ, Saramäki OR, et al. Amplification and overexpression of androgen receptor gene in hormone-refractory prostate cancer. Cancer Res 2001;61:3550–5.

35. Han G, Buchanan G, Ittmann M, et al. Mutation of the androgen receptor causes oncogenic transformation of the prostate. Proc Natl Acad Sci U S A 2005;102:1151–6.

36. Arora VK, Schenkein E, Murali R, et al. Glucocorticoid receptor confers resistance to antiandrogens by bypassing androgen receptor blockade. Cell 2013;155:1309–22.

37. Paschalis A, Sharp A, Welti JC, et al. Alternative splicing in prostate cancer. Nat Rev Clin Oncol 2018;15:663–75.

38. Antonarakis ES, Armstrong AJ, Dehm SM, et al. J. Androgen receptor variant-driven prostate cancer: clinical implications and therapeutic targeting. Prostate Cancer Prostatic Dis 2016;19:231–41.

39. Senapati D, Kumari S, Heemers HV. Androgen receptor co-regulation in prostate cancer. Asian J Urol 2020;7:219–32.

40. Dai C, Heemers H, Sharifi N. Androgen Signaling in Prostate Cancer. Cold Spring Harb Perspect Med 2017;7.

41. Burkhart DL, Morel KL, Sheahan AV, et al. The Role of RB in Prostate Cancer Progression. Adv Exp Med Biol 2019;1210:301–18.

42. Tan HL, Sood A, Rahimi HA, et al. Rb loss is characteristic of prostatic small cell neuroendocrine carcinoma. Clin Cancer Res 2014;20:890–903.

43. Chen WS, Alshalalfa M, Zhao SG, et al. Novel RB1-loss transcriptomic signature is associated with poor clinical outcomes across cancer types. Clin Cancer Res 2019;25:4290–9.

44. Sharma A, Comstock CE, Knudsen ES, et al. Retinoblastoma tumor suppressor status is a critical determinant of therapeutic response in prostate cancer cells. Cancer Res 2007;67:6192–203.

45. Sharma A, Yeow WS, Ertel A, et al. The retinoblastoma tumor suppressor controls androgen signaling and human prostate cancer progression. J Clin Invest 2010;120:4478–92.

46. McNair C, Xu K, Mandigo AC, et al. Differential impact of RB status on E2F1 reprogramming in human cancer. J Clin Invest 2018;128:341–58.

47. Mu P, Zhang Z, Benelli M, et al. SOX2 promotes lineage plasticity and antiandrogen resistance in TP53- and RB1-deficient prostate cancer. Science 2017;355:84–8.

48. Ku SY, Rosario S, Wang Y, et al. Rb1 and Trp53 cooperate to suppress prostate cancer lineage plasticity, metastasis, and antiandrogen resistance. Science 2017;355:78–83.

49. Grabowska MM, DeGraff DJ, Yu X, et al. Mouse models of prostate cancer: picking the best model for the question. Cancer Metastasis Rev 2014;33:377–97.

50. Berman-Booty LD, Knudsen KE. Models of neuroendocrine prostate cancer. Endocr Relat Cancer 2015;22:R33–49.

51. Hamid AA, Gray KP, Shaw G, et al. Compound genomic alterations of TP53, PTEN, and RB1 tumor suppressors in localized and metastatic prostate cancer. Eur Urol 2019;76:89–97.

52. Chakraborty G, Armenia J, Mazzu YZ, et al. Significance of BRCA2 and RB1 Co-loss in Aggressive Prostate Cancer Progression. Clin Cancer Res 2020;26:2047–64.

53. Mandigo AC, Knudsen KE. Double trouble: concomitant RB1 and BRCA2 depletion evokes aggressive phenotypes. Clin Cancer Res 2020; 26:1784–6.

54. Quintanal-Villalonga A, Chan JM, Yu HA, et al. Lineage plasticity in cancer: a shared pathway of therapeutic resistance. Nat Rev Clin Oncol 2020;17: 360–71.

55. Yamada Y, Beltran H. Clinical and biological features of neuroendocrine prostate cancer. Curr Oncol Rep 2021;23:15.

56. Beltran H, Hruszkewycz A, Scher HI, et al. The role of lineage plasticity in prostate cancer therapy resistance. Clin Cancer Res 2019;25:6916–24.

57. Beltran H, Rickman DS, Park K, et al. Molecular characterization of neuroendocrine prostate cancer and identification of new drug targets. Cancer Discov 2011;1:487–95.

58. Aparicio AM, Shen L, Tapia EL, et al. Combined tumor suppressor defects characterize clinically defined aggressive variant prostate cancers. Clin Cancer Res 2016;22:1520–30.

59. Berchuck JE, Viscuse PV, Beltran H, et al. Clinical considerations for the management of androgen indifferent prostate cancer. Prostate Cancer Prostatic Dis 2021. https://doi.org/10.1038/s41391-021-00332-5.

60. Dicken H, Hensley PJ, Kyprianou N. Prostate tumor neuroendocrine differentiation via EMT: The road less traveled. Asian J Urol 2019;6:82–90.

61. Tiwari R, Manzar N, Ateeq B. Dynamics of cellular plasticity in prostate cancer progression. Front Mol Biosci 2020;7:130.

62. Bishop JL, Thaper D, Vahid S, et al. The master neural transcription factor BRN2 is an androgen receptor-suppressed driver of neuroendocrine differentiation in prostate cancer. Cancer Discov 2017;7:54–71.

63. Dardenne E, Beltran H, Benelli M, et al. N-Myc induces an EZH2-mediated transcriptional program driving neuroendocrine prostate cancer. Cancer Cell 2016;30:563–77.

64. Davies A, Zoubeidi A, Selth LA. The epigenetic and transcriptional landscape of neuroendocrine prostate cancer. Endocr Relat Cancer 2020;27: R35–50.

65. Akamatsu S, Wyatt AW, Lin D, et al. The placental gene PEG10 promotes progression of neuroendocrine prostate cancer. Cell Rep 2015;12:922–36.

66. Kim S, Thaper D, Bidnur S, et al. PEG10 is associated with treatment-induced neuroendocrine prostate cancer. J Mol Endocrinol 2019;63:39–49.

67. Brennen WN, Zhu Y, Coleman IM, et al. Resistance to androgen receptor signaling inhibition does not necessitate development of neuroendocrine prostate cancer. JCI Insight 2021;6(8):146827.

68. Beltran H, Oromendia C, Danila DC, et al. A phase II trial of the aurora kinase a inhibitor alisertib for patients with castration- resistant and neuroendocrine prostate cancer: efficacy and biomarkers. Clin Cancer Res 2019;25:43–51.

69. Zhang W, Liu B, Wu W, et al. Targeting the MYCN-PARP-DNA damage response pathway in neuroendocrine prostate cancer. Clin Cancer Res 2018;24: 696–707.

70. Kwon OJ, Zhang L, Jia D, et al. De novo induction of lineage plasticity from human prostate luminal epithelial cells by activated AKT1 and c-Myc. Oncogene 2020;39:7142–51.

71. Tiwari R, Manzar N, Bhatia V, et al. Androgen deprivation upregulates SPINK1 expression and

potentiates cellular plasticity in prostate cancer. Nat Commun 2020;11:384.

72. Yasumizu Y, Rajabi H, Jin C, et al. MUC1-C regulates lineage plasticity driving progression to neuroendocrine prostate cancer. Nat Commun 2020;11:338.

73. Quaglia F, Krishn SR, Wang Y, et al. Differential expression of alphaVbeta3 and alphaVbeta6 integrins in prostate cancer progression. PLoS One 2021;16:e0244985.

74. Quaglia F, Krishn SR, Daaboul GG, et al. Small extracellular vesicles modulated by alphaVbeta3 integrin induce neuroendocrine differentiation in recipient cancer cells. J Extracell Vesicles 2020;9: 1761072.

75. Fernandes RC, Toubia J, Townley S, et al. Post-transcriptional gene regulation by microrna-194 promotes neuroendocrine transdifferentiation in prostate cancer. Cell Rep 2021;34:108585.

76. Domingo-Domenech J, Vidal SJ, Rodriguez-Bravo V, et al. Suppression of acquired docetaxel resistance in prostate cancer through depletion of notch- and hedgehog-dependent tumor-initiating cells. Cancer Cell 2012;22:373–88.

77. Vidal SJ, Rodriguez-Bravo V, Quinn SA, et al. A targetable GATA2-IGF2 axis confers aggressiveness in lethal prostate cancer. Cancer Cell 2015; 27:223–39.

78. Cyrta J, Augspach A, De Filippo MR, et al. Role of specialized composition of SWI/SNF complexes in prostate cancer lineage plasticity. Nat Commun 2020;11:5549.

79. Wu Y, Yu H, Li S, et al. Rare Germline pathogenic mutations of DNA repair genes are most strongly associated with grade group 5 prostate cancer. Eur Urol Oncol 2020;3:224–30.

80. Kaur H, Salles DC, Murali S, et al. Genomic and clinicopathologic characterization of ATM-deficient prostate cancer. Clin Cancer Res 2020; 26:4869–81.

81. Isaacsson Velho P, Silberstein JL, Markowski MC, et al. Intraductal/ductal histology and lymphovascular invasion are associated with germline DNA-repair gene mutations in prostate cancer. Prostate 2018;78:401–7.

82. Carter HB, Helfand B, Mamawala M, et al. Germline mutations in ATM and BRCA1/2 are associated with grade reclassification in men on active surveillance for prostate cancer. Eur Urol 2019;75:743–9.

83. Nguyen-Dumont T, MacInnis RJ, Steen JA, et al. Rare germline genetic variants and risk of aggressive prostate cancer. Int J Cancer 2020;147: 2142–9.

84. Darst BF, Dadaev T, Saunders E, et al. Germline sequencing DNA repair genes in 5,545 men with aggressive and non- aggressive prostate cancer. J Natl Cancer Inst 2020. https://doi.org/10.1093/jnci/djaa132.

85. Mijuskovic M, Saunders EJ, Leongamornlert DA, et al. Rare germline variants in DNA repair genes and the angiogenesis pathway predispose prostate cancer patients to develop metastatic disease. Br J Cancer 2018;119:96–104.

86. Na R, Zheng SL, Han M, et al. Germline mutations in ATM and BRCA1/2 distinguish risk for lethal and indolent prostate cancer and are associated with early age at death. Eur Urol 2017;71:740–7.

87. Antonarakis ES, Lu C, Luber B, et al. Germline DNA-repair gene mutations and outcomes in men with metastatic castration-resistant prostate cancer receiving first-line abiraterone and enzalutamide. Eur Urol 2018;74:218–25.

88. Mota JM, Barnett E, Nauseef JT, et al. Platinum-based chemotherapy in metastatic prostate cancer with DNA repair gene alterations. JCO Precis Oncol 2020;4:355–66.

89. Zafeiriou Z, Bianchini D, Chandler R, et al. Genomic analysis of three metastatic prostate cancer patients with exceptional responses to carboplatin indicating different types of DNA repair deficiency. Eur Urol 2019;75:184–92.

90. Isaacsson Velho P, Qazi F, Hassan S, et al. Efficacy of radium-223 in bone-metastatic castration-resistant prostate cancer with and without homologous repair gene defects. Eur Urol 2019;76:170–6.

91. van der Doelen MJ, Velho PI, Slootbeek PHJ, et al. Impact of DNA damage repair defects on response to radium-223 and overall survival in metastatic castration-resistant prostate cancer. Eur J Cancer 2020;136:16–24.

92. Marshall CH, Sokolova AO, McNatty AL, et al. Differential response to olaparib treatment among men with metastatic castration-resistant prostate cancer harboring BRCA1 or BRCA2 Versus ATM Mutations. Eur Urol 2019;76:452–8.

93. Abida W, Campbell D, Patnaik A, et al. Non-BRCA DNA damage repair gene alterations and response to the PARP Inhibitor rucaparib in metastatic castration-resistant prostate cancer: analysis from the Phase II TRITON2 Study. Clin Cancer Res 2020;26:2487–96.

94. Harris BRE, Zhang Y, Tao J, et al. ATM inhibitor KU-55933 induces apoptosis and inhibits motility by blocking GLUT1- mediated glucose uptake in aggressive cancer cells with sustained activation of Akt. FASEB J 2021;35:e21264.

95. Xu L, Ma E, Zeng T, et al. ATM deficiency promotes progression of CRPC by enhancing Warburg effect. Endocr Relat Cancer 2019;26:59–71.

96. Mersch J, Jackson M, Park M, et al. Cancers associated with BRCA1 and BRCA2 mutations other than breast and ovarian. Cancer 2015;121:269–75.

97. Chandrasekar T, Gross L, Gomella LG, et al. Prevalence of Suspected Hereditary Cancer Syndromes and Germline Mutations Among a Diverse Cohort of Probands Reporting a Family History of Prostate Cancer: Toward Informing Cascade Testing for Men. Eur Urol Oncol 2020;3:291–7.

98. Castro E, Goh C, Olmos D, et al. Germline BRCA mutations are associated with higher risk of nodal involvement, distant metastasis, and poor survival outcomes in prostate cancer. J Clin Oncol 2013; 31:1748–57.

99. Gallagher DJ, Gaudet MM, Pal P, et al. Germline BRCA mutations denote a clinicopathologic subset of prostate cancer. Clin Cancer Res 2010;16: 2115–21.

100. Castro E, Goh C, Leongamornlert D, et al. Effect of BRCA mutations on metastatic relapse and cause-specific survival after radical treatment for localised prostate cancer. Eur Urol 2015;68:186–93.

101. Nyberg T, Frost D, Barrowdale D, et al. Prostate Cancer Risks for Male BRCA1 and BRCA2 Mutation Carriers: A Prospective Cohort Study. Eur Urol 2020;77:24–35.

102. Castro E, Romero-Laorden N, Del Pozo A, et al. PROREPAIR-B: a prospective cohort study of the impact of germline DNA repair mutations on the outcomes of patients with metastatic castration-resistant prostate cancer. J Clin Oncol 2019;37: 490–503.

103. Akbari MR, Wallis CJD, Toi A, et al. The impact of a BRCA2 mutation on mortality from screen-detected prostate cancer. Br J Cancer 2014;111:1238–40.

104. Edwards SM, Cunningham SA, Dunlop AL, et al. Prostate cancer in BRCA2 germline mutation carriers is associated with poorer prognosis. Br J Cancer 2010;103:918–24.

105. Thorne H, Willems AJ, Niedermayr E, et al. Decreased prostate cancer-specific survival of men with BRCA2 mutations from multiple breast cancer families. Cancer Prev Res (Phila) 2011;4: 1002–10.

106. Tryggvadóttir L, Vidarsdóttir L, Thorgeirsson T, et al. Prostate cancer progression and survival in BRCA2 mutation carriers. J Natl Cancer Inst 2007;99:929–35.

107. Nyberg T, Frost D, Barrowdale D, et al. Prostate cancer risk by BRCA2 genomic regions. Eur Urol 2020;78:494–7.

108. Cheng HH, Pritchard CC, Boyd T, et al. Biallelic inactivation of brca2 in platinum-sensitive metastatic castration-resistant prostate cancer. Eur Urol 2016;69:992–5.

109. Mateo J, Porta N, Bianchini D, et al. Olaparib in patients with metastatic castration-resistant prostate cancer with DNA repair gene aberrations (TOPARP-B): a multicentre, open-label, randomised, phase 2 trial. Lancet Oncol 2020;21: 162–74.

110. Abida W, Patnaik A, Campbell D, et al. Rucaparib in men with metastatic castration-resistant prostate cancer harboring a BRCA1 or BRCA2 gene alteration. J Clin Oncol 2020;38(32):3763–72.

111. Clarke N, Wiechno P, Alekseev B, et al. Olaparib combined with abiraterone in patients with metastatic castration-resistant prostate cancer: a randomised, double-blind, placebo-controlled, phase 2 trial. Lancet Oncol 2018;19:975–86.

112. Schiewer MJ, Mandigo AC, Gordon N, et al. PARP-1 regulates DNA repair factor availability. EMBO Mol Med 2018;10:e8816.

113. Mainetti LE, Zhe X, Diedrich J, et al. Bone-induced c-kit expression in prostate cancer: a driver of intra-osseous tumor growth. Int J Cancer 2015;136: 11–20.

114. Moro L, Arbini AA, Yao JL, et al. Loss of BRCA2 promotes prostate cancer cell invasion through up-regulation of matrix metalloproteinase-9. Cancer Sci 2008;99:553–63.

115. Risbridger GP, Taylor RA, Clouston D, et al. Patient-derived xenografts reveal that intraductal carcinoma of the prostate is a prominent pathology in BRCA2 mutation carriers with prostate cancer and correlates with poor prognosis. Eur Urol 2015;67:496–503.

116. Porter LH, Hashimoto K, Lawrence MG, et al. Intraductal carcinoma of the prostate can evade androgen deprivation, with emergence of castrate-tolerant cells. BJU Int 2018;121:971–8.

117. Goodwin JF, Schiewer MJ, Dean JL, et al. A hormone-DNA repair circuit governs the response to genotoxic insult. Cancer Discov 2013;3:1254–71.

118. Polkinghorn WR, Parker JS, Lee MX, et al. Androgen receptor signaling regulates DNA repair in prostate cancers. Cancer Discov 2013;3: 1245–53.

119. Schiewer MJ, Goodwin JF, Han S, et al. Dual roles of PARP-1 promote cancer growth and progression. Cancer Discov 2012;2:1134–49.

120. Schiewer MJ, Knudsen KE. Linking DNA Damage and Hormone Signaling Pathways in Cancer. Trends Endocrinol Metab 2016;27:216–25.

121. Annala M, Struss WJ, Warner EW, et al. Treatment outcomes and tumor loss of heterozygosity in germline DNA repair- deficient prostate cancer. Eur Urol 2017;72:34–42.

122. Mateo J, Cheng HH, Beltran H, et al. Clinical outcome of prostate cancer patients with germline DNA repair mutations: retrospective analysis from an international study. Eur Urol 2018;73:687–93.

Genetic Contribution to Metastatic Prostate Cancer

Alexandra O. Sokolova, MD[a,b,c], Elias I. Obeid, MD, MPH[d], Heather H. Cheng, MD, PhD[a,b],*

KEYWORDS

- Metastatic prostate cancer • Genetic testing • Germline • *BRCA2*

KEY POINTS

- Up to 12% of men with metastatic prostate cancer carry an actionable pathogenic germline mutation in DNA damage repair genes, most frequently *BRCA2*, *ATM*, *CHEK2*, and *BRCA1*.
- Germline *BRCA2* mutations are associated with increased risk of prostate cancer and worse prostate cancer outcomes.
- The poly-(ADP-ribose) polymerase inhibitors olaparib and rucaparib have received US Food and Drug Administration approval for metastatic prostate cancer with DNA damage repair alterations.
- Platinum chemotherapy has also been reported to be effective among men with DNA damage repair alterations.

INTRODUCTION

Prostate cancer is well recognized to have a strong heritable component, but incorporation of genetic testing for germline pathogenic and likely pathogenic variants (hereafter referred to as mutations) in DNA repair genes has recently increased and is becoming more widespread (**Tables 1** and **2**). Several landmark studies have recently led to a dramatic shift in understanding and clinical practice, particularly in the setting of metastatic prostate cancer because of treatment implications. These same germline mutations in DNA repair genes may represent known or suspected autosomal dominant inherited cancer risk genes, the most notable of which is *BRCA2*. This article focuses on the current knowledge of germline (also known as inherited) genetic contributions to metastatic prostate cancer. Other articles in this issue review in greater depth the topics of therapeutic implications (including in earlier disease states), opportunities in screening and early detection of prostate cancer, genetic predisposition syndromes, multigene testing, and polygenic risk scores.

PROSTATE CANCER HAS A STRONG HERITABLE COMPONENT

Approximately 57% of prostate cancer risk can be attributable to genetic factors, based on long-term follow-up from the Norwegian Twin Cancer study, comparing monozygotic and dizygotic twin pairs.[1,2] In the Prostate Cancer Database Sweden (PCBaSe), the overall risk of developing prostate cancer for men with a brother with prostate cancer by the age 65 years was 14.9%, compared with 4.8% in men without a brother with prostate cancer, and the risk was 30.3% versus 12.9% at age 75 years. This observation held, even after exclusion of low-risk prostate cancer.[3]

EARLY SEQUENCING DISCOVERIES IN PROSTATE METASTASES INVOLVE DNA REPAIR GENES

Before 2015, understanding about molecular features of prostate cancer tumors came largely from prostatectomies and biopsies because archival tumor material due to clinical acquisition for diagnostic or treatment purposes. With the

[a] Department of Medicine (Div. Oncology), University of Washington, Seattle, WA, USA; [b] Clinical Research Division, Fred Hutchinson Cancer Research Center, Seattle, WA, USA; [c] VA Puget Sound Health Care System, Seattle, WA, USA; [d] Fox Chase Cancer Center, Philadelphia, PA, USA
* Corresponding author. 825 Eastlake Avenue East, Seattle, WA 98109.
E-mail address: hhcheng@uw.edu
Twitter: @HEATHERHCHENG (H.H.C.)

Urol Clin N Am 48 (2021) 349–363
https://doi.org/10.1016/j.ucl.2021.03.005

Table 1
Genes with current and potential clinical actionability

Gene	Association with ↑ PC Risk	Prevalence of Germline Mutations in Metastatic PC (%)	Prevalence of Germline Mutations in PC with Family History(%)	DNA Damaging Agents: PARP Inhibitors, Platinum[b]	Immune Checkpoint Inhibitors: PD-1 Inhibitors
ATM	X	1.6	2.0	XX	—
ATR	—	0.3	Not evaluated	—	—
BARD1	—	Not evaluated	Not evaluated	XX	—
BRCA1	X	0.9	0.7	XXX	—
BRCA2	X	5.4	4.7	XXXX	—
BRIP1	—	0.2	0.3	XX	—
CDK12 (somatic only)	—	—	Not evaluated	XX	X
CHEK1	—	Not evaluated	Not evaluated	XX	—
CHEK2	X	1.9	2.9	XX	—
FAM175A	—	0.2	Not evaluated	—	—
FANCA	—	—	Not evaluated	X	—
FANCL	—	Not evaluated	Not evaluated	XX	—
HOXB13 (germline only)	X	Not evaluated	1.1	—	—
MLH1	X	—	0.06	—	X
MRE11A	—	0.14	Not evaluated	—	—
MSH2	X	0.14	0.69	—	X
MSH6	X	0.14	0.45	—	X
NBN	—[a]	0.3	0.32	XX	—
PALB2	—[a]	0.4	0.56	XX	—
PMS2	X	0.3	0.54	—	X
RAD51B	—	Not evaluated	Not evaluated	XX	—
RAD51C	—	0.14	0.21	XX	—
RAD51D	—	0.4	0.15	XX	—
RAD54L	—	Not evaluated	Not evaluated	XX	—

Abbreviations: PARP, poly-(ADP-ribose) polymerase; PC, prostate cancer; PD-1 programmed cell death protein 1.
[a] Emerging/limited data.
[b] XX designation follows US Food and Drug Administration approval based on ProFOUND (Phase 3 Study of Olaparib vs. Enzalutamide or Abiraterone for Metastatic Castration-Resistant Prostate Cancer with Homologous Recombination Repair Gene Alterations) study.

Data from Cheng, H. H., Sokolova, A. O., Schaeffer, E. M., Small, E. J. & Higano, C. S. Germline and Somatic Mutations in Prostate Cancer for the Clinician. J. Natl. Compr. Cancer Netw. JNCCN 17, 515–521 (2019).

exception of a few select rapid autopsy research programs, metastatic prostate cancer tumors were largely uncharacterized until an international, multi-institutional study to obtain metastatic biopsies and characterize mutational spectra was made possible by Stand Up 2 Cancer (SU2C) and the Prostate Cancer Foundation. Results from the first 150 metastatic biopsies were reported in 2015 and identified a high proportion of actionable mutations, including 23% with mutations and other alterations in DNA repair genes such as BRCA2, ATM, and BRCA1.[4] Mounting evidence also supported that prostate cancers with BRCA2 inactivation were sensitive to platinum chemotherapy,[5,6] and the phase II trial of PARP inhibition in prostate cancer (TOPARP-A) study reported early compelling evidence from a limited number of patients that poly-(ADP-ribose)

Table 2
Selected therapeutic clinical trials in earlier stages prostate cancer with relevance to germline genetics

Phase	Title	Disease State	Trial Name	Clinicaltrials.gov
II	Olaparib Prior to Radical Prostatectomy For Patients With Locally Advanced Prostate Cancer and Defects in DNA Repair Genes	Localized disease	BrUOG 337	NCT03432897
I/II	A Multi-Center Trial of Androgen Suppression With Abiraterone Acetate, Leuprolide, PARP Inhibition and Stereotactic Body Radiotherapy in Prostate Cancer	Localized disease	ASCLEPIuS	NCT04194554
II	Niraparib Before Surgery in Treating Patients With High Risk Localized Prostate Cancer and DNA Damage Response Defects	Localized disease	—	NCT04030559
II	Olaparib in Men With High-Risk Biochemically-Recurrent Prostate Cancer Following Radical Prostatectomy, With Integrated Biomarker Analysis	BCR	—	NCT03047135
II	A Study of Olaparib and Durvalumab in Prostate Cancer	BCR	—	NCT03810105
II	Durvalumab and Olaparib for the Treatment of Prostate Cancer in Men Predicted to Have a High Neoantigen Load	BCR	—	NCT04336943
II	Rucaparib in Nonmetastatic Prostate With BRCAness	BCR	ROAR	NCT03533946
II	Trial of Rucaparib in Patients With Metastatic Hormone-Sensitive Prostate Cancer Harboring Germline DNA Repair Gene Mutations	mCSPC	TRIUMPH	NCT03413995
II	Enzalutamide Plus Talazoparib for the Treatment of Hormone Sensitive Prostate Cancer	mCSPC	ZZ-First	NCT04332744
III	A Study of Niraparib in Combination With Abiraterone Acetate and Prednisone Versus Abiraterone Acetate and Prednisone for the Treatment of Participants With Deleterious Germline or Somatic Homologous Recombination Repair (HRR) Gene-Mutated Metastatic Castration-Sensitive Prostate Cancer	mCSPC	AMPLITUDE	NCT04497844

(continued on next page)

Table 2
(continued)

Phase	Title	Disease State	Trial Name	Clinicaltrials.gov
II	Abiraterone/Prednisone, Olaparib, or Abiraterone/ Prednisone + Olaparib in Patients With Metastatic Castration-Resistant Prostate Cancer With DNA Repair Defects	First-line mCRPC	BRCAaway	NCT03012321
III	A Study of Niraparib in Combination With Abiraterone Acetate and Prednisone Versus Abiraterone Acetate and Prednisone for Treatment of Participants With Metastatic Prostate Cancer	First-line mCRPC	MAGNITUDE	NCT03748641

Abbreviations: BCR, biochemical recurrence; mCRPC, metastatic castration-resistant prostate cancer; mCSPC, metastatic castration-sensitive prostate cancer.

polymerase (PARP) inhibitors, such as olaparib, held tantalizing promise for metastatic castration-resistant prostate cancers (mCRPCs) harboring defects in genes involved in homologous recombination DNA repair (*BRCA2, ATM, CHEK2, PALB2,* and others).[7] Notably, about half of the patients with DNA repair mutations in these early studies had a germline component, representing known or suspected autosomal dominant cancer predisposition syndromes. In addition, the prevalence in the population of men with metastatic disease was much higher than previously recognized.

GERMLINE DNA REPAIR GENE MUTATIONS ENRICHED IN THE POPULATION OF PATIENTS WITH METASTATIC PROSTATE CANCER

In 2016, a definitive study of 692 men with metastatic prostate cancer was conducted with targeted germline sequencing. Importantly, the men were unselected for family history or age at diagnosis. Remarkably, 11.8% (82 out of 692) had germline mutations in DNA repair genes, most frequently *BRCA2, ATM, CHEK2,* and *BRCA1.*[8] Moreover, the presence of a germline variant (mutation) that inactivated DNA repair gene function was not correlated with either family history of prostate cancer (although there was a trend toward this) or with age at diagnosis. In the patients where tumors were available for sequencing, 67% (36 out of 61) had evidence of second allele inactivation, supporting that germline alterations were biologically relevant rather than simply bystanders. That the proportion of men with metastatic prostate cancer carrying germline mutations exceeded 10%, and was far higher than previously thought, justified consideration of genetic testing for all men with metastatic prostate cancer. These findings have been borne out in other studies with similar prevalence in various mCRPC cohorts, such as 16.2% (Spain), 12% (United States), and 7.5% (Canada),[9–12] and seem to be similar in the metastatic hormone-sensitive population: 9.4% prevalence in metastatic hormone-sensitive prostate cancer plus mCRPC in the study by Yadav and colleagues.[12]

These data, together with important treatment relevance to newly US Food and Drug Administration (FDA)–approved PARP inhibitors (discussed later and elsewhere in this issue), have led to major changes in the National Comprehensive Cancer Network (NCCN) prostate cancer guidelines for recommending genetic testing for inherited cancer risk mutations in all men with metastatic disease.[5]

Note that the prevalence in high-risk localized populations has also been determined to be greater than 5% and has led to the inclusion of men with high-risk localized disease, node-positive disease, and certain histologies (intraductal, cribriform, ductal; discussed further later)[13,14] to also be offered germline genetic testing in the guidelines.[5]

DNA REPAIR GENES: FROM PATHWAYS TO INDIVIDUAL GENES

There is great interest and enthusiasm in identifying, understanding, and improving the care for men with germline mutations in DNA repair genes. However, although collectively there is a group of genes involved in the critical biological processes of repairing errors and defects during DNA replication, the current understanding of individual genes is variable between the genes and ranges from more evidence to scant. The evidence for individual key genes of interest and for increased prostate cancer risk and enrichment in the metastatic disease setting are reviewed next, beginning with a discussion about BRCA2, for which there is greater existing literature and numbers about the increased risk of prostate cancer for germline BRCA2 mutation carriers, most of which comes from ascertainment by female relatives with breast and ovarian cancer.

EVIDENCE FOR INCREASED PROSTATE CANCER RISK AND LETHALITY AMONG MALE BRCA2 MUTATION CARRIERS

Several studies report evidence that men with germline BRCA2 mutations have increased risk of prostate cancer. For example, a study of the Icelandic BRCA2 founder mutation 999del5 showed that men presented with higher-risk disease at a younger age and had an increased risk of death from prostate cancer.[15] Specifically, they were found to present at a younger age at diagnosis (69 years vs 74 years; P = .002), more advanced tumor stage (stages 3–4; 79% vs 39%; P<.001), higher tumor grade (grades G3–G4; 84% vs 53%; P = .007), and shorter median survival time (2.1 years, 95% confidence interval CI = 1.4–3.6 years; vs 12.4 years, 95% CI = 9.9–19.7 years).[15] BRCA2 999del5 mutation carriers also had an increased risk of prostate cancer–specific mortality, even after adjusting for year of diagnosis, age, and stage.[15]

In another study by Gallagher and colleagues,[16] BRCA2 mutations were associated with a 3-fold increased risk of prostate cancer and higher Gleason score. As with the Icelandic study, after adjusting for clinical stage, prostate-specific antigen (PSA), Gleason score, and treatment, BRCA2 and BRCA1 mutation carriers had a higher risk of prostate cancer recurrence (hazard ratio [HR] [95% CI], 2.4 [1.2–4.8] and 4.3 [1.3–13.6], respectively) and prostate cancer–specific death (HR [95% CI], 5.5 [2.0–14.8] and 5.2 [1.1–24.5], respectively) than their noncarrier counterparts.[16]

A UK study by Castro and colleagues[17] reported similar findings that men with prostate cancer and germline BRCA2 and BRCA1 mutations were more frequently associated with Gleason score greater than or equal to 8 (P = .00003), T3/T4 stage (P = .003), nodal involvement (P = .00005), and metastases at diagnosis (P = .005) than their noncarrier counterparts. Prostate cancer–specific survival (CSS) was also significantly shorter for carriers compared with noncarriers (8.6 vs 15.7 years,

multivariable analyses [MVAs] P = .015; HR, 1.8). Subgroup analyses confirmed poor outcomes in BRCA2 patients, whereas findings for BRCA1 were less well defined because of limited size and follow-up.[18] In a follow-up study, the same group reported on prostate cancer metastasis-free outcomes in 67 BRCA1/2 carriers and 1235 noncarriers at 3, 5, and 10 years after definitive treatment: 90%, 72%, and 50% of carriers and 97%, 94%, and 84% of noncarriers were free from metastasis (P<.001).[17] The 3-year, 5-year, and 10-year CSS rates were significantly worse in carriers (96%, 76%, and 61%, respectively) than the noncarrier cohort (99%, 97%, and 85%, respectively; P<.001). Multivariate analysis confirmed BRCA1/2 mutations as an independent prognostic factor for metastasis-free survival (HR, 2.36; 95% CI, 1.38 to 4.03; P = .002) and CSS (HR, 2.17; 95% CI, 1.16–4.07; P = .016).[17]

Another larger, retrospective cohort study of 6902 men from the Consortium of Investigators of Modifiers of BRCA1/2 (CIMBA) also reported an increased risk of prostate cancer, greater in men carrying BRCA2 mutations compared with those carrying BRCA1 mutations.[19] A higher frequency of prostate cancers was associated with a higher probability of being a BRCA2 pathogenic variant carrier (odds ratio [OR], 1.39; 95% CI, 1.09–1.78; P = .008).[19]

ASSOCIATION WITH HIGHER GRADE AND DISTINCT HISTOLOGIC SUBTYPES

Intraductal carcinoma of the prostate is a distinct histologic entity that represents retrograde spread of invasive acinar adenocarcinoma into prostatic acini and ducts with basal cell preservation. This histologic variant is associated with an aggressive clinical course, including an increased risk of biochemical recurrence, metastasis, and mortality. These histologic features of prostate cancer are also enriched for carrying driver mutations. For example, men with germline BRCA mutations are more likely to have intraductal features in their prostate cancer, which correlate with poor outcomes.[20]

In addition, several other pathologic features in addition to intraductal, such as ductal, lymphovascular invasion, cribriform pattern 4, and presence of Gleason grade group 5, have been reported to be enriched for presence of germline alterations.[21–23]

ASSOCIATION OF BRCA2 MUTATIONS WITH MORE AGGRESSIVE MOLECULAR SIGNATURES

Taylor and colleagues[14] profiled the genomes and methylomes of localized prostate cancers from 14 carriers of germline BRCA2 mutations/pathogenic variants to understand the more aggressive phenotype of these tumors. They showed that BRCA2-mutant prostate cancers show increased genomic instability and mutational profiles that more closely resemble metastatic prostate cancer compared with localized prostate cancer. They also observed genomic and epigenomic dysregulation of the MED12L/MED12 axis, which is frequently dysregulated in mCRPC. This dysregulation is enriched in BRCA2-mutant prostate cancer harboring intraductal carcinoma. This study shows that localized BRCA2-mutant tumors are uniquely aggressive, because of de novo aberration in genes commonly observed in metastatic disease and thus justifying aggressive initial treatment of BRCA2 carriers who develop prostate cancer.[14]

HOMOLOGOUS RECOMBINATION DNA REPAIR GENES AND EMERGING UNDERSTANDING OF GERMLINE MUTATIONS IN GENES BEYOND BRCA2

Germline BRCA2 alterations are the most commonly observed and the most reported in prostate cancer. BRCA2 alterations are associated with the highest prostate cancer risk, poor outcomes, and the best responses to platinum and PARP inhibitors. Even though non-BRCA2 DNA repair genes are also involved in homologous recombination repair pathway, alterations in these genes may have a very different biological relevance for prostate cancer and require further individual characterization. Key differences are already apparent in estimated cancer risk and targeted treatment sensitivity in germline carriers. Genes that are implicated because of over-representation in metastatic disease with biological plausibility are discussed later. Increasingly clear is that each warrants individual evaluation and attention. There are likely to be differences in risk of tumor initiation, disease-modifying factors, subsequent elective advantage, and contribution to metastatic potential. This topic demands further close investigation, and will require long-term follow-up and collaborative efforts.

BRCA1

Together with BRCA2, germline BRCA1 mutations have also been associated with increased risk of prostate cancer, aggressive disease, and response to DNA damaging agents. However, the strength of association with prostate cancer risk and apparent magnitude of risk is less compared with BRCA2. In many of the studies discussed earlier, the numbers of BRCA1 mutation carriers and prostate cancer–specific events were less pronounced or findings less conclusive compared with BRCA2. For example, in a large study by LeCarpentier and colleagues,[24] the prostate cancer risk by age 80 years at the fifth and 95th percentiles of the polygenic risk score varies from 7% to 26% for carriers of BRCA1 mutations and from 19% to 61% for carriers of BRCA2 mutations, respectively. However, there is still enrichment in the metastatic setting, and it would still be considered a gene mutation of interest with respect to prostate cancer risk as well as metastatic disease treatment implications.

ATM

Germline ATM pathogenic variants are more common in the general population but are enriched in the metastatic prostate cancer setting, the second most common alteration after BRCA2.[8] Early data on response to PARP inhibitors in the setting of ATM inactivation suggest substantial differences compared with BRCA2, which is not surprising because of different functions of BRCA2 and ATM proteins. This finding raises some uncertainty as to whether absence of ATM function contributes to cancer initiation or to metastatic potential.

A study by Na and colleagues[25] evaluated BRCA2, BRCA1, and ATM germline mutations in a retrospective case-case study of 799 men with prostate cancer, including 313 who died of prostate cancer and 486 of European, African, and Chinese descent with low-risk localized prostate cancer. The combined BRCA1/2 and ATM mutation carrier rate was higher in patients with lethal prostate cancer (6.1%) than patients with localized prostate cancer (1.4%; P = .0007). The rate also differed significantly among patients with lethal prostate cancer as a function of age at death. Survival analysis in the entire cohort revealed mutation carriers remained an independent predictor of lethal prostate cancer after adjusting for race, age, PSA, and Gleason score at diagnosis (HR, 2.13; 95% CI, 1.24–3.66; P = .004). Although ATM was included here, the study did not investigate other known DNA repair mutations beyond BRCA1/2 and ATM, and the number of men with ATM mutations was small.[25]

In a study by Wokołorczyk and colleagues,[26] mutations in ATM, NBN, and BRCA2 predisposed to aggressive prostate cancer in the Polish population. To investigate the frequency of mutations and estimate gene-related prostate cancer risks and probability of aggressive disease, 14 genes were studied by exome sequencing in 390 men with familial prostate cancer and 308 cancer-free controls. Of 390 patients with prostate cancer, 76 men (19.5%) carried a mutation in *BRCA1*, *BRCA2*, *NBN*, *ATM*, *CHEK2*, *HOXB13*, *MSH2*, or *MSH6* genes. Significant associations with familial prostate cancer risk were observed for *CHEK2*, *NBN*, *ATM*, and *HOXB13*. High-grade (Gleason 8–10) tumors were seen in 56% of *BRCA2*, *NBN*, or *ATM* carriers, compared with 21% of patients who tested negative for mutations in these genes (OR, 4.7; 95% CI, 2.0–10.7; P = .0003).[26]

PALB2

PALB2 mutations, such as *BRCA1* and *ATM* and the others discussed later, are considerably less commonly observed compared with *BRCA2*, but are of clear interest, in part because of knowledge from other related cancer risk settings, such as breast and ovarian cancers. There are very limited and conflicting data for germline *PALB2* and prostate cancer risk, although it is thought that historic cohorts must be viewed with caution given the ascertainment via female relatives with breast and ovarian cancers, as well as incomplete reporting of prostate cancer and frequent lack of distinction between diagnoses of very common low-grade prostate cancer (Gleason 6) versus high-grade (Gleason 8–10) and metastatic prostate cancer. Earlier studies have reported lack of clear association between *PALB2* and hereditary prostate cancer families with prostate cancer diagnoses younger than 55 years or multiple affected kindred.[27–29] However, germline *PALB2* mutations have been reported in association with aggressive prostate cancer, and *PALB2* reversion mutations have been associated with resistance to PARP inhibitors, arguing biological relevance.[30,31] Increased use of panel testing in men with metastatic and localized disease will likely lead to greater identification of men with germline *PALB2* mutations and the potential to reveal a different picture with more advanced prostate cancer–specific ascertainment. This discussion may apply for each of the rarer prostate cancer germline gene variants associated with metastatic disease discussed here.

CHEK2

Germline mutations in the Chek2 kinase gene (*CHEK2*) have been associated with increased prostate cancer risk. In Poland, extensive work and several studies led by Cybulski have reported that certain truncating founder mutations (*CHEK2* 1100delC and *CHEK2* IVS2 + 1G>A) are associated with a moderate risk of prostate cancer. *CHEK2* IVS2 + 1G>A or 1100delC were identified in 9 of 1921 controls (0.5%) and in 11 of 690 (1.6%) unselected patients with prostate cancer (OR, 3.4;

P = .004).[32] The missense *CHEK2* variant I157T was associated with prostate cancer (OR, 1.7; P = .002).[33] A subsequent meta-analysis reviewed 12 articles that discussed *CHEK2* c.1100delC, and its association with prostate cancer was identified. Of the 12 prostate cancer studies, 5 studies had independent data from which to draw conclusive evidence. The pooled results of OR and 95% CI were 1.98 (1.23–3.18) for unselected cases and 3.39 (1.78–6.47) for familial cases, indicating that *CHEK2* c.1100delC mutation is associated with increased risk of prostate cancer.[34]

Some controversy exists about the broader applicability of some *CHEK2* variant findings across other populations, and broader associations of more aggressive disease remain under study. However, Wu and colleagues[35] found that *CHEK2*, c.1100delC, had a significantly higher carrier rate (1.28%) in patients with lethal prostate cancer compared patients of European American origin with low-risk prostate cancer (0.16%), P = .0038. The estimated OR for lethal prostate cancer was 7.86.

NBN (NBS1)

Cybulski and colleagues[36] evaluated founder mutations in *NBN* (also called *NBS1*) in association with prostate cancer risk in the Polish population. The prevalence of 657del5 *NBS1* founder allele in 56 patients with familial prostate cancer was compared with 305 patients with nonfamilial prostate cancer, and 1500 control subjects from Poland. Loss of heterozygosity analysis also was performed on DNA samples isolated from 17 microdissected prostate cancers, including 8 from carriers of the 657del5 mutation. The *NBS1* founder mutation was present in 5 of 56 (9%) patients with familial prostate cancer (OR, 16; P<.0001), 7 of 305 (2.2%) patients with nonfamilial prostate cancer (OR, 3.9; P = .01), and 9 of 1500 control subjects (0.6%). Evidence of second allele inactivation of *NBS1* was found in 7 of 8 prostate tumors from carriers of the *NBS1* 657del5 allele, whereas loss of heterozygosity was seen in only 1 of 9 tumors from noncarriers (P = .003), suggesting that heterozygous carriers of the *NBS1* founder mutation have increased susceptibility to prostate cancer.

In a subsequent study, also led by Cybulski and colleagues,[37] *NBS1* 657del5 allele was detected in 53 of 3750 unselected cases compared with 23 of 3956 (0.6%) controls (OR, 2.5; P = .0003). Mortality was worse for carriers of the *NBS1* mutation compared with noncarriers (HR, 1.85; P = .008). Five-year survival for men with the *NBS1* mutation was 49%, compared with 72% for mutation-negative patients. A founder mutation in *NBS1* predisposes to aggressive prostate cancer in the Polish population.[37]

Wokołorczyk and colleagues[26] reported a study described earlier in relation to *ATM* that also included *NBN* and found an association with higher-grade prostate cancer.

RAD51C

Other germline mutations (pathogenic variants) in genes that are newly implicated with metastatic prostate cancer are still less characterized than *BRCA1*, *ATM*, *PALB2*, and *CHEK2* because of rarity (eg, *FANCA* or *RAD51C*). Further study in the context of conferred prostate cancer risk, disease-modifying properties within tumors, and clinical response to molecularly targeted treatments, along with continue translational laboratory studies, will be needed.

DNA MISMATCH REPAIR GENES (LYNCH SYNDROME)

Lynch syndrome is an autosomal dominant disorder defined by a germline mutation (pathogenic variant) in one of several DNA mismatch repair genes: *MLH1*, *MSH2*, *MSH6*, or *PMS2*. The risk of prostate cancer in Lynch syndrome has been debated, but several recent studies provide a more compelling argument for increased risk for prostate cancer. Raymond and colleagues[38] examined 4127 men from familial cancer registries and reported the cumulative risk of prostate cancer to be significantly increased compared with the general population (6.3% vs 2.6% by age 60 years and 30% vs 18% by age 80 years). Haraldsdottir and colleagues[39] calculated an increased risk of 188 men with Lynch syndrome compared with the general population, with a standardized rate ratio of 4.87 (95% CI, 2.43–8.71). The prospective Lynch Syndrome Database recently reported 6350 men with Lynch syndrome and 51,646 years of follow-up, of whom 1808 men were prospectively observed to have cancer. Germline *MSH2* mutation carriers were noted to have a particularly higher risk of prostate cancer (23.8% incidence of prostate cancer by age 75 years vs 13.8% for *MLH1*, 8.9% for *MSH6*, and 4.6% for *PMS2* by age 75 years).[40]

The association with metastatic disease and genes involved in mismatch repair is less common than for genes in the homologous recombination repair pathway, but importance is still clear. Approximately 5% to 7% of patients with mCRPC have evidence of tumor microsatellite instability (MSI-H)/mismatch repair deficiency (MMRd).[41] In a study by Abida and colleagues,[42] 3% of prostate cancers of all stages (localized and metastatic) undergoing tumor sequencing had evidence of MSI-H/MMRd. Of those, approximately 20% had Lynch syndrome and about half that received anti-programmed cell death protein 1/programmed death-ligand 1 achieve durable benefit.

HOXB13

The germline *HOXB13* G84E variant was cloned and validated in association with hereditary prostate cancer.[43–45] Until recently, its association was primarily for prostate cancer risk, but not with increased aggressiveness of disease, treatment actionability, or risk of other cancers. However, active research is ongoing to further understand the biology of germline *HOXB13* G84E, and a recent study by Wei and colleagues[46] leveraged the UK Biobank to determine the association of *HOXB13* G84E variant in 1545 (0.34%) of 460,224 participants of European ancestry. In men, OR (95% CI) for overall cancer diagnosis was 2.19 (1.89–2.52), $P = 2.5E-19$. The association remained after excluding prostate cancer (OR, 1.4 [1.16–1.68]; $P = .003$), suggesting association with other cancers, potentially rectosigmoid cancer (OR, 2.25 [1.05–4.15]; $P = .05$) and nonmelanoma skin cancer (OR, 1.40 [1.12–1.74]; $P = .01$).[46]

TP53

Prostate cancer is not classically included in Li Fraumeni syndrome, but emerging evidence suggests a potential role for germline *TP53* mutations in contributing to some prostate cancers, especially in association with multiple primaries and with unusual histologies.[47,48] Although not part of Li Fraumeni guidelines, germline *TP53* mutation carriers are included in some of the high-genetic-risk prostate cancer screening studies discussed next.

LACK OF DIVERSITY IN DATASETS PERPETUATES HEALTH DISPARITIES

A notable health disparity in the United States is that men of African ancestry (AA) are at higher risk for prostate cancer while also experiencing worse cancer outcomes. Causes are multifactorial, but likely include genetic factors. Because AA men and other racial/ethnic subgroups are underrepresented in genetic studies to date, there are fewer examples of affected and unaffected individuals contributing to higher rates of variants of uncertain significance (VUS). The exact distribution of germline predisposition to prostate cancer in AA remains to be elucidated. As discussed earlier, prostate cancer has been implicated in a spectrum of hereditary cancer syndromes, including hereditary breast and ovarian cancer and Lynch syndrome, and associated with other pathogenic variants such as *ATM*, *CHEK2*, *NBN*, and other gene mutations. However, most of these studies have been conducted in disproportionately non–African American cohorts. Therefore, a major gap in knowledge exists in understanding the prevalence of genetic predisposition and prostate cancer development among African American men. A recent report found similar rates of pathogenic variants in known cancer risk genes among AA men with prostate cancer,[49,50] highlighting the urgency to improve access and ensure diverse representation in research efforts to address gaps in knowledge and update advances in prostate cancer treatment, screening, and prevention.

MULTIGENE PANEL TESTING AND TUMOR SEQUENCING, AND THEIR ROLE IN PROSTATE CANCER GENETICS

Targeted DNA sequencing of tumors (somatic tumor DNA testing) has become widely available in clinical oncology practice. As more next-generation sequencing testing is incorporated in clinical and research testing in oncology, the return of genomic testing results (also called actionable mutations) poses difficult questions about how it should be delivered and its interpretation by patients.[51,52] Efforts to study this are urgently needed to evaluate the perspectives and experiences of different racial and ethnic groups and how it may affect the process and outcomes of receiving genomic results.

MODIFIERS/POLYGENIC RISK OF *BRCA1/2*

A discussion of prostate cancer genetic factors would not be complete without mention of genome-wide association studies and considerable research investments in single nucleotide polymorphisms, which additively contribute to an individual's risk of prostate cancer and genetic modifiers. Although the clinical utility of these have been limited to date in the metastatic and also in the prostate cancer risk setting, the general approach of polygenic risk scores is gaining traction in the understanding of additional genetic modifiers of high-penetrance genes such as *BRCA1/2*, as well as in other high-risk populations, such as men of AA.[24,53] This topic is explored in depth elsewhere in this issue.

TREATMENT IMPLICATIONS IN METASTATIC CASTRATION-RESISTANT PROSTATE CANCER

Genetic testing in prostate cancer may affect treatment choices by revealing mutations that

are eligible for FDA-approved PARP inhibitors, platinum chemotherapy, or clinical trial participation. However, this topic is further developed elsewhere in this issue.

The PARP inhibitors olaparib and rucaparib have received FDA approval for mCRPC with DNA damage repair alterations. Rucaparib was evaluated in phase II TRITON2 study and showed 51% (50 out of 98) radiographic response rate among men with mCRPC and *BRCA1/2* alterations.[48] However, benefit among men with non-*BRCA* DNA repair gene alterations was less prominent (13%, 7 out of 55), and the rucaparib label includes only *BRCA1* and *BRCA2* alterations.[54–56] The phase III ProFOUND study compared olaparib and androgen receptor (AR)-targeted agents in men with mCRPC and DNA damage repair alterations who had progressed on at least 1 line of AR-targeted therapy. Olaparib improved radiographic progression-free survival (5.8 months vs 3.5 months) and was approved for men with mCRPC and alterations in one of these genes: *BRCA1*, *BRCA2*, *ATM*, *BRIP1*, *BARD1*, *CDK12*, *CHEK1*, *CHEK2*, *FANCL*, *PALB2*, *RAD51B*, *RAD51C*, *RAD51D*, and *RAD54L*.[57]

Platinum chemotherapy has been reported to be effective among men with homologous recombination-deficient prostate cancer.[5,6,58,59] A retrospective study reported that 75% (6 out of 8) of patients with mCRPC with *gBRCA2* mutations had 50% PSA decline from baseline (PSA$_{50}$) response to platinum chemotherapy.[6] In the study by Mota and colleagues,[59] the PSA$_{50}$ response rate to platinum chemotherapy was 53% (8 out of 15) among men with mCRPC and DNA damage repair mutations (*BRCA2*, *BRCA1*, *ATM*, *PALB2*, *FANCA*, and *CDK12*).

The optimal sequence and cross-resistance between PARP inhibitors and platinum chemotherapy in homologous recombination-deficient prostate cancer are currently under investigation.

The immune checkpoint inhibitor pembrolizumab received the first tumor-agnostic FDA approval in 2017 for metastatic solid tumors with MSI-H and MMRd and recently tumor mutational burden greater than 10 mut/Mb was included in the FDA-approved indication.[60,61] Almost 5% of mCRPC tumors have MSI-H/MMRd and could qualify for treatment with pembrolizumab.[41,42,62,63] The prospective phase II KEYNOTE-199 study reported that pembrolizumab led to a 5% radiographic response rate and 16.8 months median duration of response among non–biomarker-selected patients with mCRPC.[64] When retrospectively evaluated in men with mCRPC and MSI-H/MMRd, therapy with immune checkpoint inhibitors resulted in a 53% (8 out of

15) PSA_{50} response rate.[65] Thus, immune checkpoint inhibitors are promising therapy with a potentially durable response, although further studies for patients with prostate cancer are needed to refine predictive biomarkers. In addition, many combination approaches are also being explored.

Response to Conventional Therapies

Retrospective and prospective studies to date have not shown that conventional treatment (treatments that are not biomarker selected) for mCRPC should be withheld from men with homologous recombination-deficient prostate cancer.[9–11,66,67] The prospective PROREPAIR-B study showed that abiraterone, enzalutamide, and taxanes are similarly effective among germline BRCA2 carriers and noncarriers.[9] Radium-223 seems to be effective in homologous recombination-deficient prostate cancer. In a small retrospective cohort, patients with mCRPC with homologous recombination deficiency had a trend toward longer overall survival with radium-223 compared with those with homologous recombination-proficient tumors.[68,69]

Novel Therapeutic Strategies

Several targeted agents are in the pipeline for prostate cancer treatment. ATR and WEE1 are critical checkpoints in the cell cycle, and preclinical data suggest that ATR and WEE1 inhibitors might be effective in homologous recombination-deficient tumors as monotherapy or in combination with PARP inhibitors.[70,71] Lutetium[177] is a promising radiotherapeutic agent. Early data suggest that BRCA1/2 alterations may be associated with improved progression-free survival and overall survival with lutetium[177] therapy,[72] but more studies are needed.

APPLICATION OF KNOWLEDGE TO EARLIER DISEASE STATES

Because of the evidence of aggressive progression, studies are not only being conducted for more aggressive disease. Trials in the biochemical recurrence setting are underway or in development. For example, PARP inhibitors are being evaluated as monotherapy or in combination in the biochemically recurrent setting (NCT03047135; NCT03810105; NCT04336943; NCT0353394), metastatic hormone-sensitive (NCT03413995; NCT04332744; NCT04497844) and first-line castration-resistant prostate cancer (NCT03012321; NCT03748641).

IMPORTANCE OF CASCADE TESTING

One of the major important opportunities and responsibilities in germline genetic testing for men with metastatic prostate cancer is the possibility of identifying previously unknown inherited cancer risk within a family. As discussed earlier, many of the historical series are composed of men selected by either female relatives with breast and ovarian cancers or by multiple early-age prostate cancer diagnoses. However, the Pritchard and colleagues[8] study describing the ~12% prevalence in the metastatic population did not find associations with earlier age of onset or family history of prostate cancer. Thus, ascertainment by personal history of metastatic prostate cancer is now increasing and may exceed genetic testing based on family history indications. Attention to thoughtful implementation through different workflow strategies and research endeavors is an ongoing area of research. Increasingly, men with a personal history of metastatic prostate cancer may be the probands in their families.

Once a cancer predisposition pathogenic genetic variant is identified in a proband, the potential for cancer prevention extends from that 1 individual to multiple asymptomatic individuals within the family who may end up being carriers for this cancer predisposition gene. This process of cascade testing allows genetic counseling and testing in disease-free blood relatives of individuals in a sequential manner. This systematic process appropriately identifies family members who carry genes associated with increased cancer risk and allows the implementation of targeted interventions for cancer surveillance and risk reduction.

In addition, given the rapid integration of tumor genomic sequencing into clinical cancer care, it may uncover germline genetic information. Consequently, tumor genomic sequencing creates an additional pathway to cascade testing. In prostate cancer, some studies have shown that, among men with metastatic prostate cancer undergoing tumor sequencing, up to 12% of them carry an actionable pathogenic germline mutation.[8] Men with metastatic prostate cancer whose tumor testing shows pathogenic variants considered suspicious for being associated with a germline source should be recommended to complete germline genetic testing, because this may also have implications for the cancer risks of family members. A referral should be made for appropriate genetic counseling and germline testing. If the individual undergoes germline genetic testing as a result of findings on somatic tumor sequencing and is subsequently found to have a pathogenic variant, the cascade testing process should be triggered.

Cancer risks associated with pathogenic variants inform personalized cancer screening for probands as well as their male and female relatives. For example, as noted earlier, a pathogenic BRCA2 mutation is known to be associated with prostate cancer risk in men, in addition to an increase in the risk of male breast cancer, pancreatic cancer, and melanoma.[73,74] Identification of carrier status of a BRCA2 mutation in a man with prostate cancer diagnosis would inform other men should they be found to have the same pathogenic variant and allow early prostate cancer screening, clinical breast examinations (male breast cancer risk), discussion of pancreatic cancer screening options, and referral to dermatology for melanoma screening.[74] Female relatives with an identified BRCA2 pathogenic variant would benefit significantly from this cascade testing given the available strategies for cancer prevention or early detection should they carry the same familial identified BRCA2 mutation.

Thus, there are important, potentially lifesaving health care options for early detection and risk reduction for female relatives. For male relatives who might carry the same cancer risk mutations, there are increasing opportunities for education, testing, and prostate cancer screening clinical trials (discussed further later). However, this will not be fully actualized without systematic and careful attention to informing and facilitating cascade testing of relatives to fullest extent possible. Studies evaluating cascade testing for men with prostate cancer who may be the probands in their families are underway, including NCT04254133.

FURTHER STUDIES AND EXPANDED APPLICATIONS

In early 2020, Nyberg and colleagues[75] reported a prospective cohort study of male BRCA1 (n = 376) and BRCA2 carriers (n = 447) identified in clinical genetics centers in the United Kingdom and Ireland (median follow-up, 5.9 and 5.3 years, respectively). Sixteen BRCA1 and 26 BRCA2 mutation carriers were diagnosed with prostate cancer during follow-up. BRCA2 carriers had an standardized incidence ratio (SIR) of 4.45 (95% CI, 2.99–6.61) and absolute prostate cancer risk of 27% (95% CI, 17%–41%) and 60% (95% CI, 43%–78%) by ages 75 and 85 years, respectively. For BRCA1 carriers, the overall SIR was 2.35 (95% CI, 1.43–3.88); the corresponding SIR at age less than 65 years was 3.57 (95% CI, 1.68–7.58). However, the BRCA1 SIR varied between 0.74 and 2.83 in sensitivity analyses to assess potential screening effects. Prostate cancer risk for BRCA2 carriers increased with family history (HR per affected relative, 1.68; 95% CI, 0.99–2.85).[75]

This contemporary, prospective report is important, particularly given its calculated estimates of added risk from a family history of prostate cancer. This study builds on the retrospective studies mentioned at the beginning of this article describing the increased prostate cancer risk and aggressiveness for BRCA2 carriers and, to an important but lesser extent, BRCA1 carriers. It also emphasizes the importance of cascade genetic testing for the families of men with metastatic disease who are identified to have germline mutations, especially as related to opportunities for risk-reduction measures through early detection strategies and, in some cases, prophylactic measures.

Updated findings from the ongoing, international UK-led Identification of Men with a Genetic Predisposition to Prostate Cancer (IMPACT) study make a strong case for offering men with BRCA2 and BRCA1 mutations more intensified prostate cancer screening.[76] This topic is elaborated on further elsewhere in this issue, but does present the opportunity to discuss the importance of clinical trials and further innovation, particularly as several new genes are faced for which data are less robust. The practical complexities around implementation and management have been addressed at the biannual Philadelphia Consensus Conference, which convened in 2019 to debate and assemble consensus recommendations around implementation and recommendations for prostate cancer genetics, pending further data.[77]

The opportunities for more complete understanding of rare gene variants and VUS in underrepresented populations poses challenges, albeit surmountable, around best clinical practices. For localized disease management and/or early cancer detection approaches in germline carriers (discussed further elsewhere in this issue), clinical trials and variant registries should be encouraged whenever possible. There may be an increasing role for specialized cancer genetics clinics and tumor boards to synthesize available data (family history and somatic sequencing) and promote clinical and research advances.

LONG-TERM FOLLOW-UP REGISTRY RESEARCH

Collective registries and databases of rare variants in population-based and in metastatic settings will be essential to building new knowledge and refining current estimates. For men with metastatic disease for whom clinical trial enrollment is a major consideration, it is reasonable to take a more permissive approach of including germline gene mutations with less certainty in the testing panels, especially if standard treatment options have been exhausted. In this setting, patients should be encouraged to participate in therapeutic clinical trials and/or variant and mutation registries to understand treatment response, cancer risk, and penetrance, whenever possible. For example, the PROMISE prostate cancer registry (www.prostatecancerpromise.org) for germline mutation carriers with prostate cancer will launch in 2021 to provide better understanding of germline mutations as predictors of treatment response, cancer phenotype and penetrance, and modifiers of risk. In addition, registries of genetic testing experience such as the PROGRESS registry (www.progressregistry.com) and registries of germline VUS (PROMPT registry, www.promptstudy.info) will help refine and advance the current understanding.

In conclusion, genetic factors associated with metastatic prostate cancer have gained inclusion in clinical practice guidelines such as NCCN, because of their growing relevance to treatment and clinical trials. As important are the implications (potentially lifesaving) for relatives who may carry the same mutations. Ongoing research across many dimensions and disciplines will contribute to the continued momentum and advances.

CLINICS CARE POINTS

- Men with germline BRCA mutations are more likely to have intraductal features in their prostate cancer, which correlate with poor outcomes.

- Approximately 5% to 7% of patients with mCRPC have evidence of tumor MSI-H/MMRd and qualify for immune checkpoint blockade.

- Retrospective and prospective studies to date have not shown that conventional treatment (treatments that are not biomarker selected) for patients with mCRPC should be withheld from men with homologous recombination-deficient prostate cancer.

- Men with metastatic prostate cancer whose tumor testing show pathogenic variants considered suspicious for being associated with a germline source should be recommended to complete germline genetic testing, because this may also have implications for the cancer risks of family members.

DISCLOSURE

A.O. Sokolova receives research funding from NIH/NCI T32CA009515. E.I. Obeid receives research funding from the American Cancer Society, Eileen Jacoby Foundation, Genetech, Merck, NCCN Foundation Young Investigator Award, and Newtown Foundation; and has a consultancy or advisory role to Daiichi Sankyo, Ethos Immunomedics, Foundation Medicine, Incyte, Novartis, OncLive, Pfizer, and Puma. H.H. Cheng receives research funding from the PNW SPORE CA097186, Prostate Cancer Foundation, NIH/NCI P30 CA015704, DOD W81XWH-17-2-0043; receives research funding to institution from Clovis Oncology, Club Foundation, Janssen, Medivation and Sanofi; has a consultancy role to AstraZeneca; and receives royalties from UpToDate. The authors have nothing else to disclose

REFERENCES

1. Mucci LA, Hjelmborg JB, Harris JR, et al. Familial risk and heritability of cancer among twins in Nordic countries. JAMA 2016;315(1):68–76. https://doi.org/10.1001/jama.2015.17703.

2. Hjelmborg JB, Scheike T, Holst K, et al. The heritability of prostate cancer in the Nordic Twin Study of Cancer. Cancer Epidemiol Biomarkers Prev 2014;23(11):2303–10. https://doi.org/10.1158/1055-9965.EPI-13-0568.

3. Bratt O, Drevin L, Akre O, et al. Family history and probability of prostate cancer, differentiated by risk category: a nationwide population-based study. J Natl Cancer Inst 2016;108(10). https://doi.org/10.1093/jnci/djw110.

4. Robinson D, Van Allen EM, Wu Y-M, et al. Integrative clinical genomics of advanced prostate cancer. Cell 2015;161(5):1215–28. https://doi.org/10.1016/j.cell.2015.05.001.

5. Cheng HH, Pritchard CC, Boyd T, et al. Biallelic inactivation of BRCA2 in platinum sensitive, metastatic castration resistant prostate cancer. Eur Urol 2016;69(6):992–5. https://doi.org/10.1016/j.eururo.2015.11.022.

6. Pomerantz MM, Spisák S, Jia L, et al. The association between germline BRCA2 variants and sensitivity to platinum-based chemotherapy among men with metastatic prostate cancer. Cancer 2017;123(18):3532–9. https://doi.org/10.1002/cncr.30808.

7. Mateo J, Carreira S, Sandhu S, et al. DNA-repair defects and olaparib in metastatic prostate cancer. N Engl J Med 2015;373(18):1697–708. https://doi.org/10.1056/NEJMoa1506859.

8. Pritchard CC, Mateo J, Walsh MF, et al. Inherited DNA-repair gene mutations in men with metastatic prostate cancer. N Engl J Med 2016;375(5):443–53. https://doi.org/10.1056/NEJMoa1603144.

9. Castro E, Romero-Laorden N, Del Pozo A, et al. PROREPAIR-B: a prospective cohort study of the impact of germline DNA repair mutations on the outcomes of patients with metastatic castration-resistant prostate cancer. J Clin Oncol 2019;37(6): 490–503. https://doi.org/10.1200/JCO.18.00358.

10. Antonarakis ES, Lu C, Luber B, et al. Germline DNA-repair gene mutations and outcomes in men with metastatic castration-resistant prostate cancer receiving first-line abiraterone and enzalutamide. Eur Urol 2018;74(2):218–25. https://doi.org/10.1016/j.eururo.2018.01.035.

11. Annala M, Struss WJ, Warner EW, et al. Treatment outcomes and tumor loss of heterozygosity in germline DNA repair-deficient prostate cancer. Eur Urol 2017;72(1):34–42. https://doi.org/10.1016/j.eururo.2017.02.023.

12. Yadav S, Hart SN, Hu C, et al. Contribution of inherited DNA-repair gene mutations to hormone-sensitive and castrate-resistant metastatic prostate cancer and implications for clinical outcome. JCO Precis Oncol 2019;3. https://doi.org/10.1200/PO.19.00067.

13. Khani F, Wobker SE, Hicks JL, et al. Intraductal carcinoma of the prostate in the absence of high-grade invasive carcinoma represents a molecularly distinct type of in situ carcinoma enriched with oncogenic driver mutations. J Pathol 2019;249(1):79–89. https://doi.org/10.1002/path.5283.

14. Taylor RA, Fraser M, Livingstone J, et al. Germline BRCA2 mutations drive prostate cancers with distinct evolutionary trajectories. Nat Commun 2017;8(1): 1–10. https://doi.org/10.1038/ncomms13671.

15. Tryggvadóttir L, Vidarsdóttir L, Thorgeirsson T, et al. Prostate cancer progression and survival in BRCA2 mutation carriers. J Natl Cancer Inst 2007;99(12): 929–35. https://doi.org/10.1093/jnci/djm005.

16. Gallagher DJ, Gaudet MM, Pal P, et al. Germline BRCA mutations denote a clinicopathologic subset of prostate cancer. Clin Cancer Res 2010;16(7): 2115–21. https://doi.org/10.1158/1078-0432.CCR-09-2871.

17. Castro E, Goh C, Olmos D, et al. Germline BRCA mutations are associated with higher risk of nodal involvement, distant metastasis, and poor survival outcomes in prostate cancer. J Clin Oncol 2013; 31(14):1748–57. https://doi.org/10.1200/JCO.2012.43.1882.

18. Castro E, Goh C, Leongamornlert D, et al. Effect of BRCA mutations on metastatic relapse and cause-specific survival after radical treatment for localised prostate cancer. Eur Urol 2015;68(2):186–93. https://doi.org/10.1016/j.eururo.2014.10.022.

19. Silvestri V, Leslie G, Barnes DR, et al. Characterization of the cancer spectrum in men with germline BRCA1 and BRCA2 pathogenic variants: results from the consortium of investigators of modifiers of BRCA1/2

(CIMBA). JAMA Oncol 2020;6(8):1218–30. https://doi.org/10.1001/jamaoncol.2020.2134.

20. Risbridger GP, Taylor RA, Clouston D, et al. Patient-derived xenografts reveal that intraductal carcinoma of the prostate is a prominent pathology in BRCA2 mutation carriers with prostate cancer and correlates with poor prognosis. Eur Urol 2015;67(3):496–503. https://doi.org/10.1016/j.eururo.2014.08.007.

21. Antonarakis ES, Shaukat F, Isaacsson Velho P, et al. Clinical features and therapeutic outcomes in men with advanced prostate cancer and DNA mismatch repair gene mutations. Eur Urol 2019;75(3):378–82. https://doi.org/10.1016/j.eururo.2018.10.009.

22. Isaacsson Velho P, Silberstein JL, Markowski MC, et al. Intraductal/ductal histology and lymphovascular invasion are associated with germline DNA-repair gene mutations in prostate cancer. Prostate 2018; 78(5):401–7. https://doi.org/10.1002/pros.23484.

23. Schweizer MT, Antonarakis ES, Bismar TA, et al. Genomic characterization of prostatic ductal adenocarcinoma identifies a high prevalence of DNA repair gene mutations. JCO Precis Oncol 2019;3: 1–9. https://doi.org/10.1200/PO.18.00327.

24. Lecarpentier J, Silvestri V, Kuchenbaecker KB, et al. Prediction of breast and prostate cancer risks in male BRCA1 and BRCA2 mutation carriers using polygenic risk scores. J Clin Oncol 2017;35(20):2240–50. https://doi.org/10.1200/JCO.2016.69.4935.

25. Na R, Zheng SL, Han M, et al. Germline mutations in ATM and BRCA1/2 distinguish risk for lethal and indolent prostate cancer and are associated with early age at death. Eur Urol 2017;71(5):740–7. https://doi.org/10.1016/j.eururo.2016.11.033.

26. Wokołorczyk D, Kluźniak W, Huzarski T, et al. Mutations in ATM, NBN and BRCA2 predispose to aggressive prostate cancer in Poland. Int J Cancer 2020;147(10):2793–800. https://doi.org/10.1002/ijc.33272.

27. Yang X, Leslie G, Doroszuk A, et al. Cancer risks associated with germline PALB2 pathogenic variants: an international study of 524 families. J Clin Oncol 2020;38(7):674–85. https://doi.org/10.1200/JCO.19.01907.

28. Pakkanen S, Wahlfors T, Siltanen S, et al. PALB2 variants in hereditary and unselected Finnish prostate cancer cases. J Negat Results Biomed 2009;8:12. https://doi.org/10.1186/1477-5751-8-12.

29. Tischkowitz M, Sabbaghian N, Ray AM, et al. Analysis of the gene coding for the BRCA2-interacting protein PALB2 in hereditary prostate cancer. Prostate 2008; 68(6):675–8. https://doi.org/10.1002/pros.20729.

30. Goodall J, Mateo J, Yuan W, et al. Circulating cell-free DNA to guide prostate cancer treatment with PARP inhibition. Cancer Discov 2017;7(9):1006–17. https://doi.org/10.1158/2159-8290.CD-17-0261.

31. Horak P, Weischenfeldt J, von Amsberg G, et al. Response to olaparib in a PALB2 germline mutated

prostate cancer and genetic events associated with resistance. Cold Spring Harb Mol Case Stud 2019; 5(2). https://doi.org/10.1101/mcs.a003657.

32. Cybulski C, Huzarski T, Górski B, et al. A novel founder CHEK2 mutation is associated with increased prostate cancer risk. Cancer Res 2004;64(8):2677–9. https://doi.org/10.1158/0008-5472.can-04-0341.

33. Cybulski C, Górski B, Huzarski T, et al. CHEK2 is a multiorgan cancer susceptibility gene. Am J Hum Genet 2004;75(6):1131–5. https://doi.org/10.1086/426403.

34. Hale V, Weischer M, Park JY. CHEK2 (*) 1100delC mutation and risk of prostate cancer. Prostate Cancer 2014;2014:294575. https://doi.org/10.1155/2014/294575.

35. Wu Y, Yu H, Zheng SL, et al. A comprehensive evaluation of CHEK2 germline mutations in men with prostate cancer. Prostate 2018;78(8):607–15. https://doi.org/10.1002/pros.23505.

36. Cybulski C, Górski B, Debniak T, et al. NBS1 is a prostate cancer susceptibility gene. Cancer Res 2004;64(4):1215–9. https://doi.org/10.1158/0008-5472.can-03-2502.

37. Cybulski C, Wokołorczyk D, Kluźniak W, et al. An inherited NBN mutation is associated with poor prognosis prostate cancer. Br J Cancer 2013;108(2): 461–8. https://doi.org/10.1038/bjc.2012.486.

38. Raymond VM, Mukherjee B, Wang F, et al. Elevated risk of prostate cancer among men with Lynch syndrome. J Clin Oncol 2013;31(14):1713–8. https://doi.org/10.1200/JCO.2012.44.1238.

39. Haraldsdottir S, Hampel H, Wei L, et al. Prostate cancer incidence in males with Lynch syndrome. Genet Med 2014;16(7):553–7. https://doi.org/10.1038/gim.2013.193.

40. Dominguez-Valentin M, Sampson JR, Seppälä TT, et al. Cancer risks by gene, age, and gender in 6350 carriers of pathogenic mismatch repair variants: findings from the Prospective Lynch Syndrome Database. Genet Med 2020;22(1):15–25. https://doi.org/10.1038/s41436-019-0596-9.

41. Pritchard CC, Morrissey C, Kumar A, et al. Complex MSH2 and MSH6 mutations in hypermutated microsatellite unstable advanced prostate cancer. Nat Commun 2014;5:4988. https://doi.org/10.1038/ncomms5988.

42. Abida W, Cheng ML, Armenia J, et al. Analysis of the prevalence of microsatellite instability in prostate cancer and response to immune checkpoint blockade. JAMA Oncol 2018. https://doi.org/10.1001/jamaoncol.2018.5801.

43. Ewing CM, Ray AM, Lange EM, et al. Germline mutations in HOXB13 and prostate-cancer risk. N Engl J Med 2012;366(2):141–9. https://doi.org/10.1056/NEJMoa1110000.

44. Cai Q, Wang X, Li X, et al. Germline HOXB13 p.Gly84-Glu mutation and cancer susceptibility: a pooled analysis of 25 epidemiological studies with 145,257 participates. Oncotarget 2015;6(39):42312–21. https://doi.org/10.18632/oncotarget.5994.

45. Kote-Jarai Z, Mikropoulos C, Leongamornlert DA, et al. Prevalence of the HOXB13 G84E germline mutation in British men and correlation with prostate cancer risk, tumour characteristics and clinical outcomes. Ann Oncol 2015;26(4):756–61. https://doi.org/10.1093/annonc/mdv004.

46. Wei J, Shi Z, Na R, et al. Germline HOXB13 G84E mutation carriers and risk to twenty common types of cancer: results from the UK Biobank. Br J Cancer 2020; 123(9):1356–9. https://doi.org/10.1038/s41416-020-01036-8.

47. Spees CK, Kelleher KJ, Abaza R, et al. Prostate cancer and Li-Fraumeni syndrome: implications for screening and therapy. Urol Case Rep 2015;3(2): 21–3. https://doi.org/10.1016/j.eucr.2015.01.002.

48. Mai PL, Best AF, Peters JA, et al. Risks of first and subsequent cancers among TP53 mutation carriers in the National Cancer Institute Li-Fraumeni syndrome cohort. Cancer 2016;122(23):3673–81. https://doi.org/10.1002/cncr.30248.

49. Petrovics G, Price DK, Lou H, et al. Increased frequency of germline BRCA2 mutations associates with prostate cancer metastasis in a racially diverse patient population. Prostate Cancer Prostatic Dis 2019;22(3):406–10. https://doi.org/10.1038/s41391-018-0114-1.

50. Chandrasekar T, Gross L, Gomella LG, et al. Prevalence of suspected hereditary cancer syndromes and germline mutations among a diverse cohort of probands reporting a family history of prostate cancer: toward informing cascade testing for men. Eur Urol Oncol 2019. https://doi.org/10.1016/j.euo.2019.06.010.

51. Wolf SM, Lawrenz FP, Nelson CA, et al. Managing incidental findings in human subjects research: analysis and recommendations. J Law Med Ethics 2008;36(2):219–48. https://doi.org/10.1111/j.1748-720X.2008.00266.x, 211.

52. Wolf SM, Crock BN, Van Ness B, et al. Managing incidental findings and research results in genomic research involving biobanks and archived data sets. Genet Med 2012;14(4):361–84. https://doi.org/10.1038/gim.2012.23.

53. Darst BF, Wan P, Sheng X, et al. A germline variant at 8q24 contributes to familial clustering of prostate cancer in men of African ancestry. Eur Urol 2020; 78(3):316–20. https://doi.org/10.1016/j.eururo.2020.04.060.

54. Abida W, Bryce AH, Balar AV, et al. TRITON2: an international, multicenter, open-label, phase II study of the PARP inhibitor rucaparib in patients with metastatic castration-resistant prostate cancer (mCRPC) associated with homologous recombination deficiency (HRD). J Clin Oncol 2018;36(6_suppl):

TPS388. https://doi.org/10.1200/JCO.2018.36.6_suppl.TPS388.

55. Abida W. Non-BRCA DNA damage repair gene alterations and response to the PARP inhibitor rucaparib in metastatic castration-resistant prostate cancer. Clin Cancer Res 2020;26(11):2487–96.

56. Sokolova AO, Yu EY, Cheng HH. Honing in on PARPi response in prostate cancer: from HR pathway to gene-by-gene granularity. Clin Cancer Res 2020; 26(11):2439–40. https://doi.org/10.1158/1078-0432. CCR-20-0707.

57. de Bono J, Mateo J, Fizazi K, et al. Olaparib for metastatic castration-resistant prostate cancer. N Engl J Med 2020;382(22):2091–102. https://doi.org/10. 1056/NEJMoa1911440.

58. Mota JM, Barnett E, Nauseef J, et al. Platinum-based chemotherapy in metastatic prostate cancer with alterations in DNA damage repair genes. J Clin Oncol 2019;37(15_suppl):5038. https://doi.org/ 10.1200/JCO.2019.37.15_suppl.5038.

59. Mota JM, Barnett E, Nauseef JT, et al. Platinum-based chemotherapy in metastatic prostate cancer with DNA repair gene alterations. JCO Precis Oncol 2020;(4):355–66. https://doi.org/10.1200/PO.19. 00346.

60. FDA/CEDR resources page. Food and Drug Administration Web site. Available at: https://www.fda.gov/ drugs/resources-information-approved-drugs/fda-grants-accelerated-approval-pembrolizumab-first-tissuesite-agnostic-indication. Accessed April 18, 2021.

61. Le DT, Uram JN, Wang H, et al. PD-1 blockade in tumors with mismatch-repair deficiency. N Engl J Med 2015;372(26):2509–20. https://doi.org/10.1056/ NEJMoa1500596.

62. Rescigno P, Rodrigues DN, Yuan W, et al. Abstract 4679: mismatch repair defects in lethal prostate cancer. Cancer Res 2017;77(13 Supplement):4679. https://doi.org/10.1158/1538-7445.AM2017-4679.

63. Guedes LB, Antonarakis ES, Schweizer MT, et al. MSH2 loss in primary prostate cancer. Clin Cancer Res 2017;23(22):6863–74. https://doi.org/10.1158/ 1078-0432.CCR-17-0955.

64. Antonarakis ES, Piulats JM, Gross-Goupil M, et al. Pembrolizumab for treatment-refractory metastatic castration-resistant prostate cancer: multicohort, open-label phase II KEYNOTE-199 study. J Clin Oncol 2020;38(5):395–405. https://doi.org/10.1200/ JCO.19.01638.

65. Graham LS, Montgomery B, Cheng HH, et al. Mismatch repair deficiency in metastatic prostate cancer: response to PD-1 blockade and standard therapies. PLoS One 2020;15(5). https://doi.org/10. 1371/journal.pone.0233260.

66. Mateo J, Cheng HH, Beltran H, et al. Clinical outcome of prostate cancer patients with germline DNA repair mutations: retrospective analysis from an international study. Eur Urol 2018;73(5):687–93. https://doi.org/10.1016/j.eururo.2018.01.010.

67. Carlson AS, Acevedo RI, Lim DM, et al. Impact of mutations in homologous recombination repair genes on treatment outcomes for metastatic castration resistant prostate cancer. PLoS One 2020;15(9). https://doi.org/10.1371/journal.pone.0239686.

68. Velho PI, Qazi F, Hassan S, et al. Efficacy of radium-223 in bone-metastatic castration-resistant prostate cancer with and without homologous repair gene defects. Eur Urol 2019;76(2):170–6. https://doi.org/ 10.1016/j.eururo.2018.09.040.

69. Steinberger AE, Cotogno P, Ledet EM, et al. Exceptional duration of radium-223 in prostate cancer with a BRCA2 mutation. Clin Genitourin Cancer 2017; 15(1):e69–71. https://doi.org/10.1016/j.clgc.2016. 09.001.

70. Rafiei S, Fitzpatrick K, Liu D, et al. ATM loss confers greater sensitivity to ATR inhibition than PARP inhibition in prostate cancer. Cancer Res 2020;80(11): 2094–100. https://doi.org/10.1158/0008-5472.CAN-19-3126.

71. Yap TA, O'Carrigan B, Penney MS, et al. Phase I trial of first-in-class ATR inhibitor M6620 (VX-970) as monotherapy or in combination with carboplatin in patients with advanced solid tumors. J Clin Oncol 2020. https://doi.org/10.1200/JCO.19.02404. JCO.19.02404.

72. Conteduca V, Oromendia C, Vlachostergios PJ, et al. Clinical and molecular analysis of patients treated with prostate-specific membrane antigen (PSMA)-targeted radionuclide therapy. J Clin Oncol 2019;37(7_suppl):272. https://doi.org/10.1200/JCO. 2019.37.7_suppl.272.

73. Mersch J, Jackson MA, Park M, et al. Cancers associated with BRCA1 and BRCA2 mutations other than breast and ovarian. Cancer 2015;121(2):269–75. https://doi.org/10.1002/cncr.29041.

74. NCCN genetic/familial high-risk assessment: breast, ovarian, pancreas (version 2.2021). Available at: https://www.nccn.org/professionals/physician_gls/ pdf/genetics_bop.pdf. Accessed April 18, 2021.

75. Nyberg T, Frost D, Barrowdale D, et al. Prostate cancer risks for male BRCA1 and BRCA2 mutation carriers: a prospective cohort study. Eur Urol 2020; 77(1):24–35. https://doi.org/10.1016/j.eururo.2019. 08.025.

76. Page EC, Bancroft EK, Brook MN, et al. Interim results from the IMPACT study: evidence for prostate-specific antigen screening in BRCA2 mutation carriers. Eur Urol 2019;76(6):831–42. https://doi. org/10.1016/j.eururo.2019.08.019.

77. Giri VN, Knudsen KE, Kelly WK, et al. Implementation of germline testing for prostate cancer: Philadelphia Prostate Cancer Consensus Conference 2019. J Clin Oncol 2020;38(24):2798–811. https://doi.org/ 10.1200/JCO.20.00046.

Genetically Informed Prostate Cancer Treatment for Metastatic Disease

Aisha L. Siebert, MD, PhD, MPH[a,1], Brittany M. Szymaniak, PhD, CGC[b,1], Yazan Numan, MD[c,1], Alicia K. Morgans, MD, MPH[c,*]

KEYWORDS

- Metastatic prostate cancer • Targeted treatment • DNA-damage repair • Mismatch repair

KEY POINTS

- Patients with high-risk localized or metastatic prostate cancer should undergo germline genetic testing.
- BRCA1/2 mutations confer responsiveness to PARP inhibitor therapies including olaparib and rucaparib.
- Additional DNA damage repair (DDR) mutations may confer responsiveness to PARP inhibitor therapy, such as olaparib, although the data supporting this are less robust than for BRCA1/2 mutations.
- Pembrolizumab is approved for MSI-H tumors or prostate cancer with TMB ($\geq$10 mutations/megabase).

INTRODUCTION

Germline and somatic testing for DNA-damage repair (DDR) genes is now an integral part of the treatment decision-making process for men with metastatic prostate cancer as more genetically targeted therapies become available. It is estimated that 5% to 10% of all cancers are from an underlying hereditary cause. However, Pritchard and colleagues[1] in their landmark study identified that 11.8% of men with metastatic prostate cancer harbor a germline mutation in a DDR gene - 44% of which were in the *BRCA2* gene - as opposed to only 4.6% for men with localized prostate cancer. National Comprehensive Cancer Center (NCCN) clinical guidelines recommend germline and somatic tissue testing for men diagnosed with metastatic prostate cancer.[2] Unimodal testing may miss clinically actionable DDR mutations, possibly precluding promising systemic therapeutic options, such as poly (ADP-ribose) polymerase (PARP) inhibitors or immunotherapies. This discussion of genetically informed treatment of metastatic prostate cancer addresses the application of somatic and germline genetic testing, provides guidance on the use of specific treatment strategies, and reviews promising new research directions.

GENETIC TESTING STRATEGIES AND IMPLEMENTATION

The primary factors driving genetic testing are typically preventive cancer screening, early detection based on gene-associated risks, and cascade testing of at-risk family members. However, with the advent of genetically targeted therapies, germline and somatic mutations now play a significant

[a] Department of Urology, Feinberg School of Medicine at Northwestern University, 676 North St. Clair Street, Arkes 23-010, Chicago, IL 60611, USA; [b] Department of Urology, Feinberg School of Medicine at Northwestern University, 675 North Saint Clair Street, Suite 20-150, Chicago, IL 60611, USA; [c] Division of Hematology/Oncology, Department of Medicine, Feinberg School of Medicine at Northwestern University, 676 North St. Clair Street, Suite 850, Chicago, IL 60611, USA
[1] Authors contributed equally.
* Corresponding author.
E-mail address: Alicia.morgans@northwestern.edu

Urol Clin N Am 48 (2021) 365–371
https://doi.org/10.1016/j.ucl.2021.03.006
0094-0143/21/© 2021 Elsevier Inc. All rights reserved.

role in treatment choice and prognosis. Many genes associated with hereditary prostate cancer are involved in either homologous recombination repair (HRR) or mismatch repair (MMR), and pathogenic variants may confer sensitivity to specific therapeutic agents.

Germline Testing

The NCCN guidelines address genetic testing for prostate cancer under the Genetic/Familial High-Risk Assessment: Breast, Ovarian, and Pancreatic (v1.2021) and Prostate Cancer (v2.2020).[2] Both guidelines recommend that all men with metastatic prostate cancer, and those with high- or very-high-risk disease, should be considered for germline genetic testing, which may inform alternative treatment strategies. Men who fall into lower cancer risk groups, but with a significant family history, may also benefit from genetic testing, even when not performed primarily for treatment purposes.

Several genes have been associated with hereditary prostate cancer, but not all with clearly defined treatment, prognostic, and management implications for unaffected individuals. The NCCN guidelines and an expert panel consensus recommend prioritization of *BRCA1/2*, *MLH1*, *MSH2*, *MSH6*, and *PMS2*, with possible consideration of *ATM*, *CHEK2*, and *PALB2*.[2,3] There are multiple testing approaches available for the germline, which may range from targeted prostate-specific panels to comprehensive pan-cancer panels. Clinicians should carefully consideration which strategy may be optimal for their specific clinical application.[4]

Somatic Testing

Somatic tumor testing for prostate cancer includes analysis of either tumor tissue or circulating cell-free tumor DNA (ctDNA; eg, liquid biopsy). Next-generation sequencing entails an analysis of a targeted panel of genes (eg, FoundationOne) or a whole exome approach (eg, Tempus). Some platforms now also offer companion diagnostics (ie, HRR-specific genes) for approved therapies. These types of somatic platforms differ from those that use gene expression data to generate risk scores (ie, OncotypeDx, Decipher). Analysis of the primary tumor remains the gold standard for chemotherapy selection; however, there is a high level of concordance between ctDNA and primary tumor tissue.[5,6] Additionally, somatic testing platforms have the potential to identify underlying germline mutations; however, these tests are not clinically validated for this purpose, and confirmatory germline testing is still indicated.

Implementation

Germline genetic testing is still a new component of prostate cancer care. Implementation challenges include limited access to genetic counselors, incorporation into clinical workflow, time and space availability for adequate counseling, insurance approval, cost to the patient, and resources for interpretation of results.[7] Clinicians and their teams should familiarize themselves with the testing process and various types of genetic counseling models to determine which approach would best suit their workflows.[3,4]

Somatic and germline testing strategies should be taken into consideration during treatment planning for metastatic prostate cancer. A somatic variant in a DDR gene warrants further evaluation to determine if an underlying germline pathogenic variant is present. However, when germline testing is performed, negative results do not rule out the possibility of clinically actionable somatic variant. Clinicians should consider initiating these tests in parallel to maximize information available for treatment planning.

THERAPEUTIC APPROACH
Poly (ADP-Ribose) Polymerase Inhibitors

PARPs are a family of enzymes that catalyze transfer of ADP-ribose to target proteins to regulate DNA repair, transcription, replication, recombination, and chromatin structure. This mechanism becomes particularly important in tumors that have lost homologous recombination (HR) as the primary mechanism of DNA repair. As a result, PARP inhibitors may sensitize tumor cells to DNA-damaging agents by preventing DNA repair through the base-excision pathway.[8] Patients with *BRCA1/2* mutations have lost the ability to repair DNA damage via HR, thus cells are reliant on the base-excision pathway to repair DNA damage. On this molecular basis, PARP inhibition is a prime target for inducing cell death in tumors with *BRCA1/2* mutations.

The TOPARP-A trial included patients with metastatic castrate-resistant prostate cancer (mCRPC), who had either a germline or somatic mutation in a DDR gene, and demonstrated that these individuals were more responsive to the PARP inhibitor, olaparib.[9] In the initial cohort of 50 patients, 80% had received greater than or equal to four prior regimens for CRPC. The primary end point was the response rate, defined as either a 50% or greater reduction in prostate-specific antigen (PSA) or a reduction in the number of ctDNA. Out of the 49 patients evaluated in the trial, 16 (33%) had a response, with 14/16 (88%) of those responders identified to have either a germline or somatic mutation in a DDR gene as compared with the 2/16 (12.5%) who showed no response. In addition, the patients with a DDR mutation had a median radiologic progression-free survival (PFS) of 9.8 months versus 2.7 months for those without a DDR mutation. Furthermore, there was an improvement in overall survival for the DDR mutation cohort (13.8 months vs 7.5 months; P = .05).

The TOPARP-B phase II trial expanded on the effectiveness of PARP inhibitor olaparib in patients with mCRPC and a DDR mutation, which demonstrated that it varies depending on the gene mutation.[10] All patients had previously been treated with docetaxel and 88/96 (90%) had also been treated with abiraterone acetate and/or enzalutamide. The primary end point of a confirmed response was radiologic, 50% or greater decrease in PSA, or decrease in ctDNA, with 92 total of patients evaluable. Between the two dose groups, 43/92 (46.7%) had an overall composite response, and more specifically 25/30 (83.3%) for those with BRCA1/2 mutations, four of seven (57%) with PALB2 mutations, 7/19 (36.8%) with ATM mutations, and 5/20 (25%) with CDK12 mutations. This trial was able to provide evidence of the need for possible stratification of patients based on their specific DDR mutational profile.

The PROfound phase III trial prospectively randomized patients with DDR mutations and progression of disease during treatment with an androgen receptor (AR)-targeted agent to treatment with another AR-targeted agent (enzalutamide or abiraterone acetate) or olaparib.[11] Patients were analyzed in two separate cohorts: cohort A (162 patients on treatment) included men with BRCA1, BRCA2, or ATM mutations, whereas cohort B (94 patients on treatment) included men with other less common prespecified DDR mutations. The primary end point was radiographic PFS for patients in cohort A, which was defined as the time from randomization until soft tissue disease progression, bone lesion progression, or death. Treatment with olaparib in cohort A was associated with an improved median survival when compared with treatment with the other AR-targeted agent (7.4 vs 3.6 months; P = .001), with a confirmed objective response rate of 33% (28/84) in the olaparib group versus 2% (1/43 patients) in the control group. Across both cohorts, the median imaging-based PFS was 5.8 months for those treated with olaparib versus 3.5 months in the control groups (P = .001). Food and Drug Administration (FDA) approval has been granted for olaparib for men with mCRPC who have a deleterious or suspected deleterious germline or somatic HRR gene mutation who have had disease progression following prior treatment with enzalutamide or abiraterone. A recent analysis published by Hussain and colleagues[12] showed that olaparib, compared with control group, had improved overall survival (19.1 months vs 14.7 months; P = .02).

The ongoing phase II TRITON2 trial examined response of patients with mutations in BRCA1/2, ATM, CDK12, and other DDR genes to the PARP inhibitor, rucaparib, in patients who have failed to two lines of AR-directed therapy and one line of taxane-based chemotherapy.[13] Patients with BRCA1/2 mutations demonstrated a 44% radiographic and 51.1% PSA response, whereas those with ATM mutations had a negligible response. Follow-up data at 24 weeks demonstrated a 43.9% overall response rate among those with a BRCA1/2 mutation, and 52% PSA response (>50% reduction) with a median duration of 5.5 months. Overall response was poor among patients with ATM (9.5%), CDK12 (0%), and CHEK2 (0%) mutations, whereas the PSA response was small for ATM (3.5%), CDK12 (7.1%), and CHEK2 (14.3%).[14] Thus, men with alterations in ATM, CDK12, or CHEK2 demonstrate limited radiographic and/or PSA responses to PARP inhibition compared with other DDR mutations (BRCA1/2, PALB2). Rucaparib was granted breakthrough therapy designation by the FDA for use as monotherapy in patients specifically with BRCA1/2-positive mCRPC who have progressed on at least one AR-directed therapy and taxane-based chemotherapy.

This growing body of evidence now available showing increased effectiveness of PARP inhibitors for those with DDR mutations, with exciting new FDA approvals, suggests that there is still room for improvement in creating a more refined treatment algorithm based on a patient's genetic profile. Furthermore, the data suggest that the most robust response to PARP inhibition is seen for patients with BRCA mutations, specifically BRCA2. However, additional studies are still needed to further address the effectiveness of PARPs compared with other standard therapeutic regimens. The TRITON3 trial will be a randomized phase III study evaluating rucaparib versus physician's choice of second-line AR-directed therapy or docetaxel in patients with mCRPC and BRCA1/2 or ATM mutations who progressed on one prior AR-directed therapy and who are chemotherapy naive.

Immunotherapies/Check-Point Inhibitors

The loss of MMR proficiency through defects in the MLH1, MSH2, MSH6, or PMS2 genes is associated with a higher mutation burden, often within the microsatellite regions leading to instability (MSI), ultimately contributing to tumor development. Although this process has been well established in gastrointestinal cancers, specifically colon,[15] and has been linked to treatment benefit with immunotherapies,[16] it has been underappreciated and understudied in prostate cancer until recently.

The occurrence of MMR deficiency (MMRd) in prostate cancer is considered rare, ranging from 3% to 12%.[17,18] A prospective case series identified that 3.1% (32/1033) of prostate tumors (no specification of stage) were dMMR or high levels of MSI (MSI-H), with 21.9% of this subset having an MMR germline mutation consistent with a diagnosis of Lynch syndrome.[18] However, an analysis of advanced prostate cancer found that 12% (7/60 patients) had MMR gene mutations, predominately *MSH2* and *MSH6*, and had MSI.[18] Given the more standardized and widespread genetic testing for patients with prostate cancer, it is likely that the detection of MMRd/MSI-H tumors will increase. Furthermore, although rare, it is clinically relevant to patients because new evidence suggests that there is a therapeutic advantage of immunotherapy in these patients.

In evaluating the clinical characteristics of men with dMMR/MSI prostate cancer, Pritchard and colleagues[19] found a median time to castration resistance of 8.6 months and a median duration of treatment with first-line abiraterone or enzalutamide of 9.9 months (range, 3.0–34.5 months) for mCRPC. In regard to response to treatment, out of 11 patients with mCRPC treated with pembrolizumab, five (45.5%) achieved a durable clinical benefit, comparable with effect in other MSI-H malignant neoplasms. In addition, six (54.5%) achieved a greater than 50% decline in PSA, with four of six patients having greater than 99% decline.

Graham and colleagues[17] retrospectively evaluated the clinical outcomes and response to various therapies for men with MMRd/MSI-H metastatic prostate cancer. They identified 27 men with MMRd/MSI-H cancer, with MSH2 being the most commonly mutated gene (20%, 74%). There was an association with a high Gleason score and advanced disease at the time of diagnosis, with 13/21 (48%) having de novo metastatic disease and 19/24 (79%) men having Gleason 8 to 10 disease on biopsy. Response rates to standard therapies are comparable with those reported in unselected patients, although the response rate to checkpoint blockade was high, with 8/15 (53%) of men treated with pembrolizumab having a 50% decline in PSA, and seven of eight (87.5%) of those men remained on treatment without evidence of progression. Although this small cohort shows promising responses to immunotherapy, additional studies are needed to compare responses with other treatment regimens and further define outcomes.

The FDA has approved pembrolizumab for those with solid tumors that are unresectable or metastatic with a high mutational burden ($\geq$10 mutations/megabase) that have progressed following prior treatment and who have no satisfactory alternative treatment options. This approval was accelerated based on the findings of KEYNOTE-158 (NCT02861573). The phase II KEYNOTE-158 investigated the effectiveness of pembrolizumab in patients with previously treated, advanced noncolorectal MSI-H/MMRd cancers.[20] There were 27 tumor types represented, and only 6 out of 233 (2.6%) patients had prostate cancer. Across tumors, the objective response rate was 34.3% and the median overall survival was 23.5 months. However, given the small number of prostate cancers represented, there was not a detailed analysis of outcomes performed, so further analysis is warranted.

Keynote-365 is currently investigating pembrolizumab combination therapies in mCRPC including pembrolizumab + olaparib, pembrolizumab + docetaxel + prednisone, and pembrolizumab + enzalutamide (NCT02861573). Preliminary results show 11 out of 28 patients with reduction in tumor burden; however, no complete responses have been reported.[21] In addition, Keynote-199 is enrolling patients with mCRPC who have progressed on AR therapy or chemotherapy with two cohorts based on PDL-1 expression status. A recent report from this study showed encouraging responses. Objective response rate was 5% (95% confidence interval [CI], 2%–11%) in the PDL-1-positive group and 3% (95% CI, <1%–11%) in the PDL-1-negative group. Median duration of response was not reached (range, 1.9 to $\geq$21.8 months) and 10.6 months (range, 4.4–16.8 months), respectively.[22] Although the Keynote-365 did not report MMRd/MSI statuses for their cohorts, this study showed that none of the six complete or partial responders had MMRd/MSI-H.

Chemotherapeutic Agents

There is no head-to-head comparison of docetaxel versus platinum-based therapies in the metastatic hormone-sensitive prostate cancer population. Docetaxel is an FDA-approved, first-line agent for patients with high-volume metastatic prostate cancer, regardless of DDR status. Multiple studies have evaluated the modifying effects of DDR mutations in response to systemic chemotherapy, either by agent or sequencing of treatment with androgen-deprivation therapy (ADT).

Platinum chemotherapy is typically not used in prostate cancer, although there are some data suggesting efficacy in patients with DDR mutations. A small case series of three patients with biallelic inactivation of *BRCA1/2* and metastatic prostate cancer, who had failed or progressed on first-line therapies, demonstrated an excellent response to platinum-based therapy.[23] A subsequent retrospective study examined the response to platinum chemotherapy for men with mCRPC and a germline *BRCA2*-positive mutation (8/141 men; 5.7%).[24] In those with germline mutation, six of eight (75%) had a greater than 50% decline in PSA within 12 weeks compared with 23/133 (17%) men in the control group. Furthermore, the *BRCA2*-positive carriers had a median survival from the start of chemotherapy of 18.9 months versus 9.5 months for noncarriers.

Some data suggest that men with germline DDR mutations may have a poorer response to traditional treatment strategies, such as AR-targeted therapy.[25] Of the 319 patients with metastatic prostate cancer screened for this study, 24 (7.5%) were identified to have a germline mutation in a DDR gene. Out of the 22 included in the retrospective study, at initial diagnosis 7/22 had metastatic disease, whereas 15/22 had low- or intermediate-grade localized disease (7/15 with high-risk disease). The median time from ADT initiation to castration resistance was only 11.8 months versus 19 months in patients without a germline mutation (95% CI, 5.1–18.4). The median PSA PFS for those in the germline-positive cohort on first-line AR-targeted therapy (enzalutamide or abiraterone) was only 3.3 months versus 6.2 months in the germline-negative cohort. However, the median PFS for those first receiving docetaxel in the germline cohort was comparable with those without (7.2 vs 8.0; *P* = .12).

An international retrospective study found no association between DDR carrier status and response to first-line AR therapy versus taxane.[26] Out of the 390 patients, 60 were identified to have a germline mutation, with most having mutations in *BRCA1/2* (61%) or *ATM* (11%). In this nonrandomized cohort, 70% received docetaxel, 69% abiraterone acetate or enzalutamide, and 45% received a PARP inhibitor or platinum-based chemotherapy. There was no significant difference in PFS and overall survival benefit among different treatment modalities for the two cohorts, suggesting that similar levels of benefit are derived regardless of germline mutation status. However, this study did not take into consideration somatic mutation status and was not powered to assess differences in outcome by treatment sequencing.

The prospective PROREPAIR-B study assessed the outcomes for men with mCRPC and germline mutations in *BRCA1/2*, *ATM*, and *PALB2* who were treated with platinum-based therapies.[27] Out of the 419 patients screened, 6.2% were identified to have germline mutation in the genes of interest, which expanded to 16.2% when including other DDR genes. The median time from initiation of ADT therapy to castrate resistance was 22.8 months for those with a germline DDR mutation versus 28.4 months in the control cohort, which was more pronounced for *BRCA2*-positive men versus control subjects (22.8 vs 13.2 months; *P* = .04). They found that *BRCA2* carriers have greater survival (24.0 vs 17.0 months; *P* = .005) and more time to progression to a second therapy (18.9 vs 8.6 months; *P* = .01) when treated first with abiraterone or enzalutamide compared with taxanes.

Overall, there are still conflicting studies regarding the effectiveness of first-line AR-targeted therapies versus taxanes for those with DDR gene mutations, and no prospective randomized trials to definitively determine the optimal approach. This may be caused by factors that affect treatment sequencing in nonrandomized settings, including the disease burden. Further prospective studies are needed to better define therapeutic outcomes and treatment sequences.

SUMMARY

Patients with prostate cancer with somatic and germline mutations are increasingly recognized as a unique subset that behave differently from nonmutated counterparts. Current guidelines recommend genetic testing for all patients presenting with metastatic disease. Priority testing for genes *BRCA1/2*, *PALB2*, *ATM*, and *MSH2/6* is crucial to allow a personalized approach based on best available evidence. This approach allows a better sequencing of current and investigational therapeutics for prostate cancer with end goal of improving overall survival for these patients.

CLINICS CARE POINTS

- When seeing patients with metastatic prostate cancer, all should undergo germline genetic sequencing for priority genes (*BRCA1/2*, *PALB2*, *ATM*, and *MSH2/6*) and receive posttest counseling if a pathologic mutation associated with a cancer syndrome is identified.

- Identifying DDR mutations in a patient with prostate cancer associated with familial cancer syndromes should lead to discussions of additional cancer risk and cascade testing for interested family members.

- Clinicians should be aware that rucaparib is approved for the treatment of metastatic castration-resistant prostate cancer (mCRPC) with a *BRCA1/2* mutation after disease progression on an AR-targeted agent and a taxane.

- Clinicians should be aware that olaparib is approved for the treatment of mCRPC with one of multiple DDR mutations after disease progression on an AR-targeted agent.

- Clinicians should be aware that pembrolizumab is approved for treatment of microsatellite instability-high (MSI-H) solid tumors, cancers with high tumor mutational burden (TMB ≥ 10 mutations/megabase), and mismatch repair deficient tumors (mutations in MLH1, MSH2, MSH6, PMS2) that have progressed following prior treatment.

DISCLOSURE

A.K. Morgans: Honoraria for consulting: Astellas, AstraZeneca, Advanced Accelerator Applications, Bayer, Clovis Janssen, Myovant, and Sanofi. Research collaboration: Bayer, Seattle Genetics, and Sanofi. A.L. Siebert, Y. Numan: None to disclose. B.M. Szymaniak: Consultant for Clovis Oncology and UroGPO. Honorarium from Invitae Corp.

REFERENCES

1. Pritchard CC, Mateo J, Walsh MF, et al. Inherited DNA-repair gene mutations in men with metastatic prostate cancer. N Engl J Med 2016;375(5):443–53.
2. Available at: https://www.nccn.org/professionals/physician_gls/pdf/prostate_blocks.pdf%20/PROS-8.
3. Giri VN, Hyatt C, Gomella LG. Germline testing for men with prostate cancer navigating an expanding new world of genetic evaluation for precision therapy and precision management. J Clin Oncol 2019;37(17):1455–9.
4. Szymaniak BM, Facchini LA, Giri VN, et al. Practical considerations and challenges for germline genetic testing in patients with prostate cancer: recommendations from the Germline Genetics Working Group of the PCCTC. JCO Oncol Pract 2020;16:1–9.
5. Wyatt AW, Annala M, Aggarwal R, et al. Concordance of circulating tumor DNA and matched metastatic tissue biopsy in prostate cancer. J Natl Cancer Inst 2017;109(12):djx118.
6. Sonpavde G, Agarwal N, Pond GR, et al. Circulating tumor DNA alterations in patients with metastatic castration-resistant prostate cancer. Cancer 2019; 125(9):1459–69.
7. Paller CJ, Eisenberger MA. Progress in the systemic management of advanced prostate cancer: the hormone-sensitive paradigm. J Clin Oncol 2019; 37(32):2957–60.
8. Morales JC, Li L, Fattah FJ, et al. Review of Poly (ADP-ribose) Polymerase (PARP) mechanisms of action and rationale for targeting in cancer and other diseases. Crit Rev Eukaryot Gene Expr 2014;24(1):15–28.
9. Mateo J, Carreira S, Sandhu S, et al. DNA-repair defects and olaparib in metastatic prostate cancer. N Engl J Med 2015;373(18):1697–708.
10. Mateo J, Porta N, Bianchini D, et al. Olaparib in patients with metastatic castration-resistant prostate cancer with DNA repair gene aberrations (TOPARP-B): a multicentre, open-label, randomised, phase 2 trial. Lancet Oncol 2020;21(1):162–74.
11. de Bono J, Mateo J, Fizazi K, et al. Olaparib for metastatic castration-resistant prostate cancer. N Engl J Med 2020;382(22):2091–102.
12. Abida W, Campbell D, Patnaik A, et al. (2019). Preliminary results from the TRITON2 study of rucaparib in patients (pts) with DNA damage repair (DDR)-deficient metastatic castration-resistant prostate cancer (mCRPC): updated analyses. Annals of Oncology, 30, p327-p328.
13. Abida W, Campbell D, Patnaik A, et al. Preliminary results from the TRITON2 study of rucaparib in patients (pts) with DNA damage repair (DDR)-deficient metastatic castration-resistant prostate cancer (mCRPC): updated analyses. Ann Oncol 2019;30: v327–8.
14. Abida W, Campbell D, Patnaik A, et al. Non-BRCA DNA damage repair gene alterations and response to the PARP inhibitor rucaparib in metastatic castration-resistant prostate cancer: analysis from the phase II TRITON2 Study. Clin Cancer Res 2020;26(11):2487–96.
15. Gologan A, Krasinskas A, Hunt J, et al. Performance of the revised Bethesda guidelines for identification of colorectal carcinomas with a high level of microsatellite instability. Arch Pathol Lab Med 2005;129: 1390–7.
16. Yaghoubi N, Soltani A, Ghazvini K, et al. PD-1/PD-L1 blockade as a novel treatment for colorectal cancer. Biomed Pharmacother 2019;110:312–8.
17. Graham LS, Montgomery B, Cheng HH, et al. Mismatch repair deficiency in metastatic prostate cancer: response to PD-1 blockade and standard therapies. PLoS One 2020;15(5):e0233260.
18. Abida W, Cheng ML, Armenia J, et al. Analysis of the prevalence of microsatellite instability in prostate cancer and response to immune checkpoint blockade. JAMA Oncol 2019;5(4):471–8.

19. Pritchard CC, Morrissey C, Kumar A, et al. Complex MSH2 and MSH6 mutations in hypermutated microsatellite unstable advanced prostate cancer. Nat Commun 2014;5:4988.

20. Marabelle A, Le DT, Ascierto PA, et al. Efficacy of pembrolizumab in patients with noncolorectal high microsatellite instability/mismatch repair-deficient cancer: results from the phase II KEYNOTE-158 study. J Clin Oncol 2019;38(1):1–10.

21. De Bono JS, Goh JC, Ojamaa K, et al. KEYNOTE-199: Pembrolizumab (pembro) for docetaxel-refractory metastatic castration-resistant prostate cancer (mCRPC). ASCO-GU conference (2018): 5007-5007.

22. Antonarakis ES, Piulats JM, Gross-Goupil M, et al. Pembrolizumab for treatment-refractory metastatic castration-resistant prostate cancer: multicohort, open-label phase II KEYNOTE-199 study. Journal of Clinical Oncology 2020;38(5):395.

23. Cheng HH, Pritchard CC, Boyd T, et al. Biallelic inactivation of BRCA2 in platinum-sensitive metastatic castration-resistant prostate cancer. Eur Urol 2016; 69(6):992–5.

24. Pomerantz MM, Spisák S, Jia L, et al. The association between germline BRCA2 variants and sensitivity to platinum-based chemotherapy among men with metastatic prostate cancer. Cancer 2017; 123(18):3532–9.

25. Annala M, Struss WJ, Warner EW, et al. Treatment outcomes and tumor loss of heterozygosity in germline DNA repair–deficient prostate cancer. Eur Urol 2017;72(1):34–42.

26. Mateo J, Cheng HH, Beltran H, et al. Clinical outcome of prostate cancer patients with germline DNA repair mutations: retrospective analysis from an international study. Eur Urol 2018;73(5):687–93.

27. Castro E, Romero-Laorden N, del Pozo A, et al. PROREPAIR-B: a prospective cohort study of the impact of germline DNA repair mutations on the outcomes of patient's with metastatic castration-resistant prostate cancer. J Clin Oncol 2018;37(6): 490–503.

Genetically Informed Prostate Cancer Screening

Rohith Arcot, MD[a],*, Todd M. Morgan, MD[b], Thomas J. Polascik, MD, FACS[a]

KEYWORDS

- Prostate cancer screening ● Germline mutations ● Single nucleotide polymorphisms
- Prostate cancer ● Genetics

KEY POINTS

- The genetic basis for prostate cancer may be the result of specific high-penetrance (germline) and low-penetrance (single-nucleotide polymorphisms [SNPs]) gene variants.
- A combination of SNPs may provide evidence for an increased risk of any prostate cancer but may not identify individuals at risk for lethal prostate cancer.
- Consider early (starting at age 40) and annual screening in men with known or suspected germline mutations in BRCA1/2, ATM, CHEK2, and NBN, with the help of genetic counselors.
- Novel risk-adapted screening strategies should take advantage of traditional risk factors along with genetic predisposition, if known, to tailor screening strategies.
- Screening strategies may include the use of novel biomarkers or magnetic resonance imaging of the prostate to limit the overdiagnosis of indolent disease in those at high risk for the development of prostate cancer.

INTRODUCTION

Prior to the Food and Drug Administration approval of prostate-specific antigen (PSA) testing in the late 1980s, the early detection of prostate cancer relied on digital rectal examination (DRE) that lacked reproducibility and sensitivity. The improved sensitivity and specificity of serum PSA testing ushered in an era of routine clinical screening.[1] The result was a dramatic rise in the incidence of prostate cancer diagnoses, radical treatment, decreased prostate cancer mortality, and decreased incidence of advanced disease.[2] Although the benefits of prostate cancer screening seem obvious, the effectiveness of routine population-based screening came under fire after randomized controlled trials showed limited improvement in mortality in screened cohorts.

Currently, multiple professional organizations, including the American Urological Association (AUA), European Association of Urology (EAU), American Cancer Society (ACS), National Comprehensive Cancer Network (NCCN), and the US Preventive Services Task Force (USPSTF), provide guidelines for the early detection of prostate cancer despite the lack of agreement on an optimal strategy. All groups do agree that patients should be well informed and discuss the role of PSA screening on an individual basis with their health advocate before testing.[3–7]

Although there is a lack of agreement on when and how to screen the average risk man, it generally is believed that those populations with higher incidence, progression, and mortality stand to benefit the most from early detection. Until now, high-risk populations typically have been

Funding: None.
[a] Division of Urology, Duke University, 20 Duke Medicine Circle, Durham, NC 27710, USA; [b] Department of Urology, University of Michigan, 1500 E Medical Center Dr, Ann Arbor, MI 48109, USA
* Corresponding author. Division of Urology, Duke University, Duke Cancer Center, 20 Duke Medicine Circle, Durham, NC 27710.
E-mail address: rohith.arcot@duke.edu

Urol Clin N Am 48 (2021) 373–386
https://doi.org/10.1016/j.ucl.2021.04.001

characterized by age, race, and family history, but increasing evidence supports the use of genetic components to improve the precision of risk assessment. This article presents the current evidence for genetically informed, risk-adapted screening strategies for prostate cancer.

CONTROVERSY SURROUNDING PROSTATE-SPECIFIC ANTIGEN TESTING

To understand the controversy surrounding the implementation of PSA screening, the changes that have occurred over time in the USPSTF recommendations need to be look at. In 2008, the USPSTF determined that they were unable to recommend for or against prostate cancer screening due to a lack evidence. By 2012 the USPSTF revised their recommendations centered on 2 large population-based screening trials—the European Randomized Study of Screening for Prostate Cancer (ERSPC) and the Prostate, Lung, Colorectal and Ovarian (PLCO) trial, and issued a controversial grade D recommendation, stating that there was moderate to high certainty that prostate cancer screening has no net benefit or that the harms outweigh benefits.[8]

The ERSPC was initiated in 1994 and attempted to answer the question as to whether or not PSA-based screening could reduce prostate cancer mortality. The trial truly was a compendium of trials among 7 European countries with different eligibility, randomization schemes, screening intervals, and follow-up.[9] In 2009, initial results identified a mortality reduction of approximately 20% attributed to prostate cancer screening but with no difference in all-cause mortality between groups.[10] The overall number needed-to-screen (NNS) was greater than 1000 and the number needed-to-treat (NNT) was greater than 30 to prevent 1 death that at the time was comparatively high compared with breast cancer screening trials.[11] The results suggested that although screening may improve mortality, the overall benefit may be small and that the downstream effects of screening—invasive biopsies, overtreatment, and morbidity-associated with treatment—negate the realized mortality benefits. Longer follow-up, however, has shown steady decreases in the NNS and NNT, which now are more favorable than those associated with breast cancer screening.

The sister trial in the United States, the PLCO Cancer Screening Trial, was initiated at approximately the same time as the ERSPC and sought to answer a similar question. The trial included 10 US centers and randomized men to annual screening versus usual care. At the initial interim analysis after 7 years to 10 years, the rate of death from prostate cancer was very low in both groups, and there was no statistically significant difference between groups.[12] As reported in 2016 by Shoag and colleagues,[13] the control arm was contaminated with opportunistic screening in as many as 90% of participants, making the 2 groups nearly indistinguishable for the intervention being studied.

The nuances and limitations affecting the findings in these trials are beyond the scope of this article, but a limitation that cannot be overstated is the lack of enrichment for high-risk groups in either trial. These populations with higher prevalence of aggressive disease include black men and those with a family history of prostate cancer or other cancers, and these patients could benefit from early detection.[14–18]

From 2018 to the present, the USPSTF has revised their recommendation, stating in 2018 that well-informed patients with greater than 10 years to 15 years life expectancy may benefit from screening.[6] Among the numerous organizations providing guidance, no consensus opinion exists regarding the best strategy for early detection of prostate cancer with PSA screening in average risk individuals. All organizations do recognize, however, that high-risk populations may benefit from early and/or more frequent screening, but lack of evidence showing improved outcomes with targeted screening in these populations limit statements regarding the best approach.

GENETIC PREDISPOSITION TO PROSTATE CANCER

With advances in molecular oncology, the 1-size fits all approach to screening and treatment of cancer may be supplanted by more individualized risk-adapted pathways.[19] Many of these advances come from both studies using genome-wide association studies (GWASs), which can identify low-penetrance gene loci, known as single-nucleotide polymorphisms (SNPs), and the identification of known high-penetrance variants and their associations with various cancers.[20,21] Furthermore, as genetic testing becomes increasingly affordable and available, understanding the genetic basis of cancer incidence and phenotype is becoming increasingly essential.

Prostate cancer represents 1 of the more heritable cancers, with up to 57% of variation among individuals attributed to genetic factors.[22–24] Furthermore, men with a family history of prostate cancer are more likely to be diagnosed and die of prostate cancer than those without a family history.[15] Evidence now supports a link between aggressive cancers and the frequency of certain heritable mutations that is beginning to inform treatment decisions in advanced disease.[25–27] Genetically informed prostate cancer screening represents an important area of study and is of particular importance because PSA screening is confounded by many nonmalignant factors, limiting its utility.[28–30]

Risk-adapted approaches to prostate cancer screening are not new but until now have been limited largely to stratification by age, race, and family history that to some degree may correlate with genetic predisposition. Inherited prostate cancer can be separated into 2 groups: familial prostate cancer (FPC), representing 15% to 20% of cases and lacking detectable single germline mutations; and heritable prostate cancer (HPC) that is rare in most populations and associated with high-penetrance genetic variants, such as breast cancer gene 1 (*BRCA1*) and breast cancer gene 2 (*BRCA2*), that increase the lifetime risk of prostate and other cancers.[31] It now is recognized that the risk associated with FPC may be accounted at least partially for by SNPs. Approximately 10 million SNPs have been identified with different patterns of altered loci associated with various disease traits and cancers.[20,21] Using a combination of loci, a particular risk can be assigned to an individual by compiling the number SNPs, each of which may be associated with a very slight increase in cancer risk.

HPC, representing 10% to 15% of cases, is quite different, related to much rarer variants, each of which is associated with moderate effect size. Genes known to predispose to prostate cancer include DNA damage-repair, such as *BRCA1*, *BRCA2*, *ATM*, *CHEK2*, and *PALB2,* as well as mismatch repair (MMR) genes related to Lynch syndrome (*MSH6*, *MSH2*, *MLH1*, and *MLH2*), and homeobox protein HOXB13.[25,32–36] The importance of cancer predisposition genes to inform screening is well known in breast cancer and ovarian cancer, where there long have been guidelines incorporating this information into screening. As expected, many of the occurrences of prostate cancer in families have come from studies including those families with known hereditary breast and ovarian cancer (HBOC) or Lynch syndrome.[37–39]

Ideally, genetically informed prostate cancer screening would better align individual patient risk with initiation and frequency of screening to identify more cancers when they still are curable, while minimizing unnecessary biopsies and overdetection of clinically insignificant cancers (Gleason grade group [GGG] 1).

Germline Variants in Prostate Cancer

Current understanding of HPC comes from the identification of germline pathogenic variants and likely pathogenic variants (PVs/LPVs) found in men belonging to families with hereditary cancer syndromes.[37–40] In 1 early study, a founder mutation in BRCA2 was detected in an Iceland population of families with HBOC. Men within the affected families developed both early-onset and lethal prostate cancer. Examination of an unselected population revealed a very low frequency (<5%), limiting the perceived utility in the general population.[40] In a relatively recent report by Pritchard and colleagues,[25] however, the investigators were able to show, unexpectedly, that 12% of men with metastatic prostate cancer harbor germline pathogenic variants that was significantly higher compared with the general population and to men with localized prostate cancer. Following this report, for the first time, in 2017, the NCCN Guidelines for Prostate Cancer Early Detection began to include germline-specific language in screening recommendations.[3]

To date, the most well-studied germline mutations not only associate with prostate cancer but also with lethal prostate cancer, which include BRCA1/2 followed by ATM, CHEK2, PALB2, and NBN.[25,41,42] In primarily European American men (EAM), carriers of these genes are known to have early onset and more frequent metastasis and/or worse cancer-specific survival compared with noncarriers.[25,32–34,41,43–47] Other candidate genes associated with prostate cancer but less evidence for the risk of lethal prostate cancer include Lynch syndrome genes (MSH2, MSH6, MLH1, and PMS2), BRIP1, and RAD51C-D.[25,37,38,41,48–50] The only non-DNA repair gene consistently associated with prostate cancer is the rare missense mutation G84E variant of the HOXB13 gene, but the variant has not been shown to affect the development of lethal prostate cancer.[35,51]

The overall frequency of germline mutations in the general population and the full gamut of PVs/LPVs that have an impact on prostate cancer risk still are not fully understood and continue to grow with new studies performed (**Table 1**).[42] In addition, a majority of studies at present have not included diverse racial groups, limiting current knowledge of germline testing in those non-EAM populations.[25,41,48] Nevertheless, current data suggest that targeted screening in those with known or suspected germline variants could have an impact on long-term outcomes.

Single Nucleotide Polymorphisms in Prostate Cancer

Although family history is an important risk factor that predisposed to prostate cancer, the specific risk attributable to family history is complex

Table 1
Genetic Contribution of Prostate Cancer Risk, Aggressiveness, and Metastatic Potential

Pathogenic Variant	Association with Prostate Cancer[a]	Risk of Aggressive Prostate Cancer[a]	Prevalence in Mestatic Prostate Cancer[b]	Mechanism of Action
BRCA2	+++	+++	+++	DNA damage repair
ATM	+	++	++	DNA damage response
CHEK2	++	+	++	DNA damage repair by phosphorylation of BRCA2
HOXB13	+++	—	—	AR Repressor
BRCA1	++	+/−	+	DNA damage repair
MSH2/MSH6	++	+	+	DNA repair
MLH1/PMS2	+	+/−	+	DNA repair
NBN	+/−	+/−	+	DNA repair
PALB2	—	+	+	Tumor suppressor
RAD51C-D	—	—	+	DNA repair
BRIP1	—	—	+	DNA repair by interaction with BRCA1

[a] Evidence from case-control, familial, cohort studies: strong (+++); moderate (++); low (+); conflicting data (+/−); and not established (−).
[b] High prevalence ($\geq$4% = +++); moderate (1%–4% = ++); low prevalence (<1% = +); and not reported (−).
Adapted with permission from JCO from Giri et al. Implementation of Germline Testing for Prostate Cancer: Philadelphia Prostate Cancer Consensus Conference 2019.

because it is modified by the degree of relatedness to the affected individual, age at diagnosis, and phenotype of the cancer diagnosed.[52,53] Furthermore, comprehensive and accurate assessment of family history is constrained by patient recall. Over the past decade, GWASs have sought to unravel the genetic basis for familial prostate cancer susceptibility.

Since the late 2000s, the mapping of the human genome has allowed GWASs to query multiple loci across chromosomes and identified approximately 170 loci associated with prostate cancer.[20,54,55] Unlike high-penetrance variants, SNPs are found at higher frequencies in the population and often are found in noncoding regions of DNA that have unknown biological significance. Individually, SNPs lack a strong effect, low penetrance but taken together produce a cumulative risk of prostate cancer. In 1 study, prostate cancer risk increased by 4.5-fold and by 10-fold in those with a family history of prostate cancer compared with controls.[56] To date, most studies have included only EAM, but studies including African American men have identified new risk loci.[57,58] Thus, future studies, including diverse study populations, may help account race-specific differences in prostate cancer susceptibility.

Several different methods have been described to measure the cumulative effect of SNPs, but a commonly used approach is to calculate a polygenic risk score (PRS) that calculates the odds ratio of each SNP, providing a cumulative risk association with each SNP added. The genetic risk score (GRS) is similar but weights risk against a population standard. The score output is a relative risk from the combination of SNPs compared with the general population in which the average risk individual score is equal to 1, whereas a value greater than 1 confers increased risk and the opposite for less than 1.[59,60]

PRSs have been validated across several different study settings. The 2 largest studies in the literature are case-control series that found these scores to be significantly associated with prostate cancer risk. Specifically, men scoring in the ninetieth to ninety-ninth percentiles and men in the top 1 percentile had a 2.69-fold to 2.9-fold (95% CI, 2.55–3.1) and 5.7-fold to 5.71-fold (95% CI, 4.8–6.6) increased relative risk of prostate cancer compared with men with an average GRS, respectively. Conversely, men with a GRS less than 1 were found at particularly low risk of developing prostate cancer. When studied in a clinical trial setting using the control arm of the Reduction by Dutasteride of Prostate Cancer Events (REDUCE) and Prostate Cancer Prevention Trial (PCPT) trial, GRS scores proved to be an independent predicator of prostate cancer at biopsy with modest improvements to traditional clinic-demographic factors used to predict biopsy outcomes. Even when family history was negative, SNPs were able to accurately predict men at greater risk of cancer at biopsy.[61–63] Thus, GRS has the potential to provide a continuum of risk for men that is objective and able to supplement family history when available. These findings are of considerable interest because these scores could help identify high-risk and low-risk men who otherwise might be considered average risk for screening programs that provide a mortality benefit.

Currently, SNPs have not made their way into routine prostate cancer screening paradigms. This partly is due to lack of consensus on which SNPs provide the most information and because SNPs have yet to show a definitive ability to discriminate those at risk of any prostate cancer from clinically aggressive prostate cancer.[55,62,64] In spite of this, a recent population based diagnostic study was able to show that the Stockholm-3 model (STHLM3) algorithm combining 232 SNPs, the 4 kallikreins in the 4 kallikrein score (4Kscore), and standard clinical variables, such as PSA, age, family history, previous biopsy, DRE, and prostate volume, could improve the specificity of PSA-alone screening (area under the receiver operating characteristic curve [AUC] 0.56) for Gleason score 7 prostate cancer with an AUC of 0.72. Although the data are promising, questions remain regarding which components of this STHLM3 algorithm are needed and provide the most value.[65]

Future studies are needed to optimize which SNPs to query, which SNPs provide accurate risk assessment in different races, and if SNPs can help differentiate those at risk for aggressive disease and in turn benefit from an early and more frequent screening strategies. Multiple commercial platforms exist to test for SNPs, and although the optimal utility has yet to be determined, it is possible they could be used to refine screening in populations otherwise thought to be average risk due to lack of traditional risk factors.

CLINICAL TRIALS WITH GENETICALLY INFORMED PROSTATE CANCER SCREENING

The harms of routine serum-based PSA-only prostate cancer screening stem, in part, from an era of unreliable and poorly sensitive screening techniques that lead to the assumption that all PSA-detected disease would benefit from early detection and treatment; screen-detected prostate cancer, however, has a long natural history and some cancers may be amenable to deferred treatment.[66,67] Thus, although genetics may improve individual risk assessment, the appropriate screening strategy to match the type of risk conferred by genetic variants has not been studied systematically. To date, a few ongoing clinical trials could provide insight into the value of targeted screening in high-risk men with a genetic predisposition to prostate cancer.

IMPACT

The Identification of Men With a Genetic Predisposition to ProstAte Cancer (IMPACT) study is an international, multicenter trial targeting prostate cancer patients with known BRCA1/2 germline mutations.[68] The objective of the study is to determine the utility of yearly PSA screening in the detection of clinically significant prostate cancer in carriers of BRCA1/2 mutations compared with noncarriers using a PSA biopsy threshold of a 3 ng/mL. Men were recruited from families with known pathogenic BRCA1/2 mutations and were ages 45 to 69 in the Netherlands and ages 40 to 69 in all other countries. Annual screening is performed in all countries except the Netherlands, where biennial screening was done due to local regulations. The biopsy protocol is standard transrectal ultrasound-guided biopsy with 10 cores to 12 cores taken in systematic fashion. Patients at time of screening also are offered a 4Kscore in addition to PSA screening before biopsy.

In the initial report, a majority of participants were white (97%) and included 919 BRCA1 carriers, 709 BRCA1 noncarriers, 902 BRCA2 carriers, and 497 BRCA2 noncarriers. The investigators found the cancer incidence rate per 1000 person years was higher in BRCA2 carriers versus BRCA2 noncarriers (19.4 vs 12.0, respectively; $P = .03$). Furthermore, BRCA2 carriers were diagnosed at an earlier age (61 y vs 64 y, respectively; $P = .04$) and more likely to have clinically significant disease (77% vs 60%, respectively; $P = .01$) compared with BRCA2 noncarriers. No difference was detected, however, in age or tumor characteristics when comparing BRCA1 carriers to BRCA1 noncarriers. Lastly, the 4Kscore outperformed PSA regarding the identification of clinically significant cancer with an AUC = 0.73 compared with an AUC = 0.65 with PSA alone.

The interim results concluded that early and routine PSA screening in men with BRCA2 mutations is warranted and further follow-up is needed to identify the potential impact of the early detection program in BRCA1 carriers.[69]

PROFILE

In another approach to understand the role of genetics in prostate cancer early detection, the

Germline Genetic Profiling: Correlation With Targeted Prostate Cancer Screening and Treatment (PROFILE) study is collecting both clinical and SNP data while performing biopsies in all enrolled men. In this UK-based study, the primary objective is to determine the association between PRS and multiparametric magnetic resonance imaging of the prostate (mpMRI) plus biopsy outcomes in men with either a family history of prostate cancer or black race. The plan is to recruit a total of 700 men 40 years to 69 years of age who will be offered mpMRI and biopsy regardless of PSA, whereas those who refuse mpMRI or biopsy will undergo routine PSA testing at 6-month intervals. Currently, the pilot study results are available, and the larger prospective study powered to detect associations between SNP RPSs and biopsy outcomes started recruiting in 2015.[70]

A feasibility study was performed in 100 men aged 40 years to 69 years with a family history of prostate cancer. Men were offered biopsy regardless of PSA level and a PRS was calculated for all individuals based on 71 common prostate cancer susceptibility alleles. In total, 25 men were diagnosed with prostate cancer, of whom 12 (48%) had clinically significant disease based on National Institute for Health and Care Excellence guidelines. There was no association between PRS score and Gleason score 7 or greater tumors at biopsy ($P = .20157$). Prospective, long-term follow-up to evaluate the role of SNPs in a predictive model for prostate cancer risk assessment is eagerly awaited.[71]

CURRENT GUIDELINES THAT INCLUDE RISK-ADAPTED GENETICALLY INFORMED SCREENING

The NCCN Prostate Cancer Early Detection Guidelines recommend that men with suspected or known germline mutations should be evaluated by a genetics counselor, and those men with known germline mutations in BRCA1/2 should consider early screening after shared decision making, starting at age 40 and continuing at yearly intervals.[3] The EAU guidelines offer similar guidance with early screening starting at age 40 but do not include BRCA1 and recommend interval testing to be guided by baseline PSA level.[7]

Both the NCCN Prostate Cancer Early Detection Guidelines and the Philadelphia Prostate Cancer Consensus Conference statement do recognize that other germline mutations have been associated with prostate cancer; and when identified, should be part of any discussion regarding prostate screening, but as of now none has made its way into NCCN guideline statements. This is due to data

suggesting that other mutations may be less actionable, such as those of low penetrance or those lacking an association with aggressive or metastatic prostate cancer. The Philadelphia Prostate Cancer Consensus Conference statement does recommend early and annual screening begin at 40 years of age for those with known BRCA2 mutations and suggests that clinicians consider early screening and annual screening in those with known mutations in BRCA1, ATM, HOXB13, and MMR genes (in particular, MSH2).[3,42]

The ACS does not specifically include germline status as a part of their risk adapted screening guidelines; however, they do recommend that informed discussions regarding screening take place at 45 years of age in men with a first-degree relative diagnosed with prostate cancer younger than 65 years or at 40 years of age in men at even high risk with more than 1 first-degree relative diagnosed with prostate cancer young than 65 years.[5] As of yet, the AUA has not updated their guideline statements on early detection of prostate cancer to include germline screening recommendations.[4]

Ultimately, early and annual screening in populations with suspected or known germline mutations may be beneficial, but population-based screening trials are needed to compare affected and unaffected cohorts with long-term follow-up to understand the true impact of early detection. In addition, early and more frequent screening may lead to the diagnosis of predominantly indolent disease that could lead to overtreatment.[72] Finally, cost certainly is a factor and currently no evidence exists to support a cost-effective approach, although new modeling studies currently under development may inform this topic.

NOVEL SCREENING PARADIGMS

Contemporary screening strategies take advantage of several clinical and demographic factors to create risk-adapted screening algorithms. First, clinicians assess traditional risk factors (age, race, and family history) along with life expectancy to identify those who might benefit from an informed discussion about PSA screening. After shared decision making with patients, baseline PSA along with age and race-adjusted PSA values are used to determine the intensity of screening or need for biopsy. Given that PSA generally is an organ-specific and not a cancer-specific biomarker, further risk assessment may be warranted. Several avenues have been explored to improve the diagnostic accuracy of PSA that include magnetic resonance imaging, PSA derivatives, and novel biomarkers from blood, urine, and tissue.

In terms of screening, clinical validation studies have provided evidence that imaging and biomarkers can not only improve the diagnostic accuracy of PSA but also identify those at risk for clinically significant (GGG ≥2) prostate cancer. At present, however, no test is preferred over another due to lack of head-to-head comparisons and lack of level 1 evidence in screening trials.[73] Trials currently are under way, however, to answer some of these questions.

Although the burden of screening still lies with primary care, urologists have taken it on themselves to design and test contemporary screening strategies due to the complexity associated with screening.

Duke University Model

At Duke Health, a coordinated effort was undertaken by a multidisciplinary team, including Duke Primary Care (DPC) and the Duke Cancer Institute to develop a population-specific, risk-adapted screening algorithm.[17] Importantly, the algorithm was paired with health maintenance alerts and laboratory data within the electronic health record (EHR), EPIC (Verona, WI), and coupled with a decision support tool to create a seamless workflow for DPC practitioners. This novel approach provided DPC clinicians with contemporary guidelines incorporating best practices from the NCCN, ACS, AUA, and USPSTF guidelines for whom to screen, when to screen, and when to refer to urology. Following implementation, outcomes measured over a 1-year implementation period showed a 20% increase in men who met screening criteria and a decrease in practice variation among screening across all DPC clinicians. Although the number of men who met screening criteria increased, the number of PSA tests ordered remained stable due decreased testing in low-risk populations and increased testing in high-risk populations.[19] The long-term outcomes and cost from the impact of this screening algorithm are yet to be determined, but initial results provide evidence that a population specific, risk-adapted algorithm embedded in the EHR could provide the avenue to increase guideline adherence and limit practice variation.

Beyond routine screening, a high-risk prostate screening clinic with an advanced clinical care pathway was developed at Duke Health (Fig. 1). Men found to be at risk for prostate cancer are referred by DPC to urology for further risk-stratification prior to biopsy to mitigate the over-diagnosis and any unintended consequences of prostate biopsy. Novel biomarkers, such as the Prostate Health Index test, 4Kscore, and urine ExoDx tests, among others, along with mpMRI are selectively utilized to provide more detail for informed decision-making. Currently under development is the incorporation of genetically informed screening within this algorithm.[42] Patients presenting to this clinic already have an abnormal PSA, DRE, or both. Elevated PSA is confirmed with a Prostate Health Index test, and second-line testing is performed with either mpMRI and/or urine ExoDx or serum 4Kscore. Germline testing is discussed and recommended if appropriate. Counseling additionally is provided by dedicated genetic counselors. Prostate biopsy, either magnetic resonance imaging–directed or conventional, is offered to men at risk of cancer. By incorporating this pathway within the EHR the goal is to identify more men at high risk for clinically significant prostate cancer due to known or suspected germline mutations to be included in a separate high-risk screening category.[74] This adaptable and scalable initiative could provide the observational data needed to inform future screening paradigms.

University of Michigan Model

Patients at high genetic and familial risk in Michigan are eligible for participation in the University of Michigan Prostate Cancer Risk Clinic (Fig. 2).[75] Patients aged 35 to 70 with a known germline mutation or strong family history of breast cancer, ovarian cancer, and/or prostate cancer are eligible to participate. Patients are seen in a urologic oncology clinic and a self-administered survey is collected, including smoking history, alcohol consumption, use of medications and supplements, and patient utilization of preventative health care services. Following the survey, a history and physical examination are performed, including a DRE. Counseling includes a discussion of prostate cancer risk along with lifestyle factors, such as physical activity, obesity, and/or smoking cessation, as indicated. Prespecified indications for biopsy are (1) abnormal DRE, (2) PSA above threshold (>2 ng/mL for patients <50 years and >2.5 ng/mL for patients 50–75 years), or (3) SelectMDx (MDxHealth, Irvine, CA) urine biomarker assay above the threshold risk for GGG greater than or equal to 2 prostate cancer. For patients without an indication for a biopsy and for those with a negative biopsy, annual follow-up using the same algorithm is recommended.

University of Washington Model

A multi-institutional effort is under way to understand the impact of a targeted prostate cancer

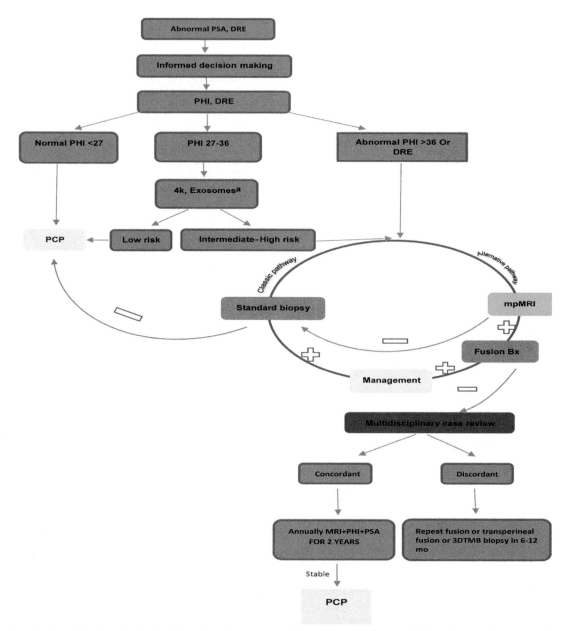

Fig. 1. Duke Health risk-stratified Prostate Cancer screening algorithm. Abnormal PSA is first confirmed via the PHI assay. Abnormal PHI or PSA can be secondarily interrogated with a serum-based 4K score or urine-based Exosomes (ExoDx) to help further stratify patient risk prior to biopsy. Other biomarker assays can similarly be used per clinician discretion in the diagnostic box containing 4k and Exosomes. For those who cannot tolerate mpMRI or those willing to simply proceed directly to prostate biopsy can take advantage of the classic biopsy pathway. Multi-disciplinary case review encompasses reconciling a suspicious MRI target to a negative targeted biopsy as part of a quality assurance program. If suspicion of cancer remains, patient is advised to consider another targeted biopsy, perhaps using a different approach (TRUS vs TP vs 3-D TMB). PCP, primary care provider; PIRADS, Prostate Imaging Reporting & Data System; PSA, prostate specific antigen; DRE, digital rectal exam; PHI, prostate Health Index; 4k, 4k score; Exosome, ExoDx; mpMRI, multiparametric MRI; MRI, magnetic resonance imaging; TRUS, transrectal ultrasound; TP, transperineal; 3D TMB, 3-dimensional template mapping biopsy; mo, months; Bx, biopsy..

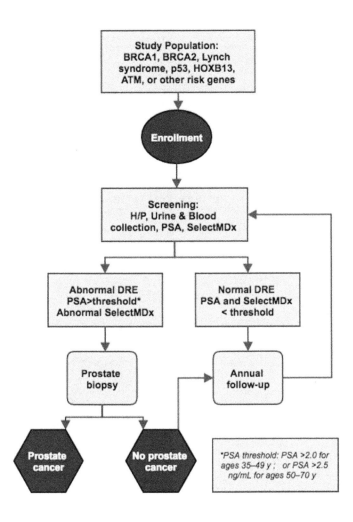

Fig. 2. Study protocol for University of Michigan Prostate Cancer Risk Clinic aimed at early detection of men with pathogenic germline mutations predisposing to prostate cancer. H/P, history and physical; PSA, prostate specific antigen; DRE, digital rectal exam.

screening program in men at increased genetic risk through enrollment in an National Cancer Institute (NCI)-funded clinical trial led by the University of Washington—Prostate Screening for Men With Inherited Risk of Developing Aggressive Prostate Cancer (PATROL) (**Fig. 3**).[76] The goal of this observational, prospective cohort study is to recruit 450 men and study blood, urine, and tissue samples at set intervals before and after diagnosis to further understand the genetics basis of prostate cancer. Men without a previous diagnosis of prostate cancer are eligible for study enrollment if greater than or equal to 40 years of age (>35 years if relative with prostate cancer diagnosis of ≤40 years) with greater than 5-year life-expectancy and have documented PVs/LPVs in known or selected suspected prostate cancer predisposing genes. The primary objective is to identify the positive predictive value of predefined age-directed PSA thresholds for biopsy. The secondary objectives include: accuracy assessment of the SelectMDx

urine biomarker for predicting prostate cancer, characterization of the prostate cancer diagnosed, and evaluation of participant reported quality of life outcomes. In addition, biospecimens will be collected to evaluate exploratory biomarkers (NCT04472338).

National Cancer Institute Model

At the NCI, a study is under way to follow men with known genetic changes with routine prostate cancer screening measures. This trial is a prospective cohort study with a target enrollment of 500 men referred to the NCI from around the United States with known germline mutations currently unaffected by prostate cancer and able to undergo magnetic resonance imaging. The primary objective of this trial is to understand the natural history of men with known germline variants or likely pathogenic variants in genes that put them at high risk of developing prostate cancer. Beyond PSA

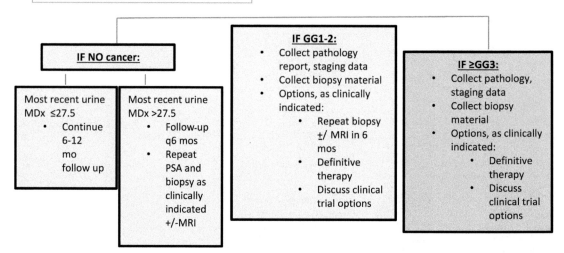

Fig. 3. University of Washington: PATROL Trial Study Protocol. Baseline information is gathered at trial enrollment and then every 6-12 months. Biopsy is performed when indicated. Treatment is based on biopsy grade group. Blood and urine are gathered routinely every 6-12 months, at biopsy, at treatment, and following treatment. (H.H. Cheng and D.W. Lin, unpublished). y, years; MO, months; DR, digital rectal exam; 5AR, 5-alpha reductase; PSA, prostate specific antigen; QOL, quality of life; GG, grade group; MRI, magnetic resonance imaging.

screening, this trial includes mpMRI with biennial follow-up that was not included in the IMPACT study. The secondary objective is to determine the potential utility of mpMRI as an adjunct to PSA screening in patients at high genetic risk of prostate cancer (NCT03805919).[77]

These novel screening algorithms represent some of the earliest attempts to evaluate the role of genetic risk and its incorporation within a high-risk screening clinic. Observations that could help inform future guidelines are awaited.

DISCUSSION

For years, pathogenic variants associated with HBOC have been used to inform target screening strategies in those with known or suspected germline variants. There is mounting evidence that the heritable predisposition to prostate cancer is an important risk factor for the development of early-onset and lethal prostate cancer. Furthermore, with the increase in commercially available multigene panel and PRS testing, there is a critical need to understand how high-penetrance and low-penetrance gene alterations have an impact on the development of prostate cancer. Despite this, few observational or randomized clinical trials exist to inform the clinical utility of prostate cancer genetic predisposition on secondary prevention. At present, multiple large institutions are working to answer this question with novel risk-adapted screening strategies in genetically high-risk groups. Ultimately, genetically informed prostate cancer screening may mitigate the risks of routine prostate cancer screening, identify those at high risk when their disease is curable, and improve long-term prostate cancer outcomes in those high-risk patients that seek to benefit the most.

Further research is needed not only to establish the scientific validity of HPC but also to identify the best approach to early detection and management of those with actionable mutations.

SUMMARY

Novel risk-adapted screening strategies are needed to mitigate the risk of routine PSA-only screening in all men based on age. As the evidence for the genetic basis of prostate cancer expands, it is possible that genetically informed screening can add traditional risk factors to tailor the age to initiate and frequency with which to screen. Observational studies and clinical trials are under way to answer the clinical utility of targeted screening in genetically high-risk groups.

CLINICS CARE POINTS

- The evidence for the genetic basis for prostate cancer is growing and includes both high-penetrance and low-penetrance gene variants
- Commercially available tests make it possible to identify pathogenic germline variants and single nucleotide polymorphisms that increase prostate cancer predisposition
- PRSs may provide evidence for increased risk of any prostate cancer, but there is limited evidence to support their use to identify increased risk of lethal prostate cancer
- Consider early (starting at age 40) and annual screening in those patients with known germline mutations in BRCA2, ATM, CHEK2, and NBN, with the help of genetic counselors
- Risk-adapted screening strategies should take advantage of traditional risk factors along with genetic predisposition, when available, to tailor screening strategies
- Targeted screening may include the use of novel biomarkers or mpMRI of the prostate to limit overdiagnosis of indolent disease in those at high risk for the diagnosis prostate cancer

DISCLOSURE

R. Arcot—none. T.M. Morgan—research funding from Myriad Genetics. T.J. Polascik—none.

REFERENCES

1. Polascik TJ, Oesterling JE, Partin AW. Prostate specific antigen: a decade of discovery–what we have learned and where we are going. J Urol 1999; 162(2):293–306.
2. Siegel RL, Miller KD, Jemal A. Cancer statistics, 2020. CA Cancer J Clin 2020;70(1):7–30.
3. National Comprehensive Cancer Network. NCCN Clinical Practice Guidelines in Oncology: Prostate Cancer Early Dectection. In: Plymouth Meeting, PA: National Comprehensive Cancer Network. 2020. Available at: https://www.nccn.org/professionals/ physician_gls/pdf/prostate_detection.pdf. Accessed October 15, 2020.
4. Carter HB, Albertsen PC, Barry MJ, et al. Early detection of prostate cancer: AUA guideline. Reviewed and validity confirmed 2018. Linthicum (MD): American Urological Association; 2013. Available at: https://www.auanet.org/guidelines/prostate-cancer-early-detection-guideline.
5. American Cancer Society. Cancer A-Z: prostate cancer early detection, diagnosis, and staging. Atlanta (GA): American Cancer Society; 2019. Available at: https://www.cancer.org/content/dam/CRC/PDF/Public/8795.00.pdf.
6. U.S Preventative Services Task Force. Prostate Cancer: Screening. 2018. Available at: https:// www.uspreventiveservicestaskforce.org/uspstf/ recommendation/prostate-cancer-screening. Accessed October 15, 2020.
7. Mottet N, Cornford P, van den Bergh RCN, et al. Prostate cancer. In: European Association of Urology, editor. EAU guidelines. Arnhem (The Netherlands): European Association of Urology; 2020. p. 1–212.
8. Moyer VA, Force USPST. Screening for prostate cancer: U.S. Preventive Services Task Force recommendation statement. Ann Intern Med 2012;157(2):120–34.
9. Miller AB. New data on prostate-cancer mortality after PSA screening. N Engl J Med 2012;366(11):1047–8.
10. Schroder FH, Hugosson J, Roobol MJ, et al. Screening and prostate-cancer mortality in a randomized European study. N Engl J Med 2009; 360(13):1320–8.
11. Hugosson J, Roobol MJ, Mansson M, et al. A 16-yr Follow-up of the European randomized study of screening for prostate cancer. Eur Urol 2019;76(1): 43–51.
12. Andriole GL, Crawford ED, Grubb RL 3rd, et al. Mortality results from a randomized prostate-cancer screening trial. N Engl J Med 2009;360(13):1310–9.
13. Shoag JE, Mittal S, Hu JC. Reevaluating PSA Testing Rates in the PLCO Trial. N Engl J Med 2016;374(18): 1795–6.
14. Shenoy D, Packianathan S, Chen AM, et al. Do African-American men need separate prostate cancer screening guidelines? BMC Urol 2016;16(1):19.
15. Liss MA, Chen H, Hemal S, et al. Impact of family history on prostate cancer mortality in white men undergoing prostate specific antigen based screening. J Urol 2015;193(1):75–9.

16. Chen YC, Page JH, Chen R, et al. Family history of prostate and breast cancer and the risk of prostate cancer in the PSA era. Prostate 2008;68(14):1582–91.

17. Patel MP, Schulman A, Shah KP, et al. Engaging the primary care community to encourage appropriate prostate cancer screening. Ther Adv Urol 2018; 10(1):11–6.

18. Aminsharifi A, Schulman A, Anderson J, et al. Primary care perspective and implementation of a multidisciplinary, institutional prostate cancer screening algorithm embedded in the electronic health record. Urol Oncol 2018;36(11):502.e1-6.

19. Shah A, Polascik TJ, George DJ, et al. Implementation and impact of a risk-stratified prostate cancer screening algorithm as a clinical decision support tool in a primary care network. J Gen Intern Med 2020;36(1):92–9.

20. Brandao A, Paulo P, Teixeira MR. Hereditary predisposition to prostate cancer: from genetics to clinical implications. Int J Mol Sci 2020;21(14):5036.

21. Benafif S, Kote-Jarai Z, Eeles RA, et al. A review of prostate cancer genome-wide association studies (GWAS). Cancer Epidemiol Biomarkers Prev 2018; 27(8):845–57.

22. Mucci LA, Hjelmborg JB, Harris JR, et al. Familial risk and heritability of cancer among twins in nordic countries. JAMA 2016;315(1):68–76.

23. Lichtenstein P, Holm NV, Verkasalo PK, et al. Environmental and heritable factors in the causation of cancer–analyses of cohorts of twins from Sweden, Denmark, and Finland. N Engl J Med 2000;343(2): 78–85.

24. Hjelmborg JB, Scheike T, Holst K, et al. The heritability of prostate cancer in the Nordic Twin Study of Cancer. Cancer Epidemiol Biomarkers Prev 2014; 23(11):2303–10.

25. Pritchard CC, Mateo J, Walsh MF, et al. Inherited DNA-repair gene mutations in men with metastatic prostate cancer. N Engl J Med 2016;375(5):443–53.

26. de Bono J, Mateo J, Fizazi K, et al. Olaparib for metastatic castration-resistant prostate cancer. N Engl J Med 2020;382(22):2091–102.

27. Abida W, Patnaik A, Campbell D, et al. Rucaparib in men with metastatic castration-resistant prostate cancer harboring a BRCA1 or BRCA2 gene alteration. J Clin Oncol 2020;38(32):3763–72.

28. Marks LS, Dorey FJ, Rhodes T, et al. Serum prostate specific antigen levels after transurethral resection of prostate: a longitudinal characterization in men with benign prostatic hyperplasia. J Urol 1996;156(3):1035–9.

29. Magklara A, Scorilas A, Stephan C, et al. Decreased concentrations of prostate-specific antigen and human glandular kallikrein 2 in malignant versus nonmalignant prostatic tissue. Urology 2000;56(3):527–32.

30. Lloyd SN, Collins GN, McKelvie GB, et al. Predicted and actual change in serum PSA following prostatectomy for BPH. Urology 1994;43(4):472–9.

31. Giri VN, Beebe-Dimmer JL. Familial prostate cancer. Semin Oncol 2016;43(5):560–5.

32. Mitra A, Fisher C, Foster CS, et al. Prostate cancer in male BRCA1 and BRCA2 mutation carriers has a more aggressive phenotype. Br J Cancer 2008; 98(2):502–7.

33. Sutcliffe EG, Stettner AR, Miller SA, et al. Differences in cancer prevalence among CHEK2 carriers identified via multi-gene panel testing. Cancer Genet 2020;246-247:12–7.

34. Hale V, Weischer M, Park JY. CHEK2 (*) 1100delC Mutation and Risk of Prostate Cancer. Prostate Cancer 2014;2014:294575.

35. Ewing CM, Ray AM, Lange EM, et al. Germline mutations in HOXB13 and prostate-cancer risk. N Engl J Med 2012;366(2):141–9.

36. Giri VN, Knudsen KE, Kelly WK, et al. Role of genetic testing for inherited prostate cancer risk: philadelphia prostate cancer consensus conference 2017. J Clin Oncol 2018;36(4):414–24.

37. Raymond VM, Mukherjee B, Wang F, et al. Elevated risk of prostate cancer among men with Lynch syndrome. J Clin Oncol 2013;31(14):1713–8.

38. Haraldsdottir S, Hampel H, Wei L, et al. Prostate cancer incidence in males with Lynch syndrome. Genet Med 2014;16(7):553–7.

39. Easton DF, Steele L, Fields P, et al. Cancer risks in two large breast cancer families linked to BRCA2 on chromosome 13q12-13. Am J Hum Genet 1997;61(1):120–8.

40. Sigurdsson S, Thorlacius S, Tomasson J, et al. BRCA2 mutation in Icelandic prostate cancer patients. J Mol Med (Berl) 1997;75(10):758–61.

41. Na R, Zheng SL, Han M, et al. Germline mutations in ATM and BRCA1/2 distinguish risk for lethal and indolent prostate cancer and are associated with early age at death. Eur Urol 2017;71(5):740–7.

42. Giri VN, Knudsen KE, Kelly WK, et al. Implementation of germline testing for prostate cancer: philadelphia prostate cancer consensus conference 2019. J Clin Oncol 2020;38(24):2798–811.

43. Cybulski C, Wokolorczyk D, Kluzniak W, et al. An inherited NBN mutation is associated with poor prognosis prostate cancer. Br J Cancer 2013;108(2):461–8.

44. Castro E, Goh C, Olmos D, et al. Germline BRCA mutations are associated with higher risk of nodal involvement, distant metastasis, and poor survival outcomes in prostate cancer. J Clin Oncol 2013; 31(14):1748–57.

45. Castro E, Goh C, Leongamornlert D, et al. Effect of BRCA mutations on metastatic relapse and cause-specific survival after radical treatment for localised prostate cancer. Eur Urol 2015;68(2):186–93.

46. Kote-Jarai Z, Leongamornlert D, Saunders E, et al. BRCA2 is a moderate penetrance gene contributing to young-onset prostate cancer: implications for genetic testing in prostate cancer patients. Br J Cancer 2011;105(8):1230–4.

47. Tryggvadottir L, Vidarsdottir L, Thorgeirsson T, et al. Prostate cancer progression and survival in BRCA2 mutation carriers. J Natl Cancer Inst 2007;99(12):929–35.

48. Nicolosi P, Ledet E, Yang S, et al. Prevalence of germline variants in prostate cancer and implications for current genetic testing guidelines. JAMA Oncol 2019;5(4):523–8.

49. Leongamornlert D, Saunders E, Dadaev T, et al. Frequent germline deleterious mutations in DNA repair genes in familial prostate cancer cases are associated with advanced disease. Br J Cancer 2014;110(6):1663–72.

50. Kote-Jarai Z, Jugurnauth S, Mulholland S, et al. A recurrent truncating germline mutation in the BRIP1/FANCJ gene and susceptibility to prostate cancer. Br J Cancer 2009;100(2):426–30.

51. Kote-Jarai Z, Mikropoulos C, Leongamornlert DA, et al. Prevalence of the HOXB13 G84E germline mutation in British men and correlation with prostate cancer risk, tumour characteristics and clinical outcomes. Ann Oncol 2015;26(4):756–61.

52. Zeegers MP, Jellema A, Ostrer H. Empiric risk of prostate carcinoma for relatives of patients with prostate carcinoma: a meta-analysis. Cancer 2003; 97(8):1894–903.

53. Brandt A, Sundquist J, Hemminki K. Risk for incident and fatal prostate cancer in men with a family history of any incident and fatal cancer. Ann Oncol 2012;23(1):251–6.

54. Schumacher FR, Al Olama AA, Berndt SI, et al. Association analyses of more than 140,000 men identify 63 new prostate cancer susceptibility loci. Nat Genet 2018;50(7):928–36.

55. Al Olama AA, Kote-Jarai Z, Berndt SI, et al. A meta-analysis of 87,040 individuals identifies 23 new susceptibility loci for prostate cancer. Nat Genet 2014; 46(10):1103–9.

56. Zheng SL, Sun J, Wiklund F, et al. Cumulative association of five genetic variants with prostate cancer. N Engl J Med 2008;358(9):910–9.

57. Haiman CA, Chen GK, Blot WJ, et al. Characterizing genetic risk at known prostate cancer susceptibility loci in African Americans. Plos Genet 2011;7(5): e1001387.

58. Bensen JT, Xu Z, Smith GJ, et al. Genetic polymorphism and prostate cancer aggressiveness: a case-only study of 1,536 GWAS and candidate SNPs in African-Americans and European-Americans. Prostate 2013;73(1):11–22.

59. Conran CA, Na R, Chen H, et al. Population-standardized genetic risk score: the SNP-based method of choice for inherited risk assessment of prostate cancer. Asian J Androl 2016;18(4):520–4.

60. Shi Z, Yu H, Wu Y, et al. Systematic evaluation of cancer-specific genetic risk score for 11 types of cancer in The Cancer Genome Atlas and Electronic Medical Records and Genomics cohorts. Cancer Med 2019;8(6):3196–205.

61. Chen H, Na R, Packiam VT, et al. Reclassification of prostate cancer risk using sequentially identified SNPs: Results from the REDUCE trial. Prostate 2017;77(11):1179–86.

62. Kader AK, Sun J, Reck BH, et al. Potential impact of adding genetic markers to clinical parameters in predicting prostate biopsy outcomes in men following an initial negative biopsy: findings from the REDUCE trial. Eur Urol 2012;62(6):953–61.

63. Chen H, Liu X, Brendler CB, et al. Adding genetic risk score to family history identifies twice as many high-risk men for prostate cancer: Results from the prostate cancer prevention trial. Prostate 2016; 76(12):1120–9.

64. Seibert TM, Fan CC, Wang Y, et al. Polygenic hazard score to guide screening for aggressive prostate cancer: development and validation in large scale cohorts. BMJ 2018;360:j5757.

65. Gronberg H, Adolfsson J, Aly M, et al. Prostate cancer screening in men aged 50-69 years (STHLM3): a prospective population-based diagnostic study. Lancet Oncol 2015;16(16):1667–76.

66. Wilt TJ, Vo TN, Langsetmo L, et al. Radical prostatectomy or observation for clinically localized prostate cancer: extended follow-up of the prostate cancer intervention versus observation trial (PIVOT). Eur Urol 2020;77(6):713–24.

67. Tosoian JJ, Mamawala M, Epstein JI, et al. Intermediate and longer-term outcomes from a prospective active-surveillance program for favorable-risk prostate cancer. J Clin Oncol 2015;33(30):3379–85.

68. Bancroft EK, Page EC, Castro E, et al. Targeted prostate cancer screening in BRCA1 and BRCA2 mutation carriers: results from the initial screening round of the IMPACT study. Eur Urol 2014;66(3): 489–99.

69. Page EC, Bancroft EK, Brook MN, et al. Interim Results from the IMPACT Study: Evidence for Prostate-specific Antigen Screening in BRCA2 Mutation Carriers. Eur Urol 2019;76(6):831–42.

70. Eeles RA. The PROFILE study: germline genetic profiling: correlation with targeted prostate cancer screening and treatment. Surrey, UK: Institute of Cancer Research and Royal Marsden Hospital; 2015. Available at: https://clinicaltrials.gov/ct2/show/study/NCT02543905. Accessed October 15, 2020.

71. Castro E, Mikropoulos C, Bancroft EK, et al. The PROFILE feasibility study: targeted screening of men with a family history of prostate cancer. Oncologist 2016;21(6):716–22.

72. Gulati R, Cheng HH, Lange PH, et al. Screening men at increased risk for prostate cancer diagnosis: model estimates of benefits and harms. Cancer Epidemiol Biomarkers Prev 2017;26(2):222–7.

73. Cucchiara V, Cooperberg MR, Dall'Era M, et al. Genomic markers in prostate cancer decision making. Eur Urol 2018;73(4):572–82.

74. Polascik TJ, Orabi H. Considerations of germline testing in prostate cancer screening. Can J Urol 2019;26(5 Suppl 2):46–7.

75. Das S, Salami SS, Spratt DE, et al. Bringing Prostate Cancer Germline Genetics into Clinical Practice. J Urol 2019;202(2):223–30.

76. Cheng HH. Prostate screening for men with inherited risk of developing aggressive prostate cancer, PATROL study. Seattle, WC: Fred Hutch/University of Washington Cancer Consortium; 2020. Available at: https://ClinicalTrials.gov/show/NCT04472338. Accessed October 15, 2020.

77. Dahut W. Men at high genetic risk for prostate cancer. Bethesda, MD: National Cancer Institute; 2019. Available at: https://ClinicalTrials.gov/show/NCT03805919. Accessed October 15, 2020.

Polygenic Risk Scores in Prostate Cancer Risk Assessment and Screening

Lindsey Byrne, MS[a], Amanda Ewart Toland, PhD[b,c],*

KEYWORDS

- Polygenic risk score • Prostate cancer • Risk prediction • Genome-wide association study
- Cancer screening

KEY POINTS

- Polygenic risk scores improve the predictive value of prostate-specific antigen screening.
- Polygenic risk scores may have utility in determining age at which prostate cancer screening should begin and identification of highest and lowest risk individuals.
- Clinical trials to evaluate the utility of polygenic risk scores for screening decision-making and risk prediction are needed.

INTRODUCTION

Prostate cancer (PCa) is the most common cancer among men with a lifetime risk of 12% and median age of diagnosis of 66.[1] In 2020, 191,930 new cases are expected to be diagnosed in the United States.[1] Established risk factors for PCa include genetic factors, African ancestry, older age, and family history of PCa (discussed in Yasin Bhanji and colleagues' article, "Prostate Cancer Predisposition," elsewhere in this issue).[2] African American (AA) men are 1.8 times more likely to be diagnosed with PCa than men of European ancestry, with one in six AA men diagnosed in their lifetime.[1] The cause of increased PCa risk for AA men is unclear; differences in biology, socioeconomic environment, exposures, lifestyle and behavior, or a combination of all these factors may contribute. Age is also strongly associated with PCa because there is a substantial increase in the rate of diagnosis after age 55.[2] There is

about an 8.5% chance to be diagnosed with PCa younger than age 55, which increases to 32.4% in ages 55 to 64 and 39.9% in ages 65 to 74.[1] A family history of PCa, especially a first-degree relative (brother or father), has been associated with two-fold to three-fold increased risk of PCa.[3] PCa risk furthermore increases with the number of affected family members and the degree of relatedness (affected brothers compared with a father and son).[3] Importantly, about 10% to 15% of families with two to three PCa diagnoses who do not have a pathogenic variant (PV) in a known high-risk gene, and the cause of the familial clustering is unknown, are called familial PCa.[4]

Of all the common cancers, PCa has the highest heritability, or genetic contribution to risk, with up to 57% of PCa risk because of genetic risk factors.[5] Approximately 5% to 10% of PCa are caused by highly penetrant PVs in genes, such as *BRCA1* and *BRCA2*, which significantly increase lifetime risk of PCa (Matthew J. Schiewer and Karen E.

a Department of Internal Medicine, Division of Human Genetics, The Ohio State University Comprehensive Cancer Center, The Ohio State University Wexner Medical Center, 2012 Kenny Road, Columbus, OH 43221, USA; b Department of Cancer Biology and Genetics, Division of Human Genetics, Comprehensive Cancer Center, The Ohio State University, 460 West 12th Avenue, Columbus, OH 43210, USA; c Department of Cancer Biology and Genetics, Comprehensive Cancer Center, The Ohio State University, 460 West 12th Avenue, Columbus, OH 43210, USA
* Corresponding author. Department of Cancer Biology and Genetics, Comprehensive Cancer Center, The Ohio State University, 460 West 12th Avenue, Columbus, OH 43210.
E-mail address: Amanda.Toland@osumc.edu

Urol Clin N Am 48 (2021) 387–399
https://doi.org/10.1016/j.ucl.2021.03.007

urologic.theclinics.com

Knudsen's article, "Basic Science and Molecular Genetics of Prostate Cancer Aggressiveness," in this issue).[4] One in 400 individuals in the general population carry a BRCA1 or BRCA2 PV.[6,7] Men with a BRCA1 PV have a 7% to 26% lifetime risk of PCa by age 80. This risk increases to 19% to 61% for men with a BRCA2 PV.[8,9]

PVs in additional genes, such as CHEK2 and ATM, increase PCa risk by 1.9- to 3.3-fold and 6.3-fold, respectively.[10–14] A rare missense founder variant in HOXB13, G84E, has a carrier frequency of 0.2% to 1.4% in Nordic populations, which confers up to a 60% lifetime risk of PCa.[15–17] Hereditary PCa is a highly active area of research currently. Further studies are needed to define cancer risk associated with genes to improve clinical management and treatment of patients with PCa and their families.

GENOME-WIDE ASSOCIATION STUDIES AND RISK VARIANTS

In addition to variants that confer moderate to high risk of PCa, some genetic variants are associated with low, but measurable risk. Genome-wide association studies (GWAS) have been used as an agnostic means to identify low-effect common genetic variants associated with disease, most of which are single-nucleotide variants (SNV). Many risk variants associated with cancer susceptibility have low effect sizes, often with odds ratios of less than 1.10 for risk. To reach the low P values (<1 × 10^{-8}) required for statistical significance when testing millions of variants, extremely large groups of cancer cases and control subjects are required.

PCa was one of the first disorders for which GWAS were performed. In 2007, three back-to-back PCa GWAS were published leading to the identification of multiple risk variants at 8q24.[18–20] Since that time more than 40 PCa GWAS have been performed with more than 170 variants identified that associate with disease.[21] Collectively, these variants are estimated to explain approximately 28% to 38% of the familial relative risk of PCa.[21,22] Unlike high-penetrant genetic variants associated with hereditary PCa, most GWAS variants are in noncoding regions and exert an effect through gene regulation. As a result, complementary approaches to identify risk variants associated with gene expression levels are being integrated with GWAS.[23–25]

Early GWAS were primarily conducted in populations of European descent. More recently, PCa GWAS in non-European populations have been published including those in AA,[26] Chinese,[27] Japanese,[28] Latino,[29] Ugandan,[30] and multiethnic populations.[31,32] In general GWAS in non-

European populations were not as well powered to detect low-risk variants because they had fewer cases and control subjects studies. However, they revealed important insights including that different ethnic and racial populations have unique PCa risk variants that are not present, or present in low frequencies, in European populations. They also uncovered variants that are associated with risk in Europeans but no other groups.[28,33] Despite these findings, there are shared risk alleles across multiple populations. For example, Du and colleagues[29] found that the shared overlap of PCa risk variants is high between men of European Latino and European non-Latino men; 83% of risk variants identified in European populations showed a similar direction of risk in Latino men. These results are not surprising because it is expected that some risk variants will occur in multiple populations.

POLYGENIC RISK SCORES

When disease-associated variants identified using GWAS are considered individually, they each have little to no impact on risk prediction. Complex disease risk prediction in a given individual depends on a combination of associated genetic, environmental, and lifestyle factors. GWAS and genetic modeling analyses indicate that many common diseases, including PCa, are likely to have hundreds to thousands of common variants associated with disease risk.[34] Furthermore, these variants may influence disease risk differentially depending on environmental or lifestyle factors.[35]

Risk prediction models for PCa and other diseases are being developed that include hundreds to thousands of independent risk-associated variants. Additive effects of the variants are generated by summing the number of risk alleles an individual carries and weighting each by their estimated effect size from GWAS data to create a polygenic risk score (PRS), also known as a genetic risk score. Potential clinical use of PRS for cancer and other diseases have been described and range from risk prediction, informing screening decision-making, informing prevention strategies, and personal understanding of risk.[36–39]

Like GWAS, large numbers of samples are needed to generate and validate PRS. For PCa, one study estimated requiring a population of 20,000 men to develop well-calibrated PRS and 10,000 men to test the models.[40] A second study evaluating 14 different cancer types predicted that there are 4530 PCa risk variants in European populations, which collectively explain 77% of the heritability for PCa.[41] The same authors estimated that greater than 750,000 cases and control subjects may be needed to definitely identify all of these risk alleles, which is about five times the current largest studies. This highlights the issue that most risk variants are not likely to be identifiable for most populations using current methodologies and available populations for study. An unanswered question is how accurate PRS using only a subset of risk variants will be. One argument in favor of using PRS with the current numbers of variants is that these variants are likely to be the ones with the highest effect sizes and that adding in variants with extremely low effects sizes is going to have exceedingly low impact on overall risk models. Because of statistical and population differences, it is important that PRS is calibrated and validated before clinical use. In comparing approaches for calibration and validation, one study suggested that downward adjustments to odds ratio used may need to be made to decrease the likelihood of providing falsely high estimates of risk.[42]

PRS scores are converted to a population distribution with lifetime risks so that scores are more easily interpreted.[37] For example, PRSs are lumped into percentiles of risk to identify the individuals at the top 1% of risk or the bottom 10% of risk with the bulk of individuals at 26% to 74% of the population mean of disease risk. This type of scaling may enable better screening recommendations for PCa. Some individuals may have a low enough PRS that they never cross a median 10-year risk of PCa of a 50-year-old man, the age at which screening for PCa begins in the United States. Conversely, men with a PRS estimating a high lifetime risk may cross this threshold at age 34.

POLYGENIC RISK SCORES FOR PROSTATE CANCER RISK PREDICTIONS

Early PCa PRSs were those for PCa risk (**Table 1**). The first PCa PRS, published in 2008, included only five SNVs and was evaluated in approximately 3000 cases and 2000 control studies.[43] A model of risk that included these variants plus family history, age, and region had an area under the curve (AUC) of 63.3 compared with 60.8 for the same risk factors without PRS. Subsequent studies increased the number of SNVs included in the models (see **Table 1**). A PRS study of 147 SNVs found that men in the top 1% of PRS had 5.71-fold increased risk compared with men in the middle 50% of risk.[22] Just 2 years later, a 2020 study of more than 48,000 men, more than 3700 with PCa, showed that those who are at the top 2.5% of risk of a 6,606,785 SNV risk score had approximately four-fold increased risks[54] compared with individuals in the middle of the distribution of risk. This translates to an approximate 50%

lifetime risk of developing PCa compared with the average in the population of 16.3%.

POLYGENIC RISK SCORES IN NON-EUROPEAN POPULATIONS

Using GWAS hits from European and non-European populations, PRS in individuals of Latino, Asian, and African ancestry have been tested and validated (see **Table 1**). Importantly, the odds ratios used in PRS developed in individuals of European ancestry may not be as predictive as odds ratios from the population for which the PRS is being applied. As an example, a 135 SNV PRS tested in 2820 Latino PCa cases and 5293 control subjects showed that men in the top 10% and 1% of PRS had more than three-fold and four-fold increased risk compared with those in the middle 26% to 74%. However, when a Latino-weighted PRS, using odds ratios derived from Latino populations was used in the model, those risks increased to nearly four- and seven-fold.[29] Similar findings were observed in Japanese populations. A PRS for PCa of 82 variants was developed specifically for men of Japanese ancestry. It included 12 SNVs that were uniquely identified as showing risk in Japanese populations and 68 variants that had been previously identified in GWAS from other populations but that also were associated with PCa risk in Japanese men. Evaluation of this PRS in 4893 PCa cases and 10,682 male control subjects showed that the age of diagnosis in men at the top 5% of risk was 2 years earlier than the men at the bottom 5% of risk.[28] The highest risk group was also more likely to have a family history of PCa. This model of 82 SNVs was more predictive of risk than a PRS of 150 SNVs that was based on findings from European populations. Helfand and colleagues[55] specifically addressed how a 105 SNV PRS would perform across multiple racial and ethnic groups. The PRS was statistically significant as predictive for risk in European, Latino, East Asian, and AA populations but performed the best in European and Latino groups. Collectively these studies suggest that racial- and ethnic-specific PRS may be more predictive than a "one size fits all" PRS but that European-developed PRS may have some utility for all racial and ethnic groups.[28,55]

POLYGENIC RISK SCORES AND PROSTATE CANCER SCREENING

In addition to lifetime risk prediction, PRS may aid in decisions on when to begin PCa screening. A United Kingdom study found that men at the top

Table 1
Polygenic risk score models for prostate cancer risk

Study	#SNV	Cases/Control Subjects (n)	Phenotype	Population	Main Finding	Ref
Genetic risk factors for PCa	32	779/1643	PCa risk	Norwegian	Top 10% of PRS had 5-fold greater risk compared with men in the bottom 10%	Chen et al,[44] 2018
Improving PPV of low PSA	49	2696 47/125	PCa in low PSA (1–3 ng/mL) patients	Swedish	37% of men in high genetic risk had PCa compared with 18% and 28% in low and intermediate	Nordström et al,[45] 2014
PracticaL	54	1583/4828	Aggressive PCa screening	Europe	HR of top 2% for aggressive PCa = 2.9 (2.2–4.0) High PPV for PSA	Seibert et al,[46] 2018
ProtecT	54	6411/8054	PRS informed screening by age	European	Age of diagnosis varies by 19 y between top 1% and bottom 1% of PRS	Huynh-Le et al,[47] 2020
Predictive value of PRS for prostate cancer	72	1579/1280	Men undergoing testing for hereditary cancer without germline pathogenic variants	European	Men in the top 10% of PRS have a lifetime risk of PCa of 30% and men in the top 1% as high as 42% Men in the bottom 1% had lifetime risks of 2.4% AUC for prostate cancer diagnosis = 0.65 (95% CI, 0.63–0.67)	Black et al,[48] 2020
Race-Specific PRS	7/76	1338 patients with a biopsy	Comparison of race-specific PRS for PCa and high-grade disease	East Asians	An East Asian–specific PRS had higher AUC (0.602 vs 0.573) than non-Asian-specific	Na et al,[49] 2016
Risk	82	4893/10,682	PCa risk	Japan	Mean diagnosis in top 5% of PRS 2.7 y younger than bottom 5% of risk	Takata et al,[28] 2019
Michigan Genomics Initiative	93	1425/9793	Risk	European	23.4% of men in the top decile of risk had PCa compared with 5.4% in the lowest risk decile	Fritsche et al,[50] 2018

Cohort	#SNV	Cases/Controls	Purpose	Population	Results	Reference
Ugandan men	97	571/485	PrCa risk	Uganda	Men in the top 10% had 4.86-fold risk (95% CI, 2.70–8.76) compared with average-risk men	Du et al,[30] 2018
BRCA carriers	103	1313/212	Does PRS for general population modify risk in BRCA carriers?	European	Odds ratio per SD of PRS 1.57 (95% CI, 1.35–1.81; P value 3.2×10^{-9}; risk by age 80 of 61% for 95% and 19% for 5%)	Lecarpentier et al,[8] 2017
PRACTICAL	65/133	1370/1239	Validation study of PRS for risk	European	AUC 0.67 for 64 SNVs (95% CI, 0.65–0.69) AUC 0.68 (95% CI, 0.66–0.70) for 133 SNVs	Szulkin et al,[51] 2015
Multi-Consortium GWAS	147	46,939/27,910	Risk	European	Men in the top 1% had 5.71-fold increased risk (95% CI, 5.04–6.48) over those in the middle 50% of risk	Schumacher et al,[22] 2018
UK Biobank	147	4430/186,376	Risk	European	HR top 5% 3.20 (2.88–3.56) HR of 2.22 (95% CI, 52.04–2.41) for highest quintile PRS compared with middle HR 0.39 (95% CI, 0.35–0.45) for those in lowest quintile	Jia et al,[52] 2020
Latino	162	2820/5293	PCa risk	Latino	Men in the top 10% had 3.19-fold (95% CI, 2.65–3.84) increased risk and those in the top 1% a 4.02-fold (95% CI, 2.46–6.55) risk relative to average-risk (25%–75%) men	Du et al,[29] 2020
UK biobank	448	379/24,722	Risk	European	AUC 0.6399 (P value 3×10^{-6}); top 1% has 4.6-fold increase over those in middle 26%–49%	Lello et al,[53] 2019
FINNRISK	6,606,785	1172/47,679	Risk	Finnish	HR 4.07 for PCa in top 2.5% of PRS	Mars et al,[54] 2020

Abbreviations: #SNV, number of SNVs in PRS model; AUC, area under the receiver operating curve; CI, confidence interval; HR, hazard ratio; PPV, positive predictive value; PSA, prostate-specific antigen; SD, standard deviation.

1% of polygenic risk were expected to reach the 50-year-old standard risk level at age 41 and men in the bottom 1% of polygenic risk did not meet this level of risk until age 60. This translates to a 19-year difference in the risk-equivalent age to begin PCa screening in men at the two extremes of risk (**Table 2**).

Although PCa screening using prostate-specific antigen (PSA) results in decreased mortality, it leads to increased numbers of biopsies and a high rate of PCa overdiagnoses that are less likely to result in mortality.[60] Thus, approaches to improve predictive value of PSA, identify men who would benefit most from screening or further diagnostic testing, and decrease biopsies in men with reduced likelihood of being diagnosed with aggressive PCa are needed. Emerging studies suggest that the PRS may improve the positive predictive value of PSA tests (see **Table 2**). A 2015 study of Finnish men showed that combining a 66-SNV PRS with PSA screening may improve sensitivity of the PSA test. In that study of approximately 1100 cases and approximately 3900 control subjects undergoing regular PSA screening, 18% of men who were higher than the median PRS had PSA of 4 ng/mL compared with 7% in the group lower than the median ($P<.001$). PCa overdiagnosis was estimated at 58% (95% confidence interval [CI], 54–65) in the lower PRS group compared with 37% (95% CI, 31–47) in the upper risk group.[58] Other studies have shown similar findings of PRS improving predictive value of PSA screening.[47] PRS for PCa is also associated with other prostate phenotypes. Evaluation of a 93 SNV PRS for PCa risk found that PRS was also associated with increased PSA levels (P value 9.33×10^{-27}) and other phenotypes including erectile dysfunction, urinary incontinence, and prostate hyperplasia, suggesting common biologic pathways between these or the result of a PCa diagnosis of these phenotypes.[50]

Not only are the risks higher for individuals at the top end of the PRS spectrum, but many studies have shown that the age of disease onset is earlier, which could impact screening using PSA. One study found that the individuals at the top 2.5% of risk had a disease onset 5.53 years earlier compared with individuals with average PRS.[54] Another study found that men at the top 1% of risk had an average age of PCa diagnosis of 41 years compared with 60 years in men in the bottom 1% of risk.[47] Additional studies are needed, but developing individual-specific recommendations for beginning PCa screening based on PRS could result in fewer men being overdiagnosed and/or overtreated for PCa.

POLYGENIC RISK SCORES AND CLINICAL OUTCOMES

Because PRS shows promise for predicting overall risk and for improving predictive value for PSA, multiple groups have tested whether PRS is informative for aggressive disease. This would be an immensely valuable clinical tool because it could potentially lead to fewer biopsies or less overtreatment of PCa that would result in less harm to the patient. There are now consistent data that higher PRS is associated with an increased risk of aggressive or high-grade PCa.[46,49,56]

PRS may also be informative for identifying men who would benefit from biopsy. A study of 105 SNVs found that 36% and 40.4% of men with the top PRS without and with a family history of PCa in the placebo arm of the Prostate Cancer Prevention Trial had a positive biopsy compared with 24.6% and 33.3% of men with an average PRS.[55] This study also suggests that men who are considered generally to be a lower risk because of a lack of a family history might benefit from PRS information.[55]

Despite the promise of PRS for risk prediction and screening decision-making, PCa PRS has not been associated with outcomes in chemoprevention trials. A 98-SNV PRS study of men in the PCPT (finasteride or placebo) or SELECT (selenium, vitamin E, or combination) chemoprevention trials, found no association of those with higher PRS and effect of chemopreventative agent[61] despite association of a higher PRS with increased cancer risk. Additionally, GWAS to date have not led to the identification of variants predictive of PCa survival following therapy.[62,63]

POLYGENIC RISK SCORES IN COMBINATION WITH OTHER PROSTATE CANCER PREDICTION TOOLS

Several models to predict PCa and aggressive PCa risk that incorporate age, sex, race, family history, PSA, and other clinical and demographic factors have been developed.[64] PRS is starting to be incorporated into existing models to determine if adding genetic information improves the predictive value of the models (**Table 3**). Although modest, PRS does improve the AUC for prediction of PCa diagnosis. One clinical predictive model that included age, family history, and benign prostate hyperplasia showed an AUC for a PCa diagnosis of 0.840 (95% CI, 0.837–0.842).[54] Adding an approximately 6 million SNV PRS to this model improved the predictive value to 0.866 (95% CI, 0.863–0.868). Adding PRS to other predictive biomarkers, such as a four-kallikrein panel, also

Table 2
Use of PRS for informing screening and treatment decisions

#SNV	Participant Characteristics	Phenotype	Population	Main Finding	Ref
29	7-y follow-up study: 1104 men of 4528 developed PCa	Identifying high-risk men for screening using family history and/or PRS	Prostate Cancer Prevention Trial	29% of men with a high PRS risk and positive family history were diagnosed compared with 23% of men with family history and PRS for risk ($P = .001$) PCa was diagnosed in 31% of men of high risk (PRS or FH) compared with 21% of men at lower risk	Chen et al,[56] 2016
35	2135 cases 3108 control subjects	Predicting need for biopsy in men with PSA >3–4 ng/mL	Swedish	PRS could result in 12% fewer biopsies	Aly et al,[57] 2011
49	172 men randomly selected from 860 genotyped with PSA 1–3 ng/mL underwent biopsy	PRS for detecting biopsy-positive PCa with PSA 1–3 ng/mL	Swedish STHLM2 cohort	37% of men in high-risk cohort had PCa compared with 28% in the intermediate and 18% in the low genetic groups	Nordström et al,[45] 2014
54	6411 men from Protect study	Effect of PRS on risk-equivalent age (PCa risk equivalent to a 50-y-old man)	ProtecT study (UK)	Age at which risk is equivalent to a 50-y-old (screening age) differs by 19 y between men at the bottom and top 1% of risk	Huynh-Le et al,[47] 2020
54	1583 men with any PCa, 632 with aggressive PCa, with 220 very aggressive PCa, 4828 control subjects all with PSA >3 ng/mL	Using PRS to improve predictive value of PSA test for aggressive PCa	ProtecT study (UK)	The PSA test had a PPV of ~0.24 for men in top 5% of the PRS and ~0.7 for men in the bottom 5% of PRS Men in the top 20% of PRS accounted for 42% of aggressive PCa cases	Seibert et al,[46] 2018

(continued on next page)

Table 2
(continued)

#SNV	Participant Characteristics	Phenotype	Population	Main Finding	Ref
66	1089 cases 3878 control subjects	Using PRS to help interpret PSA and reduce overdiagnosis	Finnish	18% of men in higher risk group had PSA $\geq$4 ng/mL compared with 7% in lower risk group Overdiagnosis was 58% in lower risk group and 37% in upper risk group	Pashayan et al,[58] 2015
110	3225 cancer-free men at enrollment with 714 diagnoses after enrollment	Age of diagnosis for family history vs PRS	REDUCE trial	Higher GRS had worse PCa-free survival (P_{trend} <0.001); combining family history further stratified genetic risk No association between GRS and age	Na et al,[59] 2019

Abbreviations: #SNV, number of SNVs in PRS model; Dx, diagnosis; GRS, genetic risk score; PPV, positive predictive value.

Table 3
Predictive value of adding PRS to clinical models

#SNV	Population	AUC/C-Index for Clinical Factors	AUC PRS Alone	AUC Clinical Factors + PRS	Ref
66/7	2310 PrCa cases 518/2441 screened	0.71 (0.696–0.707) for PSA		7 SNV PRS + PSA AUC = 0.888 (0.886–0.891); 66 SNVs + PSA AUC = 0.967 (0.965–0.969)	Li-Sheng Chen et al,[65] 2019
135	Multiethnic cohort 1776 men (1254 cases) with PSA >2 ng/mL	4K panel AUC = 0.756 (0.731–0.78) for PCa and 0.790 (0.76–0.82) for aggressive PCa		PRS + 4K panel 0.766 (0.742–0.790) for PCa; 0.801 (0.772–0.83) for aggressive PCa	Darst et al,[66] 2020
147	4430 cases 186, 376 control subjects	Family Hx 0.529 (0.522–0.535)	0.662 (0.655–0.67)	PRS + Fam Hx 0.669 (0.661–0.676)	Jia et al,[52] 2020
6,606, 785	1172 PCa cases 47,679 control subjects	Age, Fam Hx, BPH 0.840 (0.837–0.842)	0.8416	Age, Fam Hx, BPH PRS 0.866 (0.863–0.868)	Mars et al,[54] 2020

Abbreviations: 4K, four-kallikrein; #SNV, number of SNVs in PRS model; AUC, area under the receiver operating curve; BPH, benign prostate hyperplasia; Fam Hx, family history.

improves predictive values (see **Table 3**).[67] Because PRSs on their own do not have as high a predictive value as PRS in combination with other risk factors, it is likely that PRS will not be used in isolation.

RESIDUAL RISK IN INDIVIDUALS WITH HIGH- AND MODERATE-RISK PATHOGENIC VARIANTS

Predicted lifetime PCa risk with inherited PVs varies widely because there are factors that modify risk beyond the PV, such as low-penetrance risk variants. A PRS of 104 SNVs found that additional genetic modifiers impact risk in men with BRCA PVs. For *BRCA2* PV carriers, men in the top 95% of the PRS had a lifetime risk by age 80 of PCa of 61%, whereas men in the bottom 5% had a lifetime risk of 19%. For *BRCA1* men in the top 95% had a lifetime risk of 26% compared with those in the bottom 5% with a lifetime risk of 7%.[8] The AUC for PCa in this group was 0.62 (95% CI, 0.58–0.66).

Although not yet specifically studied, PRS may help to determine lifetime risks of men with PVs in moderate-risk PCa genes. *CHEK2*, a moderate-risk gene for breast cancer, confers an estimated 25% to 39% lifetime risk.[67,68] Studies using an 86-SNV PRS for breast cancer showed that women with the lowest PRS and a pathogenic risk variant in *CHEK2* had similar lifetime risks of breast cancer as the general population, whereas women at the top quintile had 29% lifetime risks.[69] Using PRS in men with PVs in moderate- and high-risk genes may inform timing of screening and prevention decisions.

CURRENT CLINICAL USE OF PROSTATE CANCER POLYGENIC RISK SCORES

Based on the studies to date, PRS may have clinical utility including: (1) identification of individuals at increased disease risk who would benefit from more intensive screening or in the interpretation of screening results; (2) identification of people at higher risk who may benefit from therapeutic-based prevention strategies; and (3) personal understanding of risk, by helping individuals understand their risk of developing a disease for making life-decisions (**Box 1**).[39] In 2018, Ambry Genetics created the only commercially available PRS for PCa to date based 72 SNVs associated with PCa, age, and ethnicity.[48] In non–peer reviewed studies, they found that the predictive performance of the model outperformed that of family history alone for White men who tested negative for a pathogenic or likely PV in a PCa-associated gene.[48,64] There is a lack of data on using PRS in men who have a PCa diagnosis. Thus, research is needed to understand if there is any value in a score after diagnosis. Additionally, the National Comprehensive Cancer

> **Box 1**
> **Potential future clinical uses of prostate cancer PRS**
>
> - Aid in prostate cancer screening decision-making
> - Assist in interpretation of prostate cancer screening results
> - Predict prostate cancer risk, age of diagnosis, and aggressiveness
> - Improve predictive value when combined with prostate cancer biologic markers and pathologic features
> - Provide refined risk estimates to individuals with pathogenic variants in high- and moderate-risk prostate cancer susceptibility genes

Network guidelines for Genetic/Familial High-Risk Assessment: Breast, Ovarian and Pancreatic does not recommend PRS usage for clinical management because of significant limitations in interpretation.[70] PRS for genetic/familial assessments is currently only recommended in the setting of a clinical trial.[70]

CLINICAL TRIALS

There are few clinical trials evaluating PRS in a PCa context. One ongoing clinical trial, PLCO-574, aims to develop and validate a model of 50 SNVs with risk factors, such as PSA, digital rectal examination, family history, and demographics, to determine high-grade PCa risk.[71] To better understand risk in AA, a $90 "Smith Polygenic Risk test" for PCa based on more than 250 SNVs, is being developed and tested in this population.[72,73]

DISCUSSION

The addition of PRS with germline genetic testing in the genetic counseling session is the next step in clinical use and PCa risk assessment. This is currently not being done routinely, although one company offers a PRS option for men undergoing germline genetic testing for PCa risk. This may improve PCa risk prediction for men and may help to explain some of the familial PCa families without known pathogenic variations. PRS incorporation is likely to become the next step added into the standard genetic risk assessment of PCa risk in unaffected men for adjustment of risk, and affected men to gather future data.

SUMMARY

Emerging data from research studies suggest that PRS for PCa is predictive for risk; may inform

timing for screening; and may improve predictive value for other risk factors, such as family history and PSA.[55,74,75] Studies are warranted to determine if PCa PRS has utility for screening decision-making and/or improving outcomes in a clinical setting.

CLINICS CARE POINTS

> - The clinical value of PRS for PCa is emerging; potential benefits include lifetime risk assessments, determining timing of screening, and improving predictive value of PSA tests for aggressive cancer and other PCa models.
> - PCa PRS for non-European populations is less well studied and validated.
> - PCa PRS is currently only available through a limited number of clinical genetic testing laboratories.

DISCLOSURES

The authors have nothing to disclose.

REFERENCES

1. National Cancer Institute SEER Cancer Statistics Factsheets. Prostate cancer. 2020. Available at: https://seer.cancer.gov/statfacts/html/prost.html. Accessed September 4, 2020.
2. Pernar C, Ebot E, Wilson K, et al. The epidemiology of prostate cancer. Cold Spring Harb Perspect Med 2018;8:1–19.
3. Kicinski M, Vangronsveld J, Nawrot T. An epidemiological reappraisal of the familial aggregation of prostate cancer: a meta-analysis. PLoS One 2011;6:1–7.
4. Das S, Salami S, Spratt D, et al. Bring prostate cancer germline genetics into clinical practice. J Urol 2019;202:223–30.
5. Mucci L, Hjelmborg J, Harris J, et al. Familial risk and heritability of cancer among twins in Nordic countries. JAMA 2016;315(1):68–76.
6. The Breast Cancer Linkage Consortium: cancer risks in BRCA2 mutation carriers. J Natl Cancer Inst 1999;91:1310–6.
7. Liede A, Karlan B, Narod S. Cancer risk for male carriers of germline mutations in BRCA1 or BRCA2 a review of the literature. J Clin Oncol 2004;22(4):735–42.
8. Lecarpentier J, Silvestri V, Kuchenbaecker KB, et al. Prediction of breast and prostate cancer risks in male BRCA1 and BRCA2 mutation carriers using polygenic risk scores. J Clin Oncol 2017;35:2240–50.

9. Nyberg T, Frost D, Barrowdale D, et al. Prostate cancer risk for male *BRCA1* and *BRCA2* carriers: a prospective cohort study. Eur Urol 2020;77:24–35.

10. Southey M, Goldgar D, Winqvist R, et al. *PALB2, CHEK2* and *ATM* rare variants and cancer risk: data from COGS. J Med Genet 2016;53:800–11.

11. Wang Y, Dai B, Dingwei Y. CHEK2 mutation and risk of prostate cancer: a systematic review and meta-analysis. Int J Clin Exp Med 2015;8(9):15708–15.

12. Wu Y, Yu H, Zheng S, et al. A comprehensive evaluation of *CHEK2* germline mutations in men with prostate cancer. Prostate 2018;78(8):607–15.

13. Carter HB, Helfand B, Mamawala M, et al. Germline mutations in *ATM* and *BRCA1/2* are associated with grade reclassification in men on active surveillance for prostate cancer. Eur Urol 2019;75(5):743–9.

14. Na R, Zheng SL, Han M, et al. Germline mutations in ATM and BRCA1/2 distinguish risk for lethal and indolent prostate cancer and are associated with early age at death. Eur Urol 2017;71:740–7.

15. Xu J, Lange E, Lu L, et al. *HOXB13* is a susceptibility gene for prostate cancer: results from the International Consortium for Prostate Cancer Genetics (ICPCG). Hum Genet 2013;132:5–14.

16. Laitinen VH, Wahlfors T, Saaristo L, et al. *HOXB13* G84E mutations in Finland population-based analysis of prostate, breast, and colorectal cancer risk. Cancer Epidemiol Biomarkers Prev 2013;22:452–60.

17. Karlsson R, Aly M, Clements M, et al. A population-based assessment of germline *HOXB13* G84E mutation and prostate cancer risk. Eur Urol 2014; 65(1):169–76.

18. Gudmundsson J, Sulem P, Manolescu A, et al. Genome-wide association study identifies a second PCa susceptibility variant at 8q24. Nat Genet 2007; 39(5):631–7.

19. Haiman CA, Patterson N, Freedman ML, et al. Multiple regions within 8q24 independently affect risk for prostate cancer. Nat Genet 2007;39(5):638–44.

20. Yeager M, Orr N, Hayes RB, et al. Genome-wide association study of prostate cancer identifies a second risk locus at 8q24. Nat Genet 2007;39:645–9.

21. Benafif S, Kote-Jarai Z, Eeles RA, et al. A review of prostate cancer genome wide association studies (GWAS). Cancer Epidemiol Biomarkers Prev 2018; 27(8):845–57.

22. Schumacher FR, Al Olama AAA, Berndt SI, et al. Association analyses of more than 140,000 men identify 63 new prostate cancer susceptibility loci. Nat Genet 2018;50(7):928–36.

23. Emami NC, Kachuri L, Meyers TJ, et al. Association of imputed prostate cancer transcriptome with disease risk reveals novel mechanisms. Nat Commun 2019;10:3107.

24. Wu L, Wang J, Cai Q, et al. Transcriptome-wide association study in over 140,000 European descendants. Cancer Res 2019;79:3192–204.

25. Wu L, Shu X, Bao J, et al. Analysis of over 140,000 European descendants identifies genetically predicted blood protein biomarkers associated with prostate cancer risk. Cancer Res 2019;79:4592–8.

26. Conti DV, Wang K, Sheng X, et al. Two novel susceptibility loci for prostate cancer in men of African ancestry. J Natl Cancer Inst 2017;109:djx084.

27. Marzec J, Mao X, Li M, et al. A genetic study and meta-analysis of the genetic predisposition of prostate cancer in a Chinese population. Oncotarget 2016;7:21393–403.

28. Takata R, Takahashi A, Fujita M, et al. 12 new susceptibility loci for prostate cancer identified by genome-wide association study in Japanese population. Nat Commun 2019;10(1):4422.

29. Du Z, Hopp H, Ingles SA, et al. A genome-wide association study of prostate cancer in Latinos. Int J Cancer 2020;146:1819–26.

30. Du Z, Lubmawa A, Gundell S, et al. Genetic risk of prostate cancer in Ugandan men. Prostate 2018; 78:370–6.

31. Al Olama AA, Kote-Jarai Z, Berndt SI, et al. A meta-analysis of 87,040 individuals identifies 23 new susceptibility loci for PCa. Nat Genet 2014;46:1103–9.

32. Hoffmann TJ, Van Den Eeden SK, Sakoda L, et al. A large multiethnic genome-wide association study of prostate cancer identifies novel risk variants and substantial ethnic differences. Cancer Discov 2015;5:878–91.

33. Han Y, Signorello LB, Strom SS, et al. Generalizability of established prostate cancer risk variants in men of African ancestry. Int J Cancer 2015;136:1210–7.

34. Visscher PM, Wray NR, Zhang Q, et al. 10 years of GWAS discovery: biology, function and translation. Am J Hum Genet 2017;101(1):5–22.

35. Carbone M, Amelio I, Affar EB, et al. Consensus report of the 8 and 9th Weinman symposis on gene x environment interaction in carcinogenesis: novel opportunities for precision medicine. Cell Death Differ 2018;25(11):1885–904.

36. Kraft P, Wacholder S, Cornelis MC, et al. Beyond odds ratios: communicating disease risk based on genetic profiles. Nat Rev Genet 2009;10:264–9.

37. Lewis CM, Vassos E. Prospects for using risk scores in polygenic medicine. Genome Med 2017;9(1):96.

38. Maher BS. Polygenic scores in epidemiology: risk prediction, etiology, and clinical utility. Curr Epidemiol Rep 2015;2(4):239–44.

39. Torkamani A, Wineinger NE, Topol EJ. The personal and clinical utility of polygenic risk scores. Nat Rev Genet 2018;19(9):581–90.

40. Karunamuni RA, Huynh-Le MP, Fan CC, et al. The effect of sample size on polygenic hazard models for prostate cancer. Eur J Hum Genet 2020;28(10): 1467–75.

41. Zhang YD, Hurson AN, Zhang H, et al. Assessment of polygenic architecture and risk prediction based

on common variants across fourteen cancers. Nat Commun 2020;11(1):3353.

42. Yu H, Shi Z, Wu Y, et al. Concept and benchmarks for assessing narrow-sense validity of genetic risk score values. Prostate 2019;79(10):1099–105.

43. Zheng SL, Sun J, Wiklund F, et al. Cumulative association of five genetic variants with prostate cancer. N Engl J Med 2008;358(9):910–9.

44. Chen H, Ewing CM, Zheng S, et al. Genetic factors influencing prostate cancer risk in Norwegian men. Prostate 2018;78(3):186–92.

45. Nordström T, Aly M, Eklund M, et al. A genetic score can identify men at high risk for prostate cancer among men with prostate-specific antigen of 1-3 ng/ml. Eur Urol 2014;65:1184–90.

46. Seibert TM, Fan CC, Wang Y, et al. Polygenic hazard score to guide screening for aggressive prostate cancer: development and validation in large scale cohorts. BMJ 2018;360:j5757.

47. Huynh-Le MP, Fan CC, Karunamuni R, et al. A genetic risk score to personalize prostate cancer screening, applied to population data. Cancer Epidemiol Biomarkers Prev 2020;29(9):1731–8.

48. Black MH, Shuwei I, LaDuca H, et al. Validation of a prostate cancer polygenic risk score. Prostate 2020; 80(15):1314–21.

49. Na R, Ye D, Qi J, et al. Race-specific genetic risk score is more accurate than nonrace-specific genetic risk score for predicting prostate cancer and high grade diseases. Asian J Androl 2016;18:525–9.

50. Fritsche LG, Gruber SB, Wu Z, et al. Association of polygenic risk scores for multiple cancers in a phenome-wide study: results from the Michigan Genomics Initiative. Am J Hum Genet 2018;102(6):1048–61.

51. Szulkin R, Whitington T, Eklund M, et al. Prediction of individual genetic risk to prostate cancer using a polygenic score. Prostate 2015;75:1467–74.

52. Jia G, Lu Y, Wen W, et al. Evaluating the utility of polygenic risk scores in identifying high-risk individuals for eight common cancers. JNCI Cancer Spectr 2020;4(3):pkaa021, 1-8.

53. Lello L, Raben TG, Yong SY, et al. Genomic prediction of 16 complex disease risks including heart attack, diabetes, breast and prostate cancer. Sci Rep 2019;9(1):15286.

54. Mars N, Koskela JT, Ripatti P, et al. Polygenic and clinical risk scores and their impact on age at onset and prediction of cardiometabolic diseases and common cancers. Nat Med 2020;26(4):549–57.

55. Helfand BT, Kearns J, Conran C, et al. Clinical validity and utility of genetic risk scores in prostate cancer. Asian J Androl 2016;18(4):509–14.

56. Chen H, Liu X, Brendler CB, et al. Adding genetic risk score to family history identifies twice as many high-risk men for prostate cancer: results from the Prostate Cancer Prevention Trial. Prostate 2016; 76(12):1120–9.

57. Aly M, Wiklund F, Xu J, et al. Polygenic risk score improves prostate cancer a risk prediction: results from the Stockholm-1 cohort study. Eur Urol 2011; 60:21–8.

58. Pashayan N, Pharoah PD, Schleutker J, et al. Reducing overdiagnosis by polygenic risk-stratified screening: findings from the Finnish section of the ERSPC. Br J Cancer 2015;113(7):1086–93.

59. Na R, Labbate C, Yu H, et al. Single-nucleotide polymorphism-based genetic risk score and patient age at prostate cancer diagnosis. JAMA Netw Open 2019;2(12):e1918145.

60. Mishra SC. A discussion on controversies and ethical dilemmas in prostate cancer screening. J Med Ethics 2021;47:152–8.

61. Ahmed M, Goh C, Saunders E, et al. Germline genetic variation in prostate cancer susceptibility does not predict outcomes in the chemoprevention trials PCPT and SELECT. Prostate Cancer Prostatic Dis 2020;23(2):333–42.

62. Szulkin R, Karlsson R, Whitington T, et al. Genome-wide association study of prostate cancer-specific survival. Cancer Epidemiol Biomarkers Prev 2015; 24(11):1796–800.

63. Aladwani M, Lophatananon A, Ollier W, et al. Prediction models for prostate cancer to be use in the primary care setting: a systematic review. BMJ Open 2020;10(7):e034661.

64. Ambry Score for Prostate Cancer. Ambry genetics. Available at: https://www.ambrygen.com/providers/ambryscore/prostate. Accessed September 4, 2020.

65. Li-Sheng Chen S, Ching-Yuan Fann J, Sipeky C, et al. Risk prediction of prostate cancer with single nucleotide polymorphisms and prostate specific antigen. J Urol 2019;201:486–95.

66. Darst BF, Chou A, Wan P, et al. The four-Kallikrein panel is effective in identifying aggressive prostate cancer in a multiethnic population. Cancer Epidemiol Biomarkers Prev 2020;29(7):1381–8.

67. Weischer M, Bojesen SE, Ellervik C, et al. CHEK2*1100delC genotyping for clinical assessment of breast cancer risk: meta-analysis of 26,000 patient cases and 27,000 controls. J Clin Oncol 2008;26(4):542–8.

68. Cybulski C, Wokolorczyk D, Jakubowska A, et al. Risk of breast cancer in women with a CHEK2 mutation with and without a family history of breast cancer. J Clin Oncol 2011;29(28):3747–52.

69. Gallagher S, Hughes E, Wagner S, et al. Association of a polygenic risk score with breast cancer among women carriers of high- and moderate-risk breast cancer genes. JAMA Netw Open 2020;3(7): e208501.

70. National Comprehensive Cancer Network Clinical Practice Guidelines in Oncology: Genetic/Familial High-Risk Assessment: Breast, Ovarian, and

Pancreatic. Version 1.2021. Available at: https://www.nccn.org/professionals/physician_gls/pdf/genetics_bop.pdf. Accessed October 5, 2020.

71. Prostate cancer risk prediction using clinical risk factors and genetics. National Cancer Institute. Available at: https://cdas.cancer.gov/approved-projects/2494/. Accessed September 4, 2020.

72. Smith polygenic risk test for prostate cancer. Prostate Cancer Foundation. Available at: https://www.pcf.org/sprt/. Accessed September 4, 2020.

73. Billionaire Robert F. Smith partners with Prostate Cancer Foundation to address racial disparities and reduce death from disease. Good Black News: The Good Things Black People Do, Give and Receive All Over The World. Available at: https://goodblacknews.org/tag/smith-polygenic-risk-test-for-prostate-cancer/. Accessed September 4, 2020.

74. Toland AE. Polygenic risk scores for prostate cancer: testing considerations. Can J Urol 2019;26(5 Suppl 2):17–8.

75. Fantus RJ, Helfand BT. Germline genetics of prostate cancer: time to incorporate genetics into early detection tools. Clin Chem 2019;65:74–9.

Germline Testing for Prostate Cancer Prognosis
Implications for Active Surveillance

Brian T. Helfand, MD, PhD*, Jianfeng Xu, MD, DrPH

KEYWORDS

- Active surveillance • Germline • Mutations • Polygenic risk score • Genetic risk score
- Tumor upgrading • Reclassification • Positive cores

KEY POINTS

- Rare germline mutations in several DNA repair genes, such as *BRCA2* and *ATM*, have been consistently associated with aggressive prostate cancer and poor clinical outcomes.
- These rare mutations are associated with a higher rate of tumor upgrading in patients undergoing active surveillance, although the number of such studies is limited.
- There is also a trend for prostate cancer polygenic risk scores, calculated from common risk-associated variants, to be associated with tumor upgrading in patients undergoing active surveillance.
- The association of polygenic risk scores with tumor upgrading in active surveillance is likely due to its association with number of positive cores at diagnostic biopsy.

INTRODUCTION

Prostate cancer (PCa) is the most common noncutaneous malignancy diagnosed among men, with more than one million new cases reported worldwide every year.[1] PCa screening has been associated with a significant reduction in tumor metastases and disease-specific mortality.[2,3] On the other hand, tumor screening has led to the diagnosis and treatment of many cancers that would not have become life-threatening during a man's lifetime.[4] Studies have shown that the prevention of 1 death from PCa may require active treatment of up to 48 men at a median follow-up of 9 years.[2] These and other findings emphasize the prevalence of overdiagnosis and overtreatment of prostate tumors.[5] To combat these problems, active surveillance (AS) was developed as a way to combat these issues. Men with cancers thought to harbor less aggressive potential and pose minimal risk to life are monitored with prostate biopsies, and intervention with definitive treatment (eg, radiation or radical surgery) is only recommended if higher-risk features are detected during follow-up. These tumor features include a grade recategorization during subsequent from Gleason grade group (GG1) to GG2 tumors or higher-stage disease. Although results from several AS studies have demonstrated a low risk of PCa-specific mortality,[5,6] about 30% to 45% of men with GG1 disease will be found to have more aggressive tumor characteristics during a 15-year surveillance that require definitive treatment.[7,8] However, a prevailing concern is that AS may lead to a delay in treatment and may miss a treatment window for cure. As such, biomarkers that can help distinguish aggressive disease are greatly needed.

Results of germline genetic tests for PCa may serve as a biomarker that may help more accurately

Program for Personalized Cancer Care, Division of Urology, NorthShore University HealthSystem, 1001 University Place, Evanston, IL 60201, USA
* Corresponding author.
E-mail address: BHelfand@northshore.org

Urol Clin N Am 48 (2021) 401–409
https://doi.org/10.1016/j.ucl.2021.04.003
0094-0143/21/

urologic.theclinics.com

distinguish those patients likely to develop aggressive tumors. PCa is recognized as one of the most of heritable of all solid tumors.[9] As such, results of twin studies have estimated that up to 58% of PCa can be explained by heritable components.[10] Therefore, it is not surprising that almost all authoritative groups currently recommend PCa screening among high-risk individuals, including those with a positive family history (FH).[11,12] Although FH is traditionally used as an indirect measurement of inherited risk, it is largely insufficient and associated with many possible errors.[13] As an example, clinicians often only gather information regarding PCa among first-degree relatives.[14,15] Some studies have presented familial risks based on PCa in extended family members, including a familial risk assessment model.[16,17] However, detailed family histories that include extended relatives are often difficult to obtain because of survival status of male relatives, recall ability, and family communication.[18] In addition, families with few male members are less informative. FH is also subject to change, as men may be recategorized from negative to positive depending on when relatives are diagnosed. Finally, although some studies have suggested an inherited component,[19] FH does not reliably predict prostate tumor aggressiveness. As such, FH has limited ability to predict (1) more aggressive disease among men undergoing AS, (2) PCa metastases, or (3) PC-specific mortality. Therefore, other risk assessment methods are required to reliably assess inherited susceptibility to PCa.

Within recent years, it has become increasingly evident that there are improved ways to estimate the inherited risk of PCa. With advances in DNA sequencing and genotyping technologies, 2 direct measurements of inherited risk are now feasible: (1) Rare pathogenic variants/mutations (RPMs) in monogenic genes, and (2) Risk-associated single-nucleotide polymorphisms (SNPs). One is sequencing for germline mutations in candidate genes, including *HOXB13* and *BRCA2*.[20–22] These RPMs are rare in the general population (<2%) but are associated with relatively high PCa susceptibility.[20–22] Another direct measure is risk-associated SNPs. To date, more than 160 inherited PCa risk-associated SNPs have been identified through genome-wide association studies (GWAS).[23] Compared with RPMs, the frequency of SNPs in the population is common, and each has a small individual effect on PCa risk. However, SNPs have a stronger cumulative effect, which can be measured by a polygenic risk score. Published studies consistently demonstrated a dose-response association between higher percentile of polygenic risk scores and higher PCa risk.[23,24]

Rare pathogenic mutations in monogenic genes and polygenic variants now make it possible to directly and more accurately measure genetic risk. Despite this progress, several major challenges exist in implementing germline genetic testing for PCa decision making. In recent years, many clinicians have become aware of the importance of genetic testing. Genetic testing is largely related to the fact that up to 25% of men with metastatic cancer will harbor gene mutations, and many of these men may show improved and sustained responses to specific therapies, including Poly (ADP-ribose) polymerase inhibitors, platinum based-therapies, and immunotherapies.[25–27] These findings have motivated many authoritative groups to now recommend genetic testing for men with high-grade cancer, metastatic tumors, and strong FH of PCa and other related cancers.[28] Despite these changes in national guidelines, most clinicians continue to lack recognition that germline testing has utility for guiding many other clinical decisions related to the management of PCa, including screening and prognosis. In addition, there is a failure to include an assessment of polygenic variants. Therefore, the remainder of this review focuses on germline testing for predicting PCa prognosis and its implications for AS. Specifically, the authors review published studies on the association between monogenic genes and disease risk and PCa progression and published data on the association of mutations in monogenic genes with tumor grade reclassification among AS patients. Finally, the authors discuss a new hypothesis and preliminary data that polygenic risk score predicts tumor grade reclassification among AS patients.

MONOGENIC MUTATIONS AND PROSTATE CANCER PROGRESSION

As mentioned above, RPMs in several genes, especially those in the DNA repair pathway, were recently reported in PCa patients and were associated with PCa risk,[21,29,30] disease progression,[22,31,32] and response to treatment.[33–35] Based on these reports, germline testing was recently recommended by the National Comprehensive Cancer Network (NCCN) for the subset of PCa patients with high-risk, very high-risk, regional, or metastatic PCa, or FH of hereditary breast and ovarian cancer and Lynch syndrome.[11] An expert consensus-driven framework was also recently developed for comprehensive genetic evaluation of rare mutations for genetically informed management.[36]

Based on available evidence from different types of study designs, germline mutations in various genes may have distinct clinical utilities, ranging from (1) predicting PCa risk among unaffected men, (2) differentiating disease aggressiveness and predicting disease progression for men at time of PCa diagnosis, and (3) predicting responses to drug therapy among metastatic PCa patients. The second type of clinical utility is highly relevant for predicting upgrading among patients undergo AS.

Multiple case-case studies on the association between rare germline mutations in a panel of genes and PCa aggressiveness and disease progression have been reported in the last decade.[20,22,31,32,37–51] For example, by comparing RPMs of 155 DNA repair genes among 5545 European-ancestry men, including 2775 nonaggressive and 2770 aggressive PCa cases (467 of which were metastatic cases) from 12 international studies, Darst and colleagues[46] found that BRCA2 and PALB2 had the most statistically significant gene-based associations, with 2.5% of aggressive and 0.8% of nonaggressive cases carrying RPMs of BRCA2 (odds ratio [OR] = 3.19; P = 8.58E-07) and 0.65% of aggressive and 0.11% of nonaggressive cases carrying RPMs of PALB2 (OR = 6.31; P = 4.79E-04). ATM had a nominal association, with 1.6% of aggressive and 0.8% of nonaggressive cases carrying RPMs (OR = 1.88; P = .02). In aggregate, RPMs within 24 literature-curated candidate PCa DNA repair genes were more common in aggressive than nonaggressive cases (carrier frequencies = 14.2% vs 10.6%, respectively; P = 5.56E-05). However, this difference was statistically nonsignificant (P = .18) upon excluding BRCA2, PALB2, and ATM.

In the recent study comparing RPMs among 1694 PCa patients who underwent radical prostatectomy at Johns Hopkins Hospital, including 706 patients with high-grade disease (GG 4 and 5) and 988 patients with low-grade disease (GG1), the authors documented that the frequency of germline RPMs in the 14 candidate PCa genes was significantly higher in high-grade patients (8.64%) than low-grade patients (3.54%; P = 9.98E-6).[51] However, at the individual gene level, significant differences were found for only 3 genes: ATM (2.12% and 0.20%, respectively; P = 9.35×10^{-5}), BRCA2 (2.55% and 0.20%, respectively; P = 8.99×10^{-6}), and MSH2 (0.57% and 0%, respectively; P = .03). Higher but not statistically significant mutation frequencies in high grade versus low grade were found for BRCA1 (0.28% and 0.10%, respectively; P = .65) and CHEK2 (1.27% and 1.01%, respectively; P = .65). The estimated carrier rate was the same (0.71%) for HOXB13 G84E between the 2 groups.

Similar findings were found in several other studies. In a case-case study comparing the prevalence of germline RPMs of 26 candidate PCa genes in 787 men with aggressive disease and 769 with nonaggressive disease from 4 consortium in Australia, Nguyen-Dumont and colleagues[48] found significantly higher carrier rates of RPMs for BRCA2 and ATM P/LP in men with aggressive PCa than nonaggressive PCa; 2.3% and 0.5% (P = .004), and 0.02% and 0.01% (P = .06), respectively. Similarly, Rantapero and colleagues[50] compared RPMs of 26 candidate DNA repair and other candidate genes between 787 aggressive and 769 nonaggressive PCa cases in Finnish and Swedish populations. They found significantly higher carrier rates of RPMs for BRCA2 in aggressive cases than nonaggressive cases (P<.01). The carrier rate of RPMs was marginally higher in aggressive cases than nonaggressive cases (P = .06).

One prospective clinical trial (PROREPAIR-B trial) assessing the impact of ATM/BRCA1/BRCA2/PALB2 germline mutations on cause-specific survival (CSS) from diagnosis of metastatic castration-resistant PCa was recently published.[42] The study identified 68 carriers (16.2%) of 419 eligible patients, including 14 with BRCA2, 8 with ATM, 4 with BRCA1, and none with PALB2 mutations. The trial did not reach its primary end point, because the difference in CSS between ATM/BRCA1/BRCA2/PALB2 carriers and noncarriers was not statistically significant (23.3 vs 33.2 months; P = .26). CSS was halved in germline BRCA2 carriers (17.4 vs 33.2 months; P = .03), and BRCA2 mutations were identified as an independent prognostic factor for CSS (hazard ratio [HR], 2.11; P = .03).

Although RPMs in several candidate genes (especially those in the DNA repair pathway) have been reported in aggressive PCa patients, it is important to note that observation of these mutations in PCa patients with clinically significant disease alone is not sufficient to implicate them as prognostic markers. Statistical evidence is required; especially in well-designed studies where phenotypes are well characterized, and sequencing/annotation methodologies as well as racial and ethnic background are comparable between groups of PCa patients. To date, evidence for significantly higher carrier rates of RPMs in aggressive than nonaggressive PCa was consistent for BRCA2 and ATM but inconsistent for PALB2, MSH2, and CHEK2. In contrast, no association for PCa aggressiveness was consistently found for BRCA1 and HOXB13. The lack of association between BRCA1 and PCa-specific mortality was also concluded in a recent meta-analysis; estimated HR was 1.06, P = .90 (in comparison, HR was 2.63, P = 0.0, for BRCA2).[52]

MONOGENIC MUTATIONS AND THEIR IMPLICATION IN ACTIVE SURVEILLANCE

On the basis on the above data demonstrating that some RPMs associate with more aggressive PCa phenotypes, the authors tested the hypothesis that mutation carriers of men undergoing AS have worse outcomes in 2 AS cohorts at North-Shore University HealthSystem and Johns Hopkins.[32] Of these 1211 PCa patients, mutation carriers in a 3-gene panel (BRCA2, ATM, and BRCA1) were more likely to experience grade reclassification (11 of 26 carriers, 42.31%) than nonmutation carriers (278 of 1185 noncarriers, 23.45%, P = .04). The results were strongest for BRCA2. Carrier rates for BRCA2 were greater for those reclassified from GG 1 at diagnosis to GG ≥3 (4.1% in upgraded vs 0.7% in nonupgraded, P = .01) versus to grade group 2 (2.1% in upgraded vs 0.6% in upgraded; P = .03). It is recognized that the results should be validated because the number of pathogenic mutation carriers was relatively low.

Halstuch and colleagues[53] described the short-term oncologic outcomes of AS in a population of men with RPMs in several candidate genes. A prospective cohort of men with germline DNA repair gene mutations was diagnosed with grade group 1 PCa. Among the 18 RPMs carriers of BRCA1 (8), BRCA2 (6), CHEK2 (2), and Lynch syndrome genes (2), 15 (83%) patients initiated AS and 3 (17%) declined. All but 1 (93%) were fully compliant with the AS protocol (prostate-specific antigen [PSA] every 3 months, multiparametric MRI, and an MRI-ultrasound fusion confirmatory biopsy within 1 year of diagnosis). Overall, 3 (20%) had upgrading at confirmatory biopsy and were treated. At a median follow-up of 28 months (interquartile range 8.5–42), 12 (80%) patients on AS are free from upgrading or radical treatment. This descriptive study suggests AS may be feasible among carriers diagnosed with low-risk PCa. They also recommend that carriers should be very carefully monitored at a specialized clinic, optimizing patient compliance, and minimizing risk.

POLYGENIC RISK SCORE, PROSTATE CANCER PROGRESSION, AND THEIR IMPLICATIONS IN ACTIVE SURVEILLANCE

To date, more than 160 inherited PCa risk-associated SNPs have been identified through GWAS.[23] Compared with rare monogenic mutations, SNPs are more common, and each has a modest individual effect on PCa risk. However, SNPs have a stronger cumulative effect that can be measured by a polygenic risk score. Published studies to date consistently demonstrated a dose-response association between higher percentile of polygenic risk scores and higher PCa risk.[23,24,54] For example, using a large prospective cohort derived from the UK Biobank where 208,685 PCa diagnosis-free participants at recruitment were followed via the UK cancer and death registries, the authors found that a genetic risk score (GRS) based on 130 known risk-associated SNPs was not only associated with PCa incidence and shorter diagnosis-free survival time, but, more importantly, also significantly associated with higher PCa mortality.[55] Furthermore, a head-to-head comparison demonstrated that GRS was more informative for stratifying inherited PCa risk than FH and RPMs. In addition to identifying more high-risk men who had comparable PCa incidence and mortality than those identified by FH and/or RPMs, GRS also identified low-risk men who had significantly lower PCa incidence and mortality than those with average GRS. Finally, the authors' study revealed that the association between GRS with PCa incidence was independent of FH and RPMs and can therefore complement FH and RPMs for inherited risk assessment. Although FH and RPMs identified 11% of men at higher PCa risk, adding GRS identified an additional 15% of men at higher PCa risk with comparable PCa incidence and mortality.[55]

Despite the consistent finding that polygenic risk scores can effectively stratify disease risk, the clinical utility of polygenic risk scores in differentiating aggressive from indolent PCa and in predicting prognosis of PCa is unclear at this stage. In fact, no significant difference was found in 2 large studies that directly compared polygenic risk score between less and more aggressive PCa patients.[56,57] In a study of 5895 PCa cases treated by radical prostatectomy at Johns Hopkins Hospital, where each tumor was uniformly graded and staged using the same protocol, there were no statistically significant differences (P>.05) in risk allele frequencies between patients with more aggressive or less aggressive disease for 18 of the 20 reported PCa risk-associated SNPs at the time.[56] For the 2 SNPs that had significant differences between more and less aggressive disease rs2735839, near KLK3 (P = 8.4 × 10^{-7}), and rs10993994 upstream of MSMB (P = .046), the alleles that are associated with increased risk for PCa were more frequent in patients with less aggressive disease. In another recently published study on European men from the Prostate Cancer Prevention Trial (N = 2434) and the Selenium and Vitamin E Cancer Prevention Trial (N = 4885), a higher polygenic score based on 98 known risk-associated SNPs was associated with PCa risk in both trials but did not predict other outcomes.[57] They concluded that the vast majority of PCa risk-associated SNPs are not associated with aggressiveness and clinicopathologic variables of PCa and have minimal utility in predicting the risk for developing more or less aggressive forms of PCa.

Three studies that directly tested association between risk-associated SNPs and PCa progression in AS patients were reported between 2012 and 2016.[58–60] The first study assessed whether the carrier status of 35 risk alleles for PCa is associated with having unfavorable pathologic features in the radical prostatectomy specimens (GG $\geq$7 and/or $\geq$ pT2b) in men with clinically low-risk PCa who fulfill commonly accepted criteria as candidates for AS (T1c, PSA <10 ng/mL, biopsy GG $\leq$1, 3 or fewer positive cores, $\leq$50% tumor involvement/core).[58] Among the 263 patients treated at Northwestern University, 58 (22.1%) had unfavorable pathologic characteristics. Significantly higher carrier rates of risk alleles were found in men with unfavorable pathologic characteristics for 3 of the 35 SNPs (P<.05). Carriers of any one of the significantly overrepresented risk alleles had twice the likelihood of unfavorable tumor features (P = .03), and carriers of any 2 had a 7-fold increased likelihood (P = .001). However, as pointed out by the authors, none of the SNPs attained statistical significance after the Bonferroni correction. Furthermore, the observed cumulative effect of these 3 SNPs (expected if they were selected based on the significance of individual SNPs in the same cohort) needs to be confirmed in additional independent cohorts.

In a second study reported by the same research group, association of 23 known PCa risk SNPs with upgrading in 2 patient cohorts was reported (950 patients who underwent surgical treatment at Northwestern University and 209 patients enrolled for AS at the NorthShore University HealthSystem).[59] PCa patients were included if they had GG1 disease on diagnostic biopsy. The surgical cohort was then categorized into those who continued to have GG1 disease (non-upgraded) and those who had higher-grade disease (GG $\geq$2; upgraded) on surgical pathologic condition. The AS cohort included very low-risk and low-risk PCa patients defined as an initial diagnosis of GG score 6 on biopsy, PSA less than 10, and 3 or fewer cores involved with cancer on a standard template 12-core prostate biopsy performed under ultrasound guidance. Confirmatory biopsies were performed within 6 to 12 months using MRI fusion biopsy. Biopsies were then repeated every 12 to 18 months or for cause.

Patients in this cohort were categorized into 2 groups based on the results of their surveillance biopsies: men who continued to have either no cancer or GG score 6 disease (non-upgraded) and those who were diagnosed with higher-grade disease (upgraded). Overall, 31% and 34% of men were upgraded in the surgical and AS cohorts, respectively. In the surgical cohort, 1 SNP (rs11568818 on chromosome 11q22) was significantly associated with the risk of upgrading after correction for multiple testing. This SNP was also significantly associated with upgrade in the AS cohort (P = .003).

In contrast, a null association was reported in the study by Goh and colleagues[60] at the Royal Marsden Hospital. This study explored the prognostic role of FH and GRS from 39 known risk-associated SNPs in patients undergoing AS. All patients had histologically confirmed PCa, stage T1/2a, N0, M0, GG1, PSA level of less than 15 ng/mL with cancer present in less than 50% of the total number of biopsy cores. GG2 was only allowed if patients were aged greater than 65 years. Of the 471 AS patients, 55 (13.6%) had adverse histology on repeat biopsies and 145 (30.8%) had deferred treatment. No significant association between FH of PCa in any degree of relation and adverse histology or time to treatment was found. Similarly, no significant association was found between the GRS and adverse histology or time to treatment (P = .57 and P = .97, respectively).

Overall, results from the published studies to date on association of PCa risk-associated SNPs and tumor upgrade in AS patients are limited and inconsistent. These pioneering studies suffered from small sample size, short follow-up time, and limited numbers of risk-associated SNPs. Studies with larger sample size of AS patients, longer follow-up time, and using more risk-associated SNPs are needed to develop and validate SNP-based polygenic risk score for predicting tumor upgrade in AS patients.

RECENT PROGRESS OF POLYGENIC RISK SCORE IN ACTIVE SURVEILLANCE: A NOVEL HYPOTHESIS

Encouraging findings are emerging on the potential role of polygenic risk scores for predicting outcomes among AS patients. It has been shown that various pathologic characteristics, including number of cores involved with cancer, are predictors of tumor upgrading among men on AS. Different from previous published studies,[58–60] the authors recently found that a GRS based on 78 risk SNPs was significantly associated with the

Biopsy Sampling Hypothesis

Higher GRS is Associated with Biopsy Upgrade in AS Because of its Association with Higher Number of Positive Cores

Prostate cancer (PCa) and its detection:

1. PCa is multifocal
2. Prostate biopsy is sampling a small amount of tissue in the gland
3. Pathological grade from surgical specimen provides more complete evaluation of the whole gland

Known genetic observations:

Higher GRS is 1) associated with higher PCa risk but 2) not associated with pathological tumor grade based on surgical specimen

Novel genetic observations: higher GRS is

Higher GRS is 1) associated with biopsy tumor upgrade in active surveillance (AS), and 2) associated with higher numbers of positive cores in biopsy

Biopsy sampling hypothesis:

Seemingly conflicting results (GRS not associated with pathological tumor grade but associated with biopsy upgrade in AS) can be explained by:

1. Higher GRS is associated with higher numbers of either high-grade or low-grade tumor foci
2. Therefore, GRS does not differentiate high- or low-grade tumors if grade is evaluated based on a complete evaluation of the gland from surgery specimen
3. GRS, however, is associated with tumor upgrade in AS because higher grade tumors are more likely to be detected from higher numbers of foci

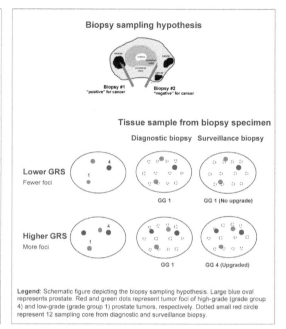

Legend: Schematic figure depicting the biopsy sampling hypothesis. Large blue oval represents prostate. Red and green dots represent tumor foci of high-grade (grade group 4) and low-grade (grade group 1) prostate tumors, respectively. Dotted small red circle represent 12 sampling core from diagnostic and surveillance biopsy.

Fig. 1. The biopsy sampling hypothesis. Large blue oval represents prostate. Red and green dots represent tumor foci of high-grade (grade group 4) and low-grade (grade group 1) prostate tumors, respectively. Dotted small red circle represents 12 sampling cores from diagnostic and surveillance biopsy.

number and laterality of tumor cores in 2 AS cohorts from NorthShore University HealthSystem and Johns Hopkins Hospital (N = 1213) (Xu, J et. al, 2021; unpublished data). Furthermore, there was a trend between higher percentile of GRS and the frequency of upgrading (GG1 to ≥GG2) on surveillance biopsy.

This association with between GRS-positive core number and tumor upgrading from surveillance biopsy is somewhat surprising considering that polygenic risk scores have been consistently shown to have no association with pathologic grade and progression of PCa from surgical specimens.[56,57] However, this discrepancy could be due to the difference between clinical grading from prostate biopsy (sampling using a small amount of tissue in the gland) and pathologic grading from surgical specimen (more complete evaluation of the whole gland) of multifocal prostate tumors, an important characteristic of PCa. Upgrading on a surveillance biopsy could reflect the detection of additional higher-grade tumors in the prostate gland that were not detected in the diagnostic biopsy, and the likelihood of upgrade increases with the presence of increased numbers of tumor foci. This reasoning is the basis of the authors' biopsy sampling hypothesis

(**Fig. 1**), that is, higher GRS is associated with biopsy upgrade in AS because of its association with higher number of positive cores. This hypothesis is supported by the authors' recent observation.

This hypothesis, however, needs to be further tested in additional large AS studies. Currently, a large multicenter study of AS patients across the United States, funded by the National Health Institute Specialized Programs of Research Excellence, is underway. If confirmed in this multicenter study, polygenic risk score could be used to supplement existing clinical and pathologic variables to predict upgrade in AS.

SUMMARY

Increased attention has been recently called to evaluate RPMs in a specific subset of genes that can predict treatment response to chemotherapies and immunotherapies for men with advanced PCa. However, given the evidence that these same monogenic gene mutations increase the risk of metastatic and lethal disease, genetic testing should not be limited to men with aggressive prostate tumors. Rather, germline testing should play a significant role in PCa screening and clinical decision making of all men with newly diagnosed PCa, including those with seemingly very-low- and low-risk tumors considering AS. Men who harbor RPMs in genes including *BRCA2* and *ATM* should consider definitive treatment and avoid strategies such as AS. In addition, emerging evidence also supports that a GRS calculated from PCa-risk SNPs can be used to identify men who are more likely to exhibit disease recategorization while undergoing AS. Although validation of these findings in other races and populations should be performed, there is sufficient evidence to support routine genetic testing at the time of PCa diagnosis.

CLINICS CARE POINTS

- Germline testing for rare pathogenic mutations in several National Comprehensive Cancer Network guideline–recommended genes should be considered for patients with newly diagnosed prostate cancer, including those managed by active surveillance.

- Although mutation carrier rate is low in patients undergoing active surveillance, carriers should be very carefully monitored because of their significantly higher risk of progressing at earlier timepoints.

- Germline testing in patients undergoing active surveillance should also include prostate cancer polygenic risk score. More than 10% of these patients have higher polygenic risk scores that are associated with an increased risk of tumor upgrading.

DISCLOSURE

Dr B.T. Helfand is an advisor and speaker for Amby Genetics. He is also a consultant for GoPath.

REFERENCES

1. Rawla P. Epidemiology of prostate cancer. World J Oncol 2019;10(2):63–89.
2. Schroder FH, Hugosson J, Roobol MJ, et al. Screening and prostate-cancer mortality in a randomized European study. N Engl J Med 2009; 360(13):1320–8.
3. Hugosson J, Carlsson S, Aus G, et al. Mortality results from the Goteborg randomised population-based prostate-cancer screening trial. Lancet Oncol 2010;11(8):725–32.
4. Draisma G, Boer R, Otto SJ, et al. Lead times and overdetection due to prostate-specific antigen screening: estimates from the European Randomized Study of Screening for Prostate Cancer. J Natl Cancer Inst 2003;95(12):868–78.
5. Welch HG, Black WC. Overdiagnosis in cancer. J Natl Cancer Inst 2010;102(9):605–13.
6. Khatami A, Aus G, Damber JE, et al. PSA doubling time predicts the outcome after active surveillance in screening-detected prostate cancer: results from the European randomized study of screening for prostate cancer, Sweden section. Int J Cancer 2007;120(1):170–4.
7. Tosoian JJ, Mamawala M, Epstein JI, et al. Active surveillance of grade group 1 prostate cancer: long-term outcomes from a large prospective cohort. Eur Urol 2020;77(6):675–82.
8. Klotz L, Vesprini D, Sethukavalan P, et al. Long-term follow-up of a large active surveillance cohort of patients with prostate cancer. J Clin Oncol 2015;33(3): 272–7.
9. Mucci LA, Hjelmborg JB, Harris JR, et al. Familial risk and heritability of cancer among twins in Nordic countries. JAMA 2016;315(1):68–76.
10. Hjelmborg JB, Scheike T, Holst K, et al. The heritability of prostate cancer in the Nordic Twin Study of Cancer. Cancer Epidemiol Biomarkers Prev 2014; 23(11):2303–10.
11. Mohler JL, Antonarakis ES, Armstrong AJ, et al. Prostate cancer, version 2.2019, NCCN clinical practice guidelines in oncology. J Natl Compr Canc Netw 2019;17(5):479–505.
12. USPST Force, Grossman DC, Curry SJ, et al. Screening for Prostate Cancer: US Preventive Services Task Force Recommendation Statement. JAMA 2018;319(18):1901–13.
13. Helfand BT, Kearns J, Conran C, et al. Clinical validity and utility of genetic risk scores in prostate cancer. Asian J Androl 2016;18(4):509–14.
14. Brandt A, Bermejo JL, Sundquist J, et al. Age-specific risk of incident prostate cancer and risk of death from prostate cancer defined by the number of affected family members. Eur Urol 2010;58(2):275–80.
15. Brandt A, Sundquist J, Hemminki K. Risk for incident and fatal prostate cancer in men with a family history of any incident and fatal cancer. Ann Oncol 2012; 23(1):251–6.
16. Amundadottir LT, Thorvaldsson S, Gudbjartsson DF, et al. Cancer as a complex phenotype: pattern of cancer distribution within and beyond the nuclear family. Plos Med 2004;1(3):e65.
17. Roudgari H, Hemminki K, Brandt A, et al. Prostate cancer risk assessment model: a scoring model based on the Swedish Family-Cancer Database. J Med Genet 2012;49(5):345–52.
18. Sun J, Na R, Hsu FC, et al. Genetic score is an objective and better measurement of inherited risk

of prostate cancer than family history. Eur Urol 2013; 63(3):585–7.

19. Albright FS, Stephenson RA, Agarwal N, et al. Relative risks for lethal prostate cancer based on complete family history of prostate cancer death. Prostate 2017;77(1):41–8.

20. Ewing CM, Ray AM, Lange EM, et al. Germline mutations in HOXB13 and prostate-cancer risk. N Engl J Med 2012;366(2):141–9.

21. Pritchard CC, Mateo J, Walsh MF, et al. Inherited DNA-repair gene mutations in men with metastatic prostate cancer. N Engl J Med 2016;375(5):443–53.

22. Na R, Zheng SL, Han M, et al. Germline mutations in ATM and BRCA1/2 distinguish risk for lethal and indolent prostate cancer and are associated with early age at death. Eur Urol 2017;71(5):740–7.

23. Schumacher FR, Al Olama AA, Berndt SI, et al. Association analyses of more than 140,000 men identify 63 new prostate cancer susceptibility loci. Nat Genet 2018;50(7):928–36.

24. Zheng SL, Sun J, Wiklund F, et al. Cumulative association of five genetic variants with prostate cancer. N Engl J Med 2008;358(9):910–9.

25. Mota JM, Barnett E, Nauseef JT, et al. Platinum-based chemotherapy in metastatic prostate cancer with DNA repair gene alterations. JCO Precis Oncol 2020;4:355–66.

26. Nizialek E, Antonarakis ES. PARP inhibitors in metastatic prostate cancer: evidence to date. Cancer Manag Res 2020;12:8105–14.

27. Graham LS, Montgomery B, Cheng HH, et al. Mismatch repair deficiency in metastatic prostate cancer: response to PD-1 blockade and standard therapies. PLoS One 2020;15(5):e0233260.

28. Mohler JL, Higano CS, Schaeffer EM, et al. Current recommendations for prostate cancer genetic testing: NCCN prostate guideline. Can J Urol 2019; 26(5 Suppl 2):34–7.

29. Kote-Jarai Z, Leongamornlert D, Saunders E, et al. BRCA2 is a moderate penetrance gene contributing to young-onset prostate cancer: implications for genetic testing in prostate cancer patients. Br J Cancer 2011;105(8):1230–4.

30. Leongamornlert DA, Saunders EJ, Wakerell S, et al. Germline DNA repair gene mutations in young-onset prostate cancer cases in the UK: evidence for a more extensive genetic panel. Eur Urol 2019;76(3): 329–37.

31. Castro E, Goh C, Olmos D, et al. Germline BRCA mutations are associated with higher risk of nodal involvement, distant metastasis, and poor survival outcomes in prostate cancer. J Clin Oncol 2013; 31(14):1748–57.

32. Carter HB, Helfand B, Mamawala M, et al. Germline mutations in ATM and BRCA1/2 are associated with grade reclassification in men on active surveillance for prostate cancer. Eur Urol 2019;75(5):743–9.

33. Mateo J, Carreira S, Sandhu S, et al. DNA-repair defects and olaparib in metastatic prostate cancer. N Engl J Med 2015;373(18):1697–708.

34. Mateo J, Cheng HH, Beltran H, et al. Clinical outcome of prostate cancer patients with germline DNA repair mutations: retrospective analysis from an international study. Eur Urol 2018;73(5):687–93.

35. Marshall CH, Sokolova AO, McNatty AL, et al. Differential response to olaparib treatment among men with metastatic castration-resistant prostate cancer harboring BRCA1 or BRCA2 Versus ATM Mutations. Eur Urol 2019;76(4):452–8.

36. Giri VN, Knudsen KE, Kelly WK, et al. Role of genetic testing for inherited prostate cancer risk: Philadelphia prostate cancer consensus conference 2017. J Clin Oncol 2018;36(4):414–24.

37. Edwards SM, Evans DG, Hope Q, et al. Prostate cancer in BRCA2 germline mutation carriers is associated with poorer prognosis. Br J Cancer 2010; 103(6):918–24.

38. Gallagher DJ, Gaudet MM, Pal P, et al. Germline BRCA mutations denote a clinicopathologic subset of prostate cancer. Clin Cancer Res 2010;16(7): 2115–21.

39. Thorne H, Willems AJ, Niedermayr E, et al. Decreased prostate cancer-specific survival of men with BRCA2 mutations from multiple breast cancer families. Cancer Prev Res (Phila) 2011;4(7): 1002–10.

40. Kote-Jarai Z, Mikropoulos C, Leongamornlert DA, et al. Prevalence of the HOXB13 G84E germline mutation in British men and correlation with prostate cancer risk, tumour characteristics and clinical outcomes. Ann Oncol 2015;26(4):756–61.

41. Mijuskovic M, Saunders EJ, Leongamornlert DA, et al. Rare germline variants in DNA repair genes and the angiogenesis pathway predispose prostate cancer patients to develop metastatic disease. Br J Cancer 2018;119(1):96–104.

42. Castro E, Romero-Laorden N, Del Pozo A, et al. PROREPAIR-B: a prospective cohort study of the impact of germline DNA repair mutations on the outcomes of patients with metastatic castration-resistant prostate cancer. J Clin Oncol 2019;37(6): 490–503.

43. Petrovics G, Price DK, Lou H, et al. Increased frequency of germline BRCA2 mutations associates with prostate cancer metastasis in a racially diverse patient population. Prostate Cancer Prostatic Dis 2019;22(3):406–10.

44. Giri VN, Hegarty SE, Hyatt C, et al. Germline genetic testing for inherited prostate cancer in practice: implications for genetic testing, precision therapy, and cascade testing. Prostate 2019;79(4):333–9.

45. Yadav S, Hart SN, Hu C, et al. Contribution of inherited DNA-repair gene mutations to hormone-sensitive and castrate-resistant metastatic prostate

cancer and implications for clinical outcome. JCO Precis Oncol 2019;3. PO.19.00067.

46. Darst BF, Dadaev T, Saunders E, et al. Germline sequencing DNA repair genes in 5,545 men with aggressive and non-aggressive prostate cancer. J Natl Cancer Inst 2020. https://doi.org/10.1093/jnci/djaa132.

47. Pritzlaff M, Tian Y, Reineke P, et al. Diagnosing hereditary cancer predisposition in men with prostate cancer. Genet Med 2020;22(9):1517–23.

48. Nguyen-Dumont T, MacInnis RJ, Steen JA, et al. Rare germline genetic variants and risk of aggressive prostate cancer. Int J Cancer 2020;147(8):2142–9.

49. Dall'Era MA, McPherson JD, Gao AC, et al. Germline and somatic DNA repair gene alterations in prostate cancer. Cancer 2020;126(13):2980–5.

50. Rantapero T, Wahlfors T, Kahler A, et al. Inherited DNA repair gene mutations in men with lethal prostate cancer. Genes (Basel). 2020;11(3):314.

51. Wu Y, Yu H, Li S, et al. Rare germline pathogenic mutations of DNA repair genes are most strongly associated with grade group 5 prostate cancer. Eur Urol Oncol 2020;3(2):224–30.

52. Oh M, Alkhushaym N, Fallatah S, et al. The association of BRCA1 and BRCA2 mutations with prostate cancer risk, frequency, and mortality: a meta-analysis. Prostate 2019;79(8):880–95.

53. Halstuch D, Ber Y, Kedar D, et al. Short-term outcomes of active surveillance for low risk prostate cancer among men with germline DNA repair gene mutations. J Urol 2020;204(4):707–13.

54. Chen H, Liu X, Brendler CB, et al. Adding genetic risk score to family history identifies twice as many high-risk men for prostate cancer: results from the prostate cancer prevention trial. Prostate 2016;76(12):1120–9.

55. Shi Z, Platz EA, Wei J, et al. Performance of three inherited risk measures for predicting prostate cancer incidence and mortality: a population-based prospective analysis. Eur Urol 2020;79(3):419–26.

56. Kader AK, Sun J, Isaacs SD, et al. Individual and cumulative effect of prostate cancer risk-associated variants on clinicopathologic variables in 5,895 prostate cancer patients. Prostate 2009;69(11):1195–205.

57. Ahmed M, Goh C, Saunders E, et al. Germline genetic variation in prostate susceptibility does not predict outcomes in the chemoprevention trials PCPT and SELECT. Prostate Cancer Prostatic Dis 2020;23(2):333–42.

58. McGuire BB, Helfand BT, Kundu S, et al. Association of prostate cancer risk alleles with unfavourable pathological characteristics in potential candidates for active surveillance. BJU Int 2012;110(3):338–43.

59. Kearns JT, Lapin B, Wang E, et al. Associations between iCOGS single nucleotide polymorphisms and upgrading in both surgical and active surveillance cohorts of men with prostate cancer. Eur Urol 2016;69(2):223–8.

60. Goh CL, Saunders EJ, Leongamornlert DA, et al. Clinical implications of family history of prostate cancer and genetic risk single nucleotide polymorphism (SNP) profiles in an active surveillance cohort. BJU Int 2013;112(5):666–73.

Germline Predisposition to Prostate Cancer in Diverse Populations

Kelly K. Bree, MD, Patrick J. Henley, MD, Curtis A. Pettaway, MD*

KEYWORDS

- Germline DNA testing • African American • Asian • Prostate cancer
- Single nucleotide polymorphisms

KEY POINTS

- Recent advances in genomic sequencing have shed light on the scarcity of racial and ethnic minority inclusion in prior clinical trials and genetic studies, underscoring the urgent need to increase diversity in genomic medicine.
- Current guidelines recommend sequencing for the homologous recombination genes *BRCA1*, *BRCA2*, *ATM*, *PALB2*, and *CHEK2*, as well as for mutations in the mismatch repair genes associated with Lynch syndrome. Although primarily studied in Caucasian men, mutations in these genes have also been identified in various minority groups.
- The importance of different variants of unknown significance (VUS) remains poorly elucidated. Given the elevated rates of VUS in minority groups compared with Caucasian men, further studies are needed to facilitate potential reclassification of VUS in these underrepresented groups.
- Among African American men, 8q24 polymorphisms have been shown to confer increased incidence of prostate cancer.
- Additional studies using the concept of polygenic risk score in analyzing the association of disease-related single-nucleotide polymorphisms with prostate cancer among underrepresented minority populations are needed to enhance early detection efforts.

INTRODUCTION

Prostate cancer (PCa) is the most common solid organ malignancy diagnosed in American men and the second leading cause of cancer-related mortality. In the United States, 192,000 new diagnoses of PCa and more than 33,000 deaths from the disease are expected in 2020.[1] Among those diagnosed with PCa, there exists significant racial disparities regarding PCa incidence and mortality. Compared with Caucasian men (CM), African American men (AAM) are more likely to be diagnosed with PCa (1 in 6 AAM vs 1 in 8 CM) and have a 2.4 times higher mortality rate.[2] Worse PCa-specific mortality compared with CM has also been demonstrated in Hispanic populations, particularly among Puerto Rican (hazard ratio [HR] = 1.71, P < .001) and Mexican American men (HR = 1.21, P = .008).[3] Conversely, although Asian American and Pacific Islanders (AAPIs) are more likely to present with advanced disease, they have better cancer-specific survival.[4] Differences in PCa burden among minority groups in the United States have previously been attributed to socioeconomic status and access to health care; however, even when socioeconomic status is controlled for, disparities in PCa incidence and mortality remain significant, highlighting the potential role of genetic factors.[5]

PCa has been identified as one of the most heritable malignancies, with 57% (95% confidence

The University of Texas MD Anderson Cancer Center, Department of Urology, 1515 Holcombe Boulevard, Houston, TX 77030, USA
* Corresponding author.
E-mail address: CPettawa@MDAnderson.org

Urol Clin N Am 48 (2021) 411–423
https://doi.org/10.1016/j.ucl.2021.03.008

interval [CI], 51–63) of variation in risk attributed to genetic factors.[6] Our knowledge of the genetics of heritable PCa is rapidly evolving, with recent studies demonstrating that 12% to 17% of men with PCa harbor germline mutations.[7,8] In 2016, the National Comprehensive Cancer Network (NCCN) guidelines began to incorporate germline mutation testing, specifically mentioning family history of BRCA1/2 mutations in regard to PCa screening. Since that time there has been significant evolution within the NCCN guidelines, with germline testing now being used throughout screening, early diagnosis, and to direct treatment decisions (eg, use of poly-ADP ribose polymerase inhibitors). As diagnostic and management paradigms continue to shift toward precision medicine in response to improved understanding of the impact of germline mutations, it is crucial that genetic differences in minority populations also be adequately evaluated to ensure appropriate risk stratification and treatment in these diverse populations.

Recent advances in genomic sequencing have shed light on the scarcity of racial and ethnic minority inclusion in prior clinical trials and genetic studies. In the study by Pritchard and colleagues[7] evaluating 692 men with metastatic PCa, inherited germline mutations were identified in 11.8% of patients. However, less than 10% of the cohort was comprised of minorities (5.8% AA, 1.7% AAPI, and 1.6% Hispanic). Similarly, a retrospective review of The Cancer Genome Atlas demonstrated that of the nearly 6000 patients, only 12% were black, 3% were Asian, and 3% were Hispanic.[9] Low enrolment of minorities within genomic sequencing studies hinders the ability to detect mutations in minority groups and, in turn, can potentially result in furthering the already disparate PCa outcomes in these populations.

HIGH-PENETRANCE GERMLINE MUTATIONS

The incorporation of genetic testing in recent NCCN guidelines, as well as recommendations from the Philadelphia Prostate Cancer Consensus and Germline Genetics Working Group of the Prostate Cancer Clinical Trials Consortium, has led to expanding use of multigene testing for various rare but highly penetrant genes associated with PCa.[10] The 2020 NCCN guidelines recommend sequencing for the homologous recombination genes BRCA1, BRCA2, ATM, PALB2, and CHEK2, as well as for mutations in the mismatch repair genes associated with Lynch syndrome (MLH1, MSH2, MSH6, and PMS2). Additional genes, including HOXB13, can be also be considered.[11] Current indications for germline testing are

outlined in **Box 1**. Such testing among diverse cohorts with the appropriate risk characteristics could prove valuable not only for the index patients but also for their family members especially in the setting of genes associated with heritable cancer syndromes (ie, BRCA1/2, Lynch syndrome, HOXB13).[12]

Herein, we review the prevalence of these high-penetrant germline mutations in various minority groups (**Table 1**). A resounding theme throughout the literature is the marked underrepresentation of minority groups undergoing genetic testing. In a retrospective review of 1351 men with PCa referred for genetic testing by Kwon and colleagues,[13] 7% of patients were from minority groups (3% African American/Canadian [AAC], 2% Hispanic, and 2% APPI). In their cohort, ethnicity was not associated with increased risk of carrying a pathogenic or likely pathogenic germline mutation. However, rates of variants of uncertain significance (VUS) were significantly higher in AAC and AAPI men (37% and 33%, respectively) when compared with CM ($P < .01$). Similarly, germline sequencing of BRCA1/2 mutations in 1235 patients with PCa, including 30% AAM, demonstrated significantly higher rates of VUS in

---

Box 1
Indications for germline testing in men with prostate cancer

High-risk and very high-risk PCa as defined by NCCN guidelines

Regional or metastatic PCa

Intraductal/cribriform pathology

Ashkenazi Jewish ancestry

Family history of high-risk germline mutations (eg, BRCA1/2)

A positive family history of cancer

• Strong history of PCa

  ○ Brother or father or multiple family members with PCa (Grade Group ≥ 2) at <60 years or who died from PCa

• More than 3 cancers on same side of family, especially if younger than or equal to 50 years

  ○ Bile duct, breast, colorectal, endometrial, gastric, kidney, melanoma, ovarian, pancreatic, prostate (≥Grade Group 2), small bowel, urothelial cancer

Data from 2020 NCCN Guidelines on Prostate Cancer. Schaeffer E SS, Antonarakis ES, et al. . NCCN Clinical Practice Guidelines in Oncology (NCCN Guidelines) Prostate Cancer Version 2.2020. . 2020.

Table 1
Multiethnic cohorts assessing the prevalence of high-penetrance germline mutations

Mutation	Population	Study size (n)	Mutation Rate in CM (n, %)	Mutation Rate in AAM (n, %)	Mutation Rate in Hispanic Men (n, %)	Mutation Rate in AAPI (n, %)	Citation
BRCA1	History of PCa	3607	29/2594, 1.1	3/227, 1.3	0/78, 0.0	2/73, 2.7	Nicolosi et al,[8] 2019
	Men with PCa referred for genetic testing	1351	8/1053, 0.8	2/41[a], 4.9	0/25, 0.0	1/24, 4.2	Kwon et al,[13] 2020
	Men with lethal or localized PCa	799	4/613[b], 0.7	0/119, 0		0/67[c], 0.0	Na et al,[14] 2017
	Men with PCa who completed Invitae panel testing	2682	29/2469, 1.2	3/213, 1.4			Sartor et al,[15] 2020
	CM and AAM <55 y with PCa	290	2/257, 0.8	0/33, 0.0			Agalliu et al,[16] 2007
BRCA2	History of PCa	3607	119/2594, 4.6	6/227, 2.6	3/78, 3.8	3/73, 4.1	Nicolosi et al,[8] 2019
	Men with PCa referred for genetic testing	1351	29/1053, 2.8	1/41[a], 2.4	0/25, 0.0	2/24, 8.3	Kwon et al,[13] 2020
	Men with lethal or localized PCa	799	12/613[b], 2.0	0/119, 0.0		3/67[c], 4.5	Na et al,[14] 2017
	Men with PCa who completed Invitae panel testing	2702	119/2488, 4.8	6/214, 2.8			Sartor et al,[15] 2020
	CM and AAM <55 y with PCa	290	2/257, 0.8	0/33, 0.0			Agalliu et al,[16] 2007
BRCA1/2	History of PCa	1235	8/770, 1.0	6/438, 1.4			Petrovics et al,[17] 2019
ATM	History of PCa	3607	48/2594, 1.9	2/227, 0.9	0/78, 0.0	2/73, 2.7	Nicolosi et al,[8] 2019
	Men with PCa referred for genetic testing	1351	22/1053, 2.1	0/41[a], 0.0	0/25, 0.0	0/24, 0.0	Kwon et al,[13] 2020
	Men with lethal or localized PCa	799	6/613[b], 1.0	1/119, 0.8		1/67[c], 1.5	Na et al,[14] 2017
	Men with PCa who completed Invitae panel testing	2508	48/2302, 2.1	2/206, 1.0			Sartor et al,[15] 2020
PALB2	History of PCa	3607	13/2594, 0.5	2/227, 0.9	0/78, 0.0	1/73, 1.4	Nicolosi et al,[8] 2019
	Men with PCa who completed Invitae panel testing	2353	13/2171, 0.6	2/182, 1.1			Sartor et al,[15] 2020

(continued on next page)

Table 1
(continued)

Mutation	Population	Study size (n)	Mutation Rate in CM (n, %)	Mutation Rate in AAM (n, %)	Mutation Rate in Hispanic Men (n, %)	Mutation Rate in AAPI (n, %)	Citation
CHEK2	History of PCa	3607	74/2594, 2.9	1/227, 0.4	0/78, 0.0	0/73, 0.0	Nicolosi et al,[8] 2019
	Men with PCa referred for genetic testing	1351	29/1053, 2.8	1/41[a], 2.4	0/25, 0.0	0/24, 0.0	Kwon et al,[13] 2020
	Men with PCa who completed Invitae panel testing	2586	74/2379, 3.1	1/207, 0.5			Sartor et al,[15] 2020
HOXB13	History of PCa	3607	24/2594, 0.9	3/227, 1.3	0/78, 0.0	0/73, 0.0	Nicolosi et al,[8] 2019
	History of PCa	1843	15/1525, 1.0	1/200, 0.5		0/101, 0.0	Akbari et al,[18] 2012
MLH1	History of PCa	3607	2/2594, 0.1	0/227, 0.0	0/78, 0.0	0/73, 0.0	Nicolosi et al,[8] 2019
	Men with PCa referred for genetic testing	1351	0/1053, 0.0	0/41[a], 0.0	0/25, 0.0	0/24, 0.0	Kwon et al,[13] 2020
	Men with PCa who completed Invitae panel testing	2614	2/2402, 0.1	0/212, 0.0			Sartor et al,[15] 2020
MSH2	History of PCa	3607	19/2594, 0.7	0/227, 0.0	0/78, 0.0	0/73, 0.0	Nicolosi et al,[8] 2019
	Men with PCa referred for genetic testing	1351	2/1053, 0.2	0/41[a], 0.0	0/25, 0.0	0/24, 0.0	Kwon et al,[13] 2020
	Men with PCa who completed Invitae panel testing	2620	19/2408, 0.8	0/212, 0.0			Sartor et al,[15] 2020
MSH6	History of PCa	3607	9/2594, 0.3	0/227, 0.0	1/78, 1.3	1/73, 1.4	Nicolosi et al,[8] 2019
	Men with PCa referred for genetic testing	1351	3/1053, 0.3	1/41[a], 2.4	0/25, 0.0	0/24, 0.0	Kwon et al,[13] 2020
	Men with PCa who completed Invitae panel testing	2616	9/2403, 0.4	0/213, 0.0			Sartor et al,[15] 2020
PMS2	History of PCa	3607	10/2594, 0.4	1/227, 0.4	0/78, 0.0	1/73, 1.4	Nicolosi et al,[8] 2019
	Men with PCa referred for genetic testing	1351	3/1053, 0.3	0/41[a], 0.0	0/25, 0.0	0/24, 0.0	Kwon et al,[13] 2020
	Men with PCa who completed Invitae panel testing	2615	10/2403, 0.4	1/212, 0.5			Sartor et al,[15] 2020

[a] African American or African Canadian.
[b] European American.
[c] Only Chinese men.

AAM compared with CM (4.6 vs 1.6%, P = .0063), whereas rates of pathologic mutations were similar across races.[17] These high rates of VUS underscore the importance of ongoing enrollment of minority groups in genetic testing studies to better elucidate whether these VUS represent truly pathogenic mutations.

BRCA1/2

Germline mutations in *BRCA1/2* have been previously linked to more aggressive PCa with higher rates of high-grade disease, nodal involvement, metastasis, and PCa-related mortality.[19] Rates of *BRCA1* mutations in multiracial cohorts have identified an incidence of 0.7% to 1.2% in CM compared with 0% to 4.9% in AAM and 0% to 4.2% in AAPI.[8,13–15] There were no *BRCA1* mutations noted among Hispanic men in the 2 individual studies. In a study of 96 AAM with early onset PCa (diagnosed at 55 years of age or earlier), a 1.0% rate of *BRCA1* was noted.[20]

BRCA2 mutations were analyzed in 5 separate multiracial studies including a total of 600 (6.9%) AAM, 103 (1.2%) Hispanic men, and 164 (1.9%) APPI men.[8,13–16] The incidence of *BRCA2* mutations in CM was 0.8% to 4.8% compared with 0% to 2.8% in AAM and 0% to 3.8% in Hispanic men. AAPI men had the highest incidence of *BRCA2* mutations with rates as high as 8.3%; however, sample size was limited. Beebe-Dimmer and colleagues evaluated AAM with early onset PCa and identified a 1% (1 of 96 patients) rate of *BRCA2* mutations.[20]

Petrovics and colleagues analyzed *BRCA1/2* mutations from 1235 patients with PCa and demonstrated similar prevalence of pathogenic mutations between CM and AAM (1.0% vs 1.4%, respectively).[17] One recent study characterized DNA repair gene alterations in men with lethal versus localized PCa—among those with lethal PCa, mutations in *BRCA1* were identified in 2 (0.8%) European Americans and mutations in *BRCA2* were noted in 8 (3.1%) European Americans and 3 (13.6%) Chinese patients. No AAM with lethal PCa had *BRCA1/2* mutations.[14] *BRCA1* and *BRCA2* mutations in localized disease ranged from 0% to 0.6% and 0% to 1.1%, respectively.

Finally, the largest study of germline mutations in men of African descent with PCa included a total of 2098 patients, composed of AAM and Ugandan men. Five patients (0.2%) harbored *BRCA1* mutations, whereas 1.0% (21 patients) harbored *BRCA2* mutations.[21] Among those with metastatic PCa, the frequency of *BRCA2* germline variants was 2.1%, compared with 5.3% previously reported in CM.[7]

ATM

ATM represents another DNA repair gene implicated in the development of aggressive PCa.[14,22] Four studies were evaluated comprising a total of 8265 patients; of these, 7.2% were AAM, 1.2% Hispanic men, and 2.0% AAPI men. Rates of pathologic *ATM* mutations were similar among CM, AAM, and AAPI men (1%–2.1%, 0%–1.0%, 0%–2.7%, respectively).[8,13–15] Of the 103 Hispanic men assessed, none harbored *ATM* mutations. A single study evaluating *ATM* mutations in AAM with early onset PCa demonstrated a 2.1% mutation rate.[20]

Although overall rates of *ATM* mutations were similar, when *ATM* mutations in men with lethal versus localized PCa were analyzed, *ATM* mutations occurred with a higher frequency in AAM and Chinese men with lethal PCa compared with European Americans (3.3% and 4.55% vs 1.53%, respectively).

Matejcic and colleagues also evaluated germline mutations in the largest cohort of AAM and Ugandan men with PCa to date (2098 patients), demonstrating an *ATM* mutation incidence rate of 0.7%.[21] Similar rates of *ATM* variants were noted in men with metastatic PCa compared with previously reported rates among CM (1.8% vs 1.6%).[7]

PALB2

In an international review of 5545 men with PCa, *PALB2* was associated with a 6.3-fold increased risk of aggressive PCa.[23] Rates of *PALB2* mutations in the literature range from 0.2% to 1.1% in AAM and 1.4% of APPI men. No *PALB2* mutations were noted in Hispanic men in a single study.[8]

In a large study of more than 2000 AAM and Ugandan men with PCa performed by Matejcic and colleagues, rates of *PALB2* mutations were 0.2%.[21]

CHEK2

The presence of *CHEK2* mutations has previously been associated with a significantly increased prevalence in men with metastatic PCa compared with localized PCa.[7] Three multiracial cohorts evaluated the incidence of *CHEK2* mutations identifying variants in 2.8% to 3.1% of CM and 0.4% to 2.4% of AAM.[8,13,15] No mutations were noted in the 2 studies that included Hispanic and AAPI men.

Low rates of *CHEK2* mutations (0.2%) were also noted in AAM and Ugandan men in a large study of 2098 men of African descent.[21]

Given the association of DNA repair gene alterations with aggressive PCa, Matejcic found that alterations in specific genes such as *ATM, BRCA2, PALB2,* and *NBN* genes among African American and Ugandan men were associated with aggressive phenotype as defined by nonlocalized, disease, Gleason score greater than 7, or death from PCa.[21] The *NBN* gene alteration finding is of note, as this is not currently listed under the NCCN guidelines as a genetic alteration to test for but may be included on commercially available multigene testing panels.[8,11] Pritchard and colleagues noted the presence of DNA repair gene alterations in 4/40 AAM (10%), 1/12 AAPI (8.3%), and 3/11 Hispanic (27%) men with castrate resistant PCa.[7] These data provide evidence for determining the presence of rare DNA repair gene alterations among diverse populations.

HOXB13

HOXB13 was the first PCa-specific susceptibility gene identified with the rare missense mutation G34E. Although presence of this mutation has been associated with earlier age of diagnosis and family history of PCa, especially among those of Swedish and Finnish ancestry, this mutation is extremely uncommon in African Americans.[24] When compared with homologous DNA repair gene alterations, *HOXB13* alterations seem to be associated with the full spectrum of PCa disease from low risk to metastatic disease.[24] Rare, novel germline mutations in *HOXB13* associated with PCa have also been recently identified in Japanese, Chinese, and Martinican men,[25–27] with others potentially yet to be discovered.

In a recent multiracial study in which 3706 PCa patients underwent germline testing, *HOXB13* mutations were noted in 0.9% of CM and 1.3% of AAM. No Hispanic or AAPI men were found to have mutations. The cohort consisted of 227 AAM (6.1%), 78 Hispanic (2.1%), and 73 AAPI men (2.0%).[8] Akbari and colleagues also evaluated the incidence of *HOXB13* mutations in 1843 Canadian men with PCa—82.7% white, 10.9% African Canadian, 5.4% Asian, and 0.1% other.[18] Twelve white men (1%) harbored the G34E mutation, whereas one African Canadian (0.5%) man harbored one rare deletion mutation (c.853delT). No AAPI patients were noted to have *HOXB13* mutations.

Lynch syndrome

Lynch syndrome is an inherited cancer predisposition syndrome with increased risk of numerous malignancies, including PCa, caused by germline mutations in the mismatch repair genes *MLH1, MSH2, MSH6,* and *PMS2.* Men with Lynch

syndrome have an approximately 2-fold higher lifetime risk of PCa.[28]

Three multiethnic cohorts evaluated the incidence of the 4 mismatch repair genes. Three AAM (0.6%), 1 Hispanic (1.0%), and 2 AAPI men (2.1%) had mutations in either *MSH6* or *PMS2.* There were no mutations identified in *MLH1* or *MSH2* in these minority groups.

Matejcic and colleagues identified *MLH1, MSH6,* and *PMS2* mutations in 0.1%, 0.2%, and 0.1%, respectively, in their large cohort of AAM and Ugandan men with PCa.[21] No patients with *MSH2* mutations were identified.

LOW PENETRANT GERMLINE SINGLE-NUCLEOTIDE POLYMORPHISMS

Genome-wide association studies (GWAS) have been fundamental in characterizing genetic influences in PCa risk and adverse pathologic characteristics, and more than 100 susceptibility loci have been identified. It can be difficult to differentiate true genetic versus environmental and epigenetic influences in alleles with low penetrance or mutational frequency, and this is certainly true for mutations associated with introns or noncoding regions of genes, with unclear downstream expression or functional manifestations. Unfortunately, ethnic minorities were underrepresented in many of the early GWAS or were excluded altogether to eliminate confounding.

The 8q24 region

The most completely characterized genetic locus with regard to PCa incidence is chromosome 8q24. In AAM, mutational frequency within 8q24 has been shown to confer increased incidence of PCa, earlier age of onset, and more clinically aggressive disease. In addition, these mutations manifest in a clinical phenotype that indicate inherited PCa compared with sporadic disease.[29] In 2 independent, large GWAS studies, including more than 5000 PCa and more than 3000 controls, the rs1447295 single-nucleotide polymorphism (SNP) at the 8q24 locus was significantly associated with PCa diagnosis.[30,31] Within the subgroup of nearly 1500 affected AAMs there was a roughly 40% incidence in the rs1447295 SNP in affected individuals with an odds ratio (OR) for developing PCa of 1.60. Notably, common mutations within a specified 3.8 Mb region on 8p24 primarily associated with the diagnosis of PCa in younger AAM, with an attenuated association in AAM older than 71 years; this has been postulated as an underlying genetic mechanism for aggressive PCa in young AAM. This region codes for 9 known genes, including the *c-MYC* oncogene.[30]

Several additional loci on 8q24 have been associated with PCa diagnosis. Yeager and colleagues identified rs6983267 as having a higher population attributable risk of PCa association than the aforementioned rs1447295 SNP (21% vs 9%, respectively), but this was not subanalyzed within AA patients.[32] In a study of more than 3400 AAM with PCa, fine mapping of the 8q24 locus was performed. Nine SNPs were preferentially expressed in AAM with PCa compared with men from European decent.[33] Similar studies have subsequently identified novel SNPs within the 8q24 locus specifically associated with PCA in AAM.[34,35] African men with West African ancestry also express 8q24 SNPs at relatively high frequency.[36] A case control study of AAM and Puerto Rican men established rs7824364 as an ancestry informative marker of West African ancestry associated with PCa in men from both ethnicities.[37] **Table 2** includes 8q24 SNPs with associated allelic frequencies expressed significantly higher in AA men with PCA compared with controls. Despite in-depth characterization of the 8q24 locus, studies to date have been limited by association in most cases with PCa incidence. Further analysis of SNPs associated with disease aggressiveness (stage, grade, response to systemic therapy) would help to establish their potential role as biomarkers with predictive and prognostic capacity.

OTHER PROGNOSTIC SINGLE-NUCLEOTIDE POLYMORPHISMS IN AFRICAN AMERICAN MEN

Table 3 outlines SNPs preferentially expressed in AAM with PCa identified in large GWAS and subsequent fine mapping of well-characterized loci. Bensen and colleagues investigated more than 1500 SNPs derived from GWAS, including several ancestral informative markers, to correlate these germline polymorphisms with PCa disease aggressiveness in more than 1000 AAM from the North Carolina-Louisiana Prostate Cancer Project.[55] This study provides unique data in this regard. They identified 5 SNPs within the 8q24 locus preferentially associated with PCa in AAM compared with European American men. These were located within the *FAM84B*, *POU5F1P1*, and *c-MYC* coding regions. Two additional SNPs within *KLK2/3*, encoding prostate-specific antigen (PSA), were also identified to be preferentially expressed in AAM with PCa. Altogether 7 SNPs were associated with PCa aggressiveness based on Gleason score greater than or equal to 8, PSA greater than 20 ng/mL, or cT3-T4 disease. Notably, the *KLK3* SNPs associated with serum PSA only in AAM, and this aligns with emerging

Table 2
8q24 single-nucleotide polymorphism allelic alteration with significantly higher incidence in African American men with prostate cancer compared with controls

8q24 SNP	AA Allelic Frequency (%)	Citation
rs6983267	88	Haiman et al,[33] 201
	87	Irizarry-Ramírez et al,[37] 2017
	95	Murphy et al,[36] 2012
rs7008482	86	Xu et al,[35] 2009
	91	Murphy et al,[36] 2012
rs7824364	82	Irizarry-Ramírez et al,[37] 2017
rs4871005	71	Xu et al,[35] 2009
rs6981122	72	Xu et al,[35] 2009
rs10086908	75	Haiman et al,[33] 201
rs16901979	55	Chung et al,[34] 2014
rs6983561	44	Haiman et al,[33] 201
	35	Murphy et al,[36] 2012
	53	Chung et al,[34] 2014
rs1456315	47	Chung et al,[34] 2014
rs13254738	60	Haiman et al,[33] 201
	34	Chung et al,[34] 2014
rs16901966	30	Chung et al,[34] 2014
DG8S737	23	Amundadottir et al,[31] 2006
rs1016343	25	Chung et al,[34] 2014
rs6987409	17	Chung et al,[34] 2014
rs13252298	10	Chung et al,[34] 2014
rs11986220	5	Haiman et al,[33] 201

evidence that poorly differentiated tumors in AAM secrete relatively less PSA than stage- and grade-matched European American tumors and that AAM exhibit inherently lower PSA density.[56,57]

Additional deleterious SNPs in AAM have been identified in *VDR*, encoding the vitamin D receptor.

Table 3
Select low-penetrance allelic single-nucleotide polymorphisms associated with prostate cancer in African American men

Associated Gene(s)	Locus	SNP ID (% Allele Frequency in AA Men with PCa)	Reference
	2p11	rs1561198 (32%)	38
EHBP1	2p15	rs6545977 (48%), rs721048 (4%), rs58235267 (44%)	33,38
	2p21	rs13017478 (80%)	38
	2p24	rs340623 (17%), rs9306894 (12%)	33,38
	2p25	rs7575106 (9%)	38
	2q21	rs12620581 (75%)	33
FARP2	2q37	rs2771570 (1%)	39
MIR4795	3p12	rs17181170 (12%), rs76668454 (5%), rs2660753 (50%–51%)	35,38,39
	3q21	rs7641133 (29%), rs4857837 (30%)	33,38
ZBTB38	3q23	rs6763931 (91%)	39
	4q13	rs4694176 (79%)	38
TET2	4q24	rs7679673 (60%)	39
	5p15	rs7726159 (81%), rs4975758 (33%)	38
HLA-DRB6	6p21	rs115306967 (65%)	40
NEDD9	6p24	rs4713266 (78%)	40
RFX6	6q22	rs339331 (17%–75%), rs12202378 (70%)	33,39
	6q25	rs2076828 (56%), rs4646284 (37%)	33,41
JAZF1	7p15	rs10486567 (71%–77%), rs7808935 (70%)	33,42,43
	8p21	rs11782388 (70%), rs1160267 (72%)	33,38
MSR1	8p22	rs4333601 (43%), rs351572 (34%)	44
	9q31	rs1746824 (48%)	38
MSMB, CTBP2	10q11	rs10993994 (40%–62%), rs4962416 (16%–27%), rs4630243 (76%)	33,42,43
CYP17	10q24	rs6163 (19%–41%), rs6162 (19%–41%), rs743572 (18%–41%)	45
TPCN2, MYEOV	11q13	rs10896449 (67%–79%), rs7931342 (78%)	33,39,42,43,46
RP1, VDR	12q13	rs80130819 (98%), rs731236 (71%), rs7975232 (37%)	40,47
PAWR	12q21	rs8176882 (21%), rs8176908 (10%), rs12827748 (54%–66%)	48
KLF5	12q22	rs9600079 (54%)	39
IGF1	12q23	rs148371593 (3%), rs78360701 (<1%)	49
ERCC5	13q33	rs2296148 (17%)	50
IRS2	13q34	rs75823044 (2%–3%)	51
HNF1B	17p12	rs4430796 (72%–85%)	43,52
ZNF652	17q21	rs7210100 (8%)	39,53
	17q25	rs6465657 (45%–89%)	54
KLK2/3	19q13	rs3760722 (72%), rs2735839 (30%–69%), rs2659124 (37%)	33,41,46,52,55
CHEK2	22q12	rs78554043 (2%)	51
NUDT10/11	Xp11	rs5945572 (14%–31%), rs4907796 (13%)	33,42,46
SLC7A	Xp13	rs6625711 (83%)	40

Nine GWAS-associated SNPs in *VDR* were investigated in a case-control study of more than 800 AAM.[47] rs731236 was associated with both PCa risk and elevated PSA levels at diagnosis, whereas rs1544410 and rs2239185 showed a statistically significant association with high Gleason score. In a fine-mapping study of *VDR* in a racially admixed cohort, SNPs within a VDR-5132 haplotype was associated with increased risk of PCa exclusively in AA men (OR = 1.83).[58] Furthermore, the specific T/C SNP at this locus eliminates a GATA-1 transcription factor binding site. GATA-1 is a transcriptional activator of *VDR*, and the investigators conclude that SNP-related downregulation of *VDR* may lead to decreased vitamin D inhibition on cell proliferation.

An additional study comparing germline SNPs with disease aggressiveness performed whole exome sequencing on more than 4000 AA affected men and controls.[59] SNPs identified within coding regions of *CYFIP1*, *FBXW9*, *MYH7*, *C9orf47*, *SERPINB9*, and *ASH1L* were exclusively associated with aggressive PCas. The allelic frequencies for each of these SNPs was less than 0.002. An additional GWAS was performed on West African men in the Ghana Prostate Study, including nearly 1000 PCa cases and controls.[39] The investigators identified 9 SNPs at the 5q31 locus highly associated with Gleason 7 to 10 disease.

There is emerging evidence to suggest that genetic linkages play a pivotal role in PCa heritability in AAM. Although the aforementioned studies were primarily characterized by association analysis, focusing on the association between a specific allele and the disease trait (PCa), genetic linkage analysis investigates the relationship between the heritable transmission of a locus and the disease trait within a lineage. Genotyping of 129 individuals from 15 large, high-risk AA families native to Southern Louisiana with homogenous pedigrees revealed preserved generational SNPs at 12q24 and 2p16 strongly associated with PCa. These specific mutations have not been recapitulated in large GWAS but represent promising biomarkers in heritable PCa in AA families.

PROSTATE CANCER SINGLE-NUCLEOTIDE POLYMORPHISMS AMONG ASIAN AND HISPANIC MEN

The presence of low-penetrant germline SNPs have been less well characterized in other ethnic monitories. It is estimated that roughly half of PCa-associated SNPs identified in GWAS have association in Chinese men.[60] A large GWAS including more than 14,000 Chinese men identified many SNPs conserved between men of African and European descent associated with PCa but reported 2 unique PCa-associated alleles on 9q31 (rs817826) and 19q13 (rs103294).[61] The latter SNP was associated with loss of expression of the inflammatory regulator *LILRA3*, and this has bene proposed as a biomarker for inheritable disease in Chinese men. A large, population-based GWAS in Japanese men identified more than 100 SNPs associated with PCa, the largest concentration of which was located in the *FAM84B/POUF1B* region on 8q24.[62] An additional unique functional deleterious SNP in *NKX3-1*, a well-characterized tumor suppressor, was highly associated with PCa (rs4872174). Notably, in a large metanalysis of polymorphisms in the DNA repair enzyme ERCC2, the only significant SNP associated with PCa was rs1799793 in Asians.[63]

Although often considered as a single ethnic group, the Latino population is characterized by considerable genetic diversity making genetic association studies difficult. GWAS performed in more than 8000 Latino men with PCa and healthy controls identified 84 allelic variants at the 10q11 and 8q24 loci, with the latter exhibiting strong association with local African ancestry.[64] This finding confirms prior reports of strong allelic conservation with West African ancestry in 8q24 in a radically admixed Latino cohort.[37] Hoffmann and colleagues generated a risk score in a large, racially admixed cohort using 105 known PCa-related SNPs.[41] Latinos exhibited the second highest risk score decile, behind non-Hispanic whites, indicating a relatively high-rate PCa is attributable to heritable germline mutations in this population.

POLYGENIC RISK SCORE

Given the knowledge of the association of (higher frequency but low penetrant) SNPs with PCa, various SNPs have been combined that collectively have shown an increased prognostication for PCa when compared with a single SNP.[65,66] Such SNP panels have been shown in largely Caucasian cohorts to be independent predictors of PCa and have improved the predictive capacity of serum PSA testing even among men with low serum PSA levels. These data could prove valuable in selecting men for early detection of PCa. Unfortunately to our knowledge such studies have not been performed in underrepresented minority populations.

FUTURE DIRECTIONS

Although inclusion of racially admixed populations adds considerable heterogeneity to GWAS and

Table 4
Clinical trials investigating genetic predispositions in prostate cancer in ethnic monitories (clinicaltrials.gov)

NCT Number	Title	Status
NCT03232411	Biobank for African American Prostate Cancer Research in Florida	Active, not recruiting
NCT02229565	Molecular Mechanisms Underlying Prostate Cancer Disparities	Suspended
NCT02723734	Validation Study on the Impact of Decipher Testing—VANDAAM Study	Recruiting
NCT02543905	The PROFILE Study: Germline Genetic Profiling: Correlation with Targeted Prostate Cancer Screening and Treatment	Recruiting
NCT00584792	Diet, Genetic Variation and Prostate Cancer Among African Americans	Completed (2007)
NCT00342771	An Epidemiological Study of Genetic Risk Factors for Prostate Cancer in African American and Caucasian Males	Completed (2020)
NCT00900185	Study of a Polymorphism in Patients with Prostate Cancer	Completed (2015)
NCT00342784	Identification of Prostate Cancer Genes	Completed (2018)

fine-mapping studies of loci attributable to PCa risk, it is imperative to include such populations to truly define the genetic basis of heritable PCa. Statistical rigor, utilization of ancestry informative markers, and robust studies with sufficient power can overcome confounding results associated with ethnicity.

There is a tremendous need for clinical and tissue archived registries with longitudinal, generational follow-up for ethnic minorities. Such studies have previously been limited by barriers to health care access and technology among these underserved populations, even in industrialized nations.

Table 4 lists clinical trials designed to study genetic predisposition for PCa in minorities, either wholly or as a dedicated aim of the study. The study titled "An Epidemiological Study of Genetic Risk Factors for Prostate Cancer in African-American and Caucasian Males" is a case-control study of PCa in men in the Baltimore, MD area. More than 2000 participants were recruited from 2004 to 2020 for whom clinical, demographic, and pathologic data were obtained, as well as blood, urine, and tissue for biomarker studies. Men were enrolled by frequency matching age and race, with a primary focus of the study to identify mechanisms in tumor biology underlying aggressive disease in AAM.

PROFILE (NCT02543905) is a European study actively recruiting in which men with family history of PCa will undergo PSA screening and prostate biopsy for genetic profiling. As a separate investigational arm, African men or those with Caribbean ancestry may be enrolled without a positive family history to better understand population-based genetic risks in these high-risk minorities who have been relatively underrepresented in historical studies. Such large-scale investigational efforts are necessary to identify genetic alterations associated with PCa and with prognostic capacity with regard to cancer-specific outcomes. In addition, further germline and somatic characterization are necessary to establish biomarkers predictive of response to therapy in organ-confined and metastatic disease states.

SUMMARY

Studies to date confirm that germline mutations are present in diverse minority groups with PCa. Prior studies are composed of small cohorts of underrepresented patients, but more recently larger more robust data are being reported. With the advent of precision medicine, components of PCa screening and treatment will likely be shaped by germline testing. Both high- and low-penetrant germline mutations have been identified in diverse populations; however, data remain very limited, and further research is needed to better elucidate the prognostic impact and prevalence of various germline mutations in non-Caucasian men and their families.

CLINICS CARE POINTS

- There remains a lack of racial and ethnic diversity in genomic PCa studies—efforts should be made to increase diversity in future clinical trials and genetic studies.

- Current guidelines recommend sequencing for the homologous recombination genes *BRCA1, BRCA2, ATM, PALB2,* and *CHEK2,* as well as for mutations in the mismatch repair genes associated with Lynch syndrome in high-risk or metastatic patients, as well as those with strong family history. Increasing the access to such testing should be a priority for underrepresented minorities. This is especially the case for those of African Ancestry who suffer disproportionate mortality from PCa.

- Polymorphisms on 8q24 have been associated with increased PCa risk and aggressiveness in AAM. Further GWAS studies are needed to evaluate the relationship of other SNPs with PCa risk and aggressiveness in both African Americans and other minority groups to determine their prognostic value.

DISCLOSURE

The authors have nothing to disclose.

REFERENCES

1. Siegel RL, Miller KD, Jemal A. Cancer statistics, 2020. CA Cancer J Clin 2020;70(1):7–30.
2. DeSantis CE, Siegel RL, Sauer AG, et al. Cancer statistics for African Americans, 2016: Progress and opportunities in reducing racial disparities. CA Cancer J Clin 2016;66(4):290–308.
3. Chinea FM, Patel VN, Kwon D, et al. Ethnic heterogeneity and prostate cancer mortality in Hispanic/Latino men: a population-based study. Oncotarget 2017;8(41):69709–21.
4. Chao GF, Krishna N, Aizer AA, et al. Asian Americans and prostate cancer: A nationwide population-based analysis. Urol Oncol 2016;34(5):233. e237-215.
5. Cheng I, Witte JS, McClure LA, et al. Socioeconomic status and prostate cancer incidence and mortality rates among the diverse population of California. Cancer Causes Control 2009;20(8):1431–40.
6. Mucci LA, Hjelmborg JB, Harris JR, et al. Familial risk and heritability of cancer among Twins in Nordic Countries. JAMA 2016;315(1):68–76.
7. Pritchard CC, Mateo J, Walsh MF, et al. Inherited DNA-repair gene mutations in men with metastatic prostate cancer. N Engl J Med 2016;375(5):443–53.
8. Nicolosi P, Ledet E, Yang S, et al. Prevalence of germline variants in prostate cancer and implications for current genetic testing guidelines. JAMA Oncol 2019;5(4):523–8.
9. Spratt DE, Chan T, Waldron L, et al. Racial/ethnic disparities in genomic sequencing. JAMA Oncol 2016;2(8):1070–4.
10. Carlo MI, Giri VN, Paller CJ, et al. Evolving intersection between inherited cancer genetics and therapeutic clinical trials in prostate cancer: a white paper from the germline genetics working group of the prostate cancer clinical trials consortium. JCO Precis Oncol 2018;2018.
11. National Comprehensive Cancer Network. Prostate Cancer (Version 2.2020). Available at: https://www.nccn.org/professionals/physician_gls/pdf/prostate.pdf.
12. Chandrasekar T, Gross L, Gomella LG, et al. Prevalence of suspected hereditary cancer syndromes and germline mutations among a diverse cohort of probands reporting a family history of prostate cancer: toward informing cascade testing for men. Eur Urol Oncol 2020;3(3):291–7.
13. Kwon DH, Borno HT, Cheng HH, et al. Ethnic disparities among men with prostate cancer undergoing germline testing. Urol Oncol 2020;38(3):80.e81–7.
14. Na R, Zheng SL, Han M, et al. Germline Mutations in ATM and BRCA1/2 distinguish risk for lethal and indolent prostate cancer and are associated with early age at death. Eur Urol 2017;71(5):740–7.
15. Sartor O, Yang S, Ledet E, et al. Inherited DNA-repair gene mutations in African American men with prostate cancer. Oncotarget 2020;11(4):440–2.
16. Agalliu I, Karlins E, Kwon EM, et al. Rare germline mutations in the BRCA2 gene are associated with early-onset prostate cancer. Br J Cancer 2007;97(6):826–31.
17. Petrovics G, Price DK, Lou H, et al. Increased frequency of germline BRCA2 mutations associates with prostate cancer metastasis in a racially diverse patient population. Prostate Cancer Prostatic Dis 2019;22(3):406–10.
18. Akbari MR, Trachtenberg J, Lee J, et al. Association between germline HOXB13 G84E mutation and risk of prostate cancer. J Natl Cancer Inst 2012;104(16):1260–2.
19. Castro E, Goh C, Olmos D, et al. Germline BRCA mutations are associated with higher risk of nodal involvement, distant metastasis, and poor survival outcomes in prostate cancer. J Clin Oncol 2013;31(14):1748–57.
20. Beebe-Dimmer JL, Zuhlke KA, Johnson AM, et al. Rare germline mutations in African American men diagnosed with early-onset prostate cancer. Prostate 2018;78(5):321–6.

21. Matejcic M, Patel Y, Lilyquist J, et al. Pathogenic variants in cancer predisposition genes and prostate cancer risk in men of African ancestry. JCO Precis Oncol 2020;4:32–43.

22. Robinson D, Van Allen EM, Wu YM, et al. Integrative clinical genomics of advanced prostate cancer. Cell 2015;162(2):454.

23. Darst BF, Dadaev T, Saunders E, et al. Germline sequencing DNA repair genes in 5,545 men with aggressive and non-aggressive prostate cancer. J Natl Cancer Inst 2020.

24. Isaacs WB, Cooney KA, Xu J. Updated insights into genetic contribution to prostate cancer predisposition: focus on HOXB13. Can J Urol 2019;26(5 Suppl 2):12–3.

25. Momozawa Y, Iwasaki Y, Hirata M, et al. Germline pathogenic variants in 7636 Japanese patients with prostate cancer and 12 366 controls. J Natl Cancer Inst 2020;112(4):369–76.

26. Lin X, Qu L, Chen Z, et al. A novel germline mutation in HOXB13 is associated with prostate cancer risk in Chinese men. Prostate 2013;73(2):169–75.

27. Marlin R, Creoff M, Merle S, et al. Mutation HOXB13 c.853delT in Martinican prostate cancer patients. Prostate 2020;80(6):463–70.

28. Raymond VM, Mukherjee B, Wang F, et al. Elevated risk of prostate cancer among men with Lynch syndrome. J Clin Oncol 2013;31(14):1713–8.

29. Ledet EM, Sartor O, Rayford W, et al. Suggestive evidence of linkage identified at chromosomes 12q24 and 2p16 in African American prostate cancer families from Louisiana. Prostate 2012;72(9):938–47.

30. Freedman ML, Haiman CA, Patterson N, et al. Admixture mapping identifies 8q24 as a prostate cancer risk locus in African-American men. Proc Natl Acad Sci U S A 2006;103(38):14068–73.

31. Amundadottir LT, Sulem P, Gudmundsson J, et al. A common variant associated with prostate cancer in European and African populations. Nat Genet 2006;38(6):652–8.

32. Yeager M, Orr N, Hayes RB, et al. Genome-wide association study of prostate cancer identifies a second risk locus at 8q24. Nat Genet 2007;39(5):645–9.

33. Haiman CA, Chen GK, Blot WJ, et al. Characterizing genetic risk at known prostate cancer susceptibility loci in African Americans. PLoS Genet 2011;7(5):e1001387.

34. Chung CC, Hsing AW, Edward Y, et al. A comprehensive resequence-analysis of 250 kb region of 8q24.21 in men of African ancestry. Prostate 2014;74(6):579–89.

35. Xu J, Kibel AS, Hu JJ, et al. Prostate cancer risk associated loci in African Americans. Cancer Epidemiol Biomarkers Prev 2009;18(7):2145–9.

36. Murphy AB, Ukoli F, Freeman V, et al. 8q24 risk alleles in West African and Caribbean men. Prostate 2012;72(12):1366–73.

37. Irizarry-Ramírez M, Kittles RA, Wang X, et al. Genetic ancestry and prostate cancer susceptibility SNPs in Puerto Rican and African American men. Prostate 2017;77(10):1118–27.

38. Han Y, Hazelett DJ, Wiklund F, et al. Integration of multiethnic fine-mapping and genomic annotation to prioritize candidate functional SNPs at prostate cancer susceptibility regions. Hum Mol Genet 2015;24(19):5603–18.

39. Cook MB, Wang Z, Yeboah ED, et al. A genome-wide association study of prostate cancer in West African men. Hum Genet 2014;133(5):509–21.

40. Al Olama AA, Kote-Jarai Z, Berndt SI, et al. A meta-analysis of 87,040 individuals identifies 23 new susceptibility loci for prostate cancer. Nat Genet 2014;46(10):1103–9.

41. Hoffmann TJ, Van Den Eeden SK, Sakoda LC, et al. A large multiethnic genome-wide association study of prostate cancer identifies novel risk variants and substantial ethnic differences. Cancer Discov 2015;5(8):878–91.

42. Chang BL, Spangler E, Gallagher S, et al. Validation of genome-wide prostate cancer associations in men of African descent. Cancer Epidemiol Biomarkers Prev 2011;20(1):23–32.

43. Thomas G, Jacobs KB, Yeager M, et al. Multiple loci identified in a genome-wide association study of prostate cancer. Nat Genet 2008;40(3):310–5.

44. Beuten J, Gelfond JA, Franke JL, et al. Single and multivariate associations of MSR1, ELAC2, and RNASEL with prostate cancer in an ethnic diverse cohort of men. Cancer Epidemiol Biomarkers Prev 2010;19(2):588–99.

45. Sarma AV, Dunn RL, Lange LA, et al. Genetic polymorphisms in CYP17, CYP3A4, CYP19A1, SRD5A2, IGF-1, and IGFBP-3 and prostate cancer risk in African-American men: the Flint Men's Health Study. Prostate 2008;68(3):296–305.

46. Hooker S, Hernandez W, Chen H, et al. Replication of prostate cancer risk loci on 8q24, 11q13, 17q12, 19q33, and Xp11 in African Americans. Prostate 2010;70(3):270–5.

47. Jingwi EY, Abbas M, Ricks-Santi L, et al. Vitamin D receptor genetic polymorphisms are associated with PSA level, Gleason score and prostate cancer risk in African-American men. Anticancer Res 2015;35(3):1549–58.

48. Bonilla C, Hooker S, Mason T, et al. Prostate cancer susceptibility Loci identified on chromosome 12 in African Americans. PLoS One 2011;6(2):e16044.

49. Giorgi EE, Stram DO, Taverna D, et al. Fine-mapping IGF1 and prostate cancer risk in African Americans: the multiethnic cohort study. Cancer Epidemiol Biomarkers Prev 2014;23(9):1928–32.

50. Hooker S, Bonilla C, Akereyeni F, et al. NAT2 and NER genetic variants and sporadic prostate cancer

susceptibility in African Americans. Prostate Cancer Prostatic Dis 2008;11(4):349–56.

51. Conti DV, Wang K, Sheng X, et al. Two novel susceptibility loci for prostate cancer in men of African Ancestry. J Natl Cancer Inst 2017;109(8).

52. Helfand BT, Roehl KA, Cooper PR, et al. Associations of prostate cancer risk variants with disease aggressiveness: results of the NCI-SPORE Genetics Working Group analysis of 18,343 cases. Hum Genet 2015;134(4):439–50.

53. Haiman CA, Chen GK, Blot WJ, et al. Genome-wide association study of prostate cancer in men of African ancestry identifies a susceptibility locus at 17q21. Nat Genet 2011;43(6):570–3.

54. Jiang X, Zhang M, Bai XY, et al. Association between 17q25.3-rs6465657 polymorphism and prostate cancer susceptibility: a meta-analysis based on 19 studies. Onco Targets Ther 2016;9:4491–503.

55. Bensen JT, Xu Z, Smith GJ, et al. Genetic polymorphism and prostate cancer aggressiveness: a case-only study of 1,536 GWAS and candidate SNPs in African-Americans and European-Americans. Prostate 2013;73(1):11–22.

56. Kryvenko ON, Balise R, Soodana Prakash N, et al. African-American men with gleason score 3+3=6 prostate cancer produce less prostate specific antigen than caucasian men: a potential impact on active surveillance. J Urol 2016;195(2):301–6.

57. Shenoy D, Packianathan S, Chen AM, et al. Do African-American men need separate prostate cancer screening guidelines? BMC Urol 2016;16(1):19.

58. Kidd LC, Paltoo DN, Wang S, et al. Sequence variation within the 5' regulatory regions of the vitamin D binding protein and receptor genes and prostate cancer risk. Prostate 2005;64(3):272–82.

59. Rand KA, Rohland N, Tandon A, et al. Whole-exome sequencing of over 4100 men of African ancestry and prostate cancer risk. Hum Mol Genet 2016; 25(2):371–81.

60. Na R, Liu F, Zhang P, et al. Evaluation of reported prostate cancer risk-associated SNPs from genome-wide association studies of various racial populations in Chinese men. Prostate 2013;73(15): 1623–35.

61. Xu J, Mo Z, Ye D, et al. Genome-wide association study in Chinese men identifies two new prostate cancer risk loci at 9q31.2 and 19q13.4. Nat Genet 2012;44(11):1231–5.

62. Ishigaki K, Akiyama M, Kanai M, et al. Large-scale genome-wide association study in a Japanese population identifies novel susceptibility loci across different diseases. Nat Genet 2020;52(7):669–79.

63. Liu Y, Hu Y, Zhang M, et al. Polymorphisms in ERCC2 and ERCC5 and risk of prostate cancer: a meta-analysis and systematic review. J Cancer 2018;9(16):2786–94.

64. Du Z, Hopp H, Ingles SA, et al. A genome-wide association study of prostate cancer in Latinos. Int J Cancer 2020;146(7):1819–26.

65. Nordstrom T, Aly M, Eklund M, et al. A genetic score can identify men at high risk for prostate cancer among men with prostate-specific antigen of 1-3 ng/ml. Eur Urol 2014;65(6):1184–90.

66. Sipeky C, Talala KM, Tammela TLJ, et al. Prostate cancer risk prediction using a polygenic risk score. Sci Rep 2020;10(1):17075.